Lecture Notes in Computer Science 6159

Commenced Publication in 1973
Founding and Former Series Editors:
Gerhard Goos, Juris Hartmanis, and Jan van Leeuwen

Yeunsook Lee Z. Zenn Bien
Mounir Mokhtari Jeong Tai Kim
Mignon Park Jongbae Kim Heyoung Lee
Ismail Khalil (Eds.)

Aging Friendly Technology for Health and Independence

8th International Conference on Smart Homes and Health Telematics, ICOST 2010
Seoul, Korea, June 22-24, 2010
Proceedings

Springer

Volume Editors

Yeunsook Lee
Yonsei University, Seoul, Korea, yeunsooklee@yonsei.ac.kr

Z. Zenn Bien
Ulsan National Institute of Science and Technology, Korea, zbien@unist.ac.kr

Mounir Mokhtari
Institut Télécom SudParis, Evry, France, mounir.mokhtari@it-sudparis.eu

Jeong Tai Kim
Kyung Hee University, Yongin, Korea, jtkim@khu.ac.kr

Mignon Park
Yonsei University, Seoul, Korea, mignpark@yonsei.ac.kr

Jongbae Kim
National Rehabilitation Center Research Institute, Seoul, Korea, jbkim@nrc.go.kr

Heyoung Lee
Seoul National University of Technology, Korea, leehy@snut.ac.kr

Ismail Khalil
Johannes Kepler University Linz, Austria, ismail.khalil@jku.at

Library of Congress Control Number: 2010928341

CR Subject Classification (1998): C.3, C.2, I.2, H.4, H.5, I.4

LNCS Sublibrary: SL 3 – Information Systems and Application, incl. Internet/Web and HCI

ISSN 0302-9743
ISBN-10 3-642-13777-6 Springer Berlin Heidelberg New York
ISBN-13 978-3-642-13777-8 Springer Berlin Heidelberg New York

springer.com

Printed in Germany

Typesetting: Camera-ready by author, data conversion by Scientific Publishing Services, Chennai, India
Printed on acid-free paper 06/3180

Preface

We are living in a world full of innovations for the elderly and people with special needs to use smart assistive technologies and smart homes to more easily perform activities of daily living, to continue in social participation, to engage in entertainment and leisure activities, and to enjoy living independently. These innovations are inspired by new technologies leveraging all aspects of ambient and pervasive intelligence with related theories, technologies, methods, applications, and services on ubiquitous, pervasive, AmI, universal, mobile, embedded, wearable, augmented, invisible, hidden, context-aware, calm, amorphous, sentient, proactive, post–PC, everyday, autonomic computing from the engineering, business and organizational perspectives. In the field of smart homes and health telematics, significant research is underway to enable aging and disabled people to use smart assistive technologies and smart homes to foster independent living and to offer them an enhanced quality of life.

A smart home is a vision of the future where computers and computing devices will be available naturally and unobtrusively anywhere, anytime, and by different means in our daily living, working, learning, business, and infotainment environments. Such a vision opens tremendous opportunities for numerous novel services/applications that are more immersive, more intelligent, and more interactive in both real and cyber spaces.

Initiated in 2003, the International Conference on Smart Homes and Health Telematics (ICOST) has become the premier forum for researchers, scientists, students, professionals, and practioners to discuss and exchange information and ideas on the current advances in enabling technologies coupled with evolving care paradigms to allow the development of novel applications and services for improving the quality of life for aging and disabled people both inside and outside of their homes. Each year ICOST has a specific theme. The theme of ICOST 2003 was "Independent Living for Persons with Disabilities and Elderly People." The theme for ICOST 2004 was "Towards a Human-Friendly Assistive Environment." ICOST 2005 focused on "From Smart Homes to Smart Care." For ICOST 2006, it was "Smart Homes and Beyond" and ICOST 2007 had the theme of "Pervasive Computing Perspectives for Quality of Life Enhancement." The theme of ICOST 2008 was "Gerontechnology: Enhancing the Quality of Life for Rural Elders." Last year the theme of ICOST 2009 was "Ambient Assistive Health and Wellness Management in the Heart of the City," which sought to address the latest approaches and technical solutions in the area of smart homes, health telematics, and emerging enabling technologies with a special emphasis on presenting the latest results in the successes of real deployment of systems and services.

This year the conference was organized under the theme of "Aging Friendly Technology for Health and Independence." At present, the absolute number and proportion of the elderly population has been increasing globally, and especially very rapidly in several countries, while the numbers of human resources that could care for the elderly have been significantly diminishing. Due to this, a burden on the elderly and on society has been pressing. Thus, information and communication technology (ICT) is a promising and pioneering field that mitigates the burden in everyday life settings and broadens beneficial opportunities. It has been expected that various technologies ranging from simple ICT to complex ICT, fixed service to mobile service, services for relatively healthy elderly to services for frail elderly are to be extended and the technology is also expected to be developed in a more ambient and user–friendly way. This ICT growth would contribute to enhancing people's life quality by being merged into diverse life environments. Moreover environmental characteristics are also considered very important in accommoding ICT and producing the synergistic effects. ICT deals with major alternatives to secure the quality of life of the elderly who can make up the majority of our society in the "aged era." In this context, this year the theme was extended to three subthemes: Smart Home and Village, Health Telematics and Healthcare Technology (including a medical part), and Aging Friendly and Enabling Technology.

We are pleased to present, gathered in these proceedings, the papers presented at the conference, which were stringently refereed and carefully selected by a Program Committee of 39 internationally renowned researchers. We would like to thank the members of the Program Committee and the authors for shaping this conference.

We are very grateful to the Scientific Committee members for their dedication to improving the scientific quality and research value of ICOST 2010. We would also like to thank the Local Organizing Committee and the publicity team for the successful organization of an internationally reputable event. We are very grateful that all these people and others behind the scenes accepted to put their academic and professional experience as well as their reputation of excellence at the service of the success of this event. We hope that we have succeeded in disseminating new ideas and results that stem from the presentations and discussions.

June 2010

Yeunsook Lee
Z. Zenn Bien
Mounir Mokhtari
Jeong Tai Kim
Mignon Park
Jongbae Kim
Heyoung Lee
Ismail Khalil

Organization

General Chair

Yeunsook Lee	Yonsei University/The Korean Gerontological Society, Korea

General Co-chairs

Z. Zenn Bien	Ulsan National Institute of Science and Technology, Korea
Mounir Mokhtari	Institut TELECOM/TELECOM SudParis, France/CNRS IPAL (UMI 2955), Singapore

Scientific Committee

Chair

Ismail Khail	Johannes Kepler University, Austria

Members

Z. Zenn Bien	Ulsan National Institute of Science and Technology, Korea
Keith Chan	The Hong Kong Polytechnic University, Hong Kong
Carl K. Chang	Iowa State University, USA
Sylvain Giroux	Université de Sherbrooke, Canada
Sumi Helal	University of Florida, USA
Jongbae Kim	National Rehabilitation Center, Korea
Hyun-Soo Lee	Yonsei University, Korea
Yeunsook Lee	Yonsei University/The Korean Gerontological Society, Korea
Mounir Mokhtari	Institut TELECOM/TELECOM SudParis, France/CNRS IPAL (UMI 2955), Singapore
Chris Nugent	University of Ulster, UK
Toshiyo Tamura	Chiba University, Japan
Tatsuya Yamazaki	National Institute of Information and Communications Technology, Japan
Daqing Zhang	Institut TELECOM/TELECOM SudParis, France

Program Committee

Chair

Mignon Park	Yonsei University, Korea

Co-chairs

Jongbae Kim	National Rehabilitation Center, Korea
Heyoung Lee	Seoul National University of Technology, Korea

Members

Bessam Abdulrazak	Université de Sherbrooke, Canada
Jeremy Bauchet	Institut TELECOM/TELECOM SudParis, France
Jit Biswas	Institute for Infocomm Research, Singapore
Keith Chan	The Hong Kong Polytechnic University, Hong Kong
Liming Chen	University of Ulster, UK
Junho Choi	Yonsei University, Korea
Jong-moon Chung	Yonsei University, Korea
Diane Cook	Washington State University, USA
Kaori Fujinami	Tokyo University of Agriculture and Technology, Japan
Sumi Helal	University of Florida, USA
Jin-Woo Jung	Dongguk University, Korea
Euntai Kim	Yonsei University, Korea
Mi Jeong Kim	Kyung Hee University, Korea
Choonhwa Lee	Hanyang University, Korea
Deok Gyu Lee	Electronics & Telecommunications Research Institute, Korea
Ji-Hyun Lee	Korea Advanced Institute of Science and Technology, Korea
Jeong Taeg Lim	Yonsei University, Korea
Fulvio Mastrogiovanni	University of Genova, Italy
Abdallah M'hamed	Institut TELECOM/TELECOM SudParis, France
Taketoshi Mori	University of Tokyo, Japan
Hongbo Ni	Université de Sherbrooke, Canada
Chris Nugent	University of Ulster, United Kingdom
Venet Osmani	Ubiquitous Interaction Group (UBiNT), CREATE-NET, Italy
Hun-Kuk Park	Kyung Hee University, Korea
Kwang-Hyun Park	Kwangwoon University, Korea
Gilles Privat	Orange Labs, France
Helene Pigot	Université de Sherbrooke, Canada
Seong Dae Sagong	Korea Institute of Science and Technology, Korea
Rich Simpson	University of Pittsburgh, USA

Jeong-Hwa Song	Namseoul University, Korea
Won-Kyung Song	National Rehabilitation Center, Korea
Toshiyo Tamura	Chiba University, Japan
Manfred Wojciechowski	Fraunhofer Institute for Software and System Engineering (ISST), Germany
Zhiwen Yu	Northwestern Polytechnical University, China
Yan Zhang	Simula Research Laboratory, Norway
Bosheng Zhou	Queen's University Belfast, UK

Organizing Committee

Chair

Gahyoun Yoon	Chonnam University/The Korean Gerontological Society, Korea

Co-chair

Jeong Tai Kim	Center for Sustainable Healthy Buildings, Korea

Preparatory Committee Members

Jin-Woo Jung	Dongguk University, Korea
Jongbae Kim	National Rehabilitation Center Research Institute, Korea
Mi Jeong Kim	Kyung Hee University, Korea
Geum-Yong Lee	Sangmyung University, Korea
Heyoung Lee	Seoul National University of Technology, Korea
Yeunsook Lee	Yonsei University/The Korean Gerontological Society, Korea
Soohyun Lim	Yonsei University, Korea
Hun-Kuk Park	Kyung Hee University, Korea
Kwang-Hyun Park	Kwangwoon University, Korea
Mignon Park	Yonsei University, Korea
Seong Dae Sagong	Korea Institute of Science and Technology, Korea
Jeong-Hwa Song	Namseoul University, Korea
Won-Kyung Song	National Rehabilitation Center Research Institute, Korea
Hye Gyung Yoon	Yonsei University, Korea

Publicity

Bessam Abdulrazak	Université de Sherbrooke, Canada
Ismail Khalil	Johannes Kepler University, Austria
Choonhwa Lee	Hanyang University, Korea
Young-Sook Park	Australian Embassy, Korea
Tatsuya Yamazaki	National Institute of Information & Communications Technology, Japan

Administrative and Financial

Hye Gyung Yoon	Yonsei University, Korea
Jung-Hyun Kim	The Korean Gerontological Society, Korea
Geum-Yong Lee	Sangmyung University, Korea
Jung-Keun Oh	Konkuk University, Korea

Communication

Soohyun Lim	Yonsei University, Korea

Conference Implemented by

KGS, The Korean Gerontological Society, Korea
MEDR, Institute of Millennium Environmental Design and Research at Yonsei University, Korea
CSHeB, Center for Sustainable Healthy Buildings, Kyung Hee University ,Korea

Conference Co-organized by

KGS, The Korean Gerontological Society, Korea
CSHeB, Center for Sustainable Healthy Buildings, Kyung Hee University, Korea
MEDR, Institute of Millennium Environmental Design and Research at Yonsei University, Korea
ET, The Electronic Times, Korea
SWF, Seoul Welfare Foundation, Korea

Conference Endorsed by

Institut TELECOM, France
UNIST, Ulsan National Institute of Science and Technology, Korea
NRC, National Rehabilitation Center, Korea

Table of Contents

Smart Home and Village

Health Telematics and Healthcare Technology

Aging Friendly and Enabling Technology

Short Papers

A Supplementary Automatic Door Device for Hybrid Support of Humans and Robots

Rui Fukui, Keita Kadowaki, Hiroshi Noguchi, Taketoshi Mori, and Tomomasa Sato

Intelligent Cooperative Systems Laboratory, the University of Tokyo
Eng. bldg. 2nd, Room 81C1. 7-3-1 Hongo, Bunkyo-ku, Tokyo, Japan
http://www.ics.t.u-tokyo.ac.jp

Abstract. This paper describes the development of Automatic Door Device as a part of intelligent environment. This device, Robo-Door, can release home robots from door opening/closing task and serve for handicapped humans as well. The characteristics of the device are (a) easy installation via wheel actuation and (b) compatibility of automatic motion and human manual handling by clutch mechanism.

Keywords: Service robot, Automatic door, Intelligent environment, Ubiquitous robot.

1 Introduction

Recently, robots are hoped to provide services for humans in living spaces, and as a strategy, structured or intelligent environment is proposed by several research groups, where sensors and actuators are distributed [1–4]. For example, Tomokuni et al. developed a caster type actuator (Active caster), which can be easily attached to a piece of furniture [5]. In addition to the purpose of supporting humans, those intelligent environments can play a role of providing infrastructures for service robots and may promote rapid introduction of current robot systems into our living spaces.

As a part of such approaches, this paper describes the development of a device to open/close a door automatically (Robo-Door, Fig. 1). For home robots, door opening/closing is an essential task [6, 7]. However, it is not practicable for robots without arms (ex. Roomba) to operate a door by themselves. By installing a door actuating device, the environment improves those robots' performances. In addition, automatic opening/closing of a door is also helpful for humans with physical handicap, especially when they use wheel chairs.

Therefore, the aim of our research is the development of a door opening/closing device which realizes (a) the support for physically handicapped persons and (b) the environmental arrangement for home robots.

The framework of this paper is as below; Implementation methodology for automatic opening/closing of a door and required specifications for the device are discussed in section 2. In section 3, design and implementation of the device are described. Experimental Results of the prototype are analyzed in Section 4, followed by conclusions and a discussion on future work in Section 5.

Y. Lee et al. (Eds.): ICOST 2010, LNCS 6159, pp. 1–8, 2010.

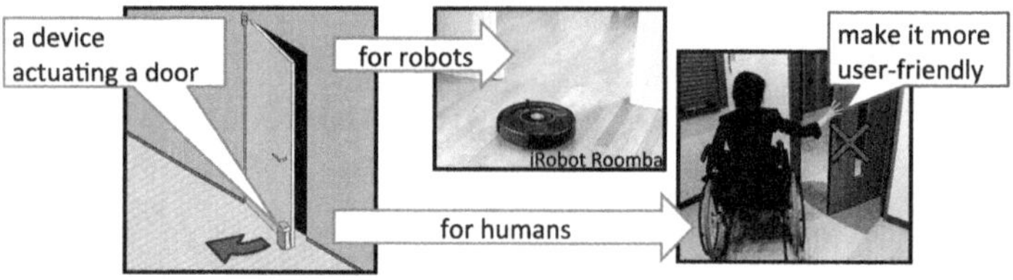

Fig. 1. Conceptual image of automatic door device

2 Required Specifications and Design of Mechanisms

In this section, required specifications for Robo-Door and implementation methodology to satisfy the requirements are discussed.

2.1 Required Specifications for Automatic Door Opening/Closing

Required specifications for Robo-Door are as below; (1) stable door operation, (2) ensuring safety and (3) low resistance for manual handling of a door. By def- inition, Robo-Door must open/close a door properly in order to enable humans and robots to go through. For ensuring safety, a function to stop operation is also required, ex. when a man/woman is caught in a door. In addition, manual usability of a door should be retained. This is because when the device is down (ex. electric outage) and if the door cannot be opened manually, the device may obstruct evacuation attempts. Moreover, it is stressful for most general users to wait for automatic opening/closing motion. Because not only the handicapped and robots but also healthy individuals use the same door, low resistance for manual operation is necessary.

Besides the described above, Robo-Door should solve a problem of doorknobs. It is enough, however, to just install a knob which can be unlocked by applying a certain extent of force, for example. This paper is discussed based on an assumption that such a doorknob has already been installed.

2.2 Methodology to Realize Robo-Door

To satisfy the requirements described above, various methods can be listed. In Section 2.2, the way to realize automatic opening/closing of a door is considered especially focusing on (1) installation to an existing living environment and (2) co-existing of humans and robots.

Consideration of door automatizing methodology. First of all, there are two schemes in order to realize automatic opening/closing of a door; (a) installation of a device to an existing door and (b) exchange of a door with easily automated one (ex. slide type, folding type and roller blind type). Fig. 2 shows the advantages and disadvantages of each scheme.

In the case of equipping a device, it is needless to exchange a door of course. Considering installation to an existing environment, this is a big advantage. As an disadvantage, interference with passersby or other objects could happen especially if the door is hinged type.

On the other hand, each alternative candidate has some advantages and disadvantages shown in the right side of Fig. 2. Their advantages, especially no interference of slide and roller blind types, are attractive. But in addition to the disadvantages depicted in Fig. 2, they have a common problem of the exchange cost. In the case of new buildings suited to the handicapped or installation of robots, these doors might be installed at the initial stage. Considering installation to an existing environment, however, a costly approach is not likely to be accepted.

As shown above, (b) exchange of a door does not exceed (a) installation of a device, taking the cost and other disadvantages into consideration. Therefore, it is valid to automatize a door by installing a new device, Robo-Door.

	(a) installing a device to a static door	(b) replacing to full automatic door		
	a hinged door and slide door	slide type	folding type	roller blind type
types of door	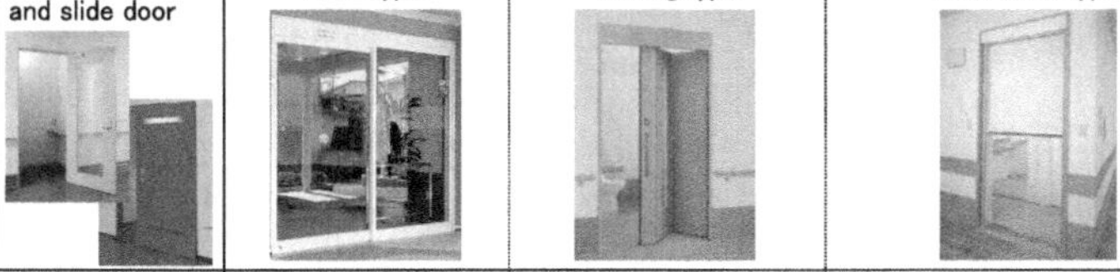			
advantages	・no need of door's exchange	・no interference ・easy manual open/close	・installation compatible with a hinged door	・no interference ・small space to install
disadvantages	・interference by opening /closing	・large space for door	・low usability for manual open/close	・low usability for hand motion ・low sound/heat insulation

Fig. 2. Comparison of two methods, installing a special device or exchange of a door

Consideration of door actuation type. Some supplementary automatic door devices have been produced (Fig. 3) [8, 9]. These commercial products adopt mechanical links to actuate a door. One advantage of this method is that the device does not interfere with human's living space. Moreover, it is easy to control because the degree of motor's rotation corresponds with the state of a door. However, most of these products need a high power motor and fabrication for installation, ex. punching on a wall. In addition to mechanical links, wires, wheels and magnetic force (like linear motors) can be listed for actuation candidates.

From these candidates, Robo-Door selects a method of actuation by a wheel. One advantage of actuation by a wheel is simplicity of its mechanism. Moreover, it could be installed to both hinged and slide doors by changing the direction of the device.

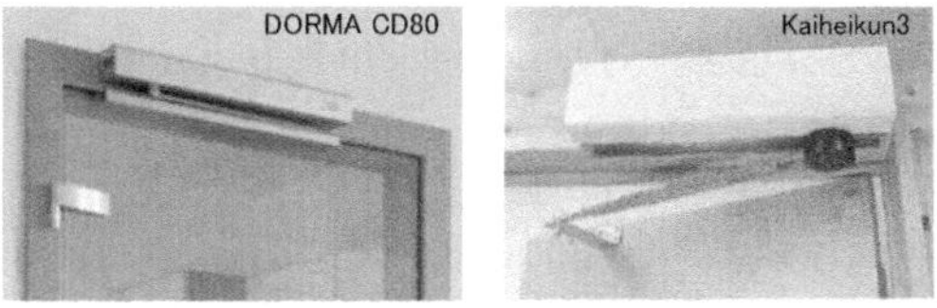

Fig. 3. Commercial products which opens/closes a door automatically by mechanical links

Additionally, as described below, the equipping method to a door is taken into account for realizing installation without fabrication. In the case of installing a new system or device into human living environment, easy installation is one of the important factors. Furthermore, Robo-Door starts operation when it receives a command by wireless communication, therefore an user is supposed to carry a remote controller.

Analysis of functions required for door actuation by a wheel. Robo-Door needs following 5 functions; (1) **Detection of collision;** Considering automation of a door, the device must ensure safety. Therefore, if humans, robots and other objects collide with a door, Robo-Door must detect the collision and stop immediately. (2) **Reduction of resistance in manual operation;** As described in Section 2.1, Robo-Door should not interrupt manual opening/closing. (3) **Easy installation;** For reduction of the installation cost, Robo-Door should be equipped with as little fabrication as possible. (4) **Sufficient door driving force;** One unique problem of the wheel actuation is that a floor state have influence on the device's performance. A floor of living space might be waving slightly, and the friction coefficient varies according to the material of the floor. To avoid slipping, it is essential to press the wheel to the floor. (5) **Recognition of door state;** One more problem is state recognition of a door. Just measuring rotation numbers of a wheel or a motor lacks accuracy, because a slip between the wheel and the floor, though it might be a little, causes error of the door position estimation.

3 Design and Implementation of Mechanism

Based on the discussion in the former section, design and implementation for satisfying the required specifications are described in this section. First, the whole structure of Robo-Door is depicted in Fig. 4. It consists of 3 units, (1) driving unit, (2) fixing unit and (3) slider guide unit.

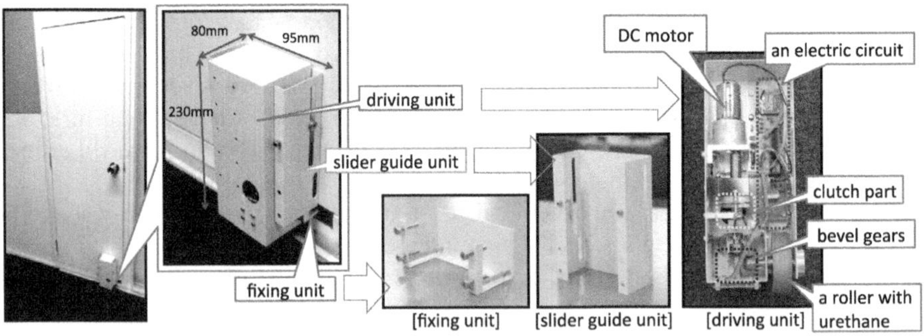

Fig. 4. Whole structure of Robo-Door

3.1 Collision Detecting Function by a Current Sensor

Robo-Door is supposed to stop its motion rapidly if the door bumps into humans or robots. Then, Robo-Door detects collision by measuring motor current, which increases as the load of the motor rises up. The current sensor installed in our prototype is "HPS-3-AS" produced by U_RD.

3.2 Resistance Reduction Function by a Pin Clutch Mechanism

In order to reduce resistance in manual opening/closing of a door, a clutch mechanism is installed into the driving unit as shown in Fig. 5. Upper side of the two pins is shifted down by a DC solenoid, and mating of the two pins achieves transmission of power from the motor to the wheel. Normally, the upper pin is pushed up by springs. Using photo interrupters, it is ensured that the two pins do not interfere with each other when the clutch makes connected.

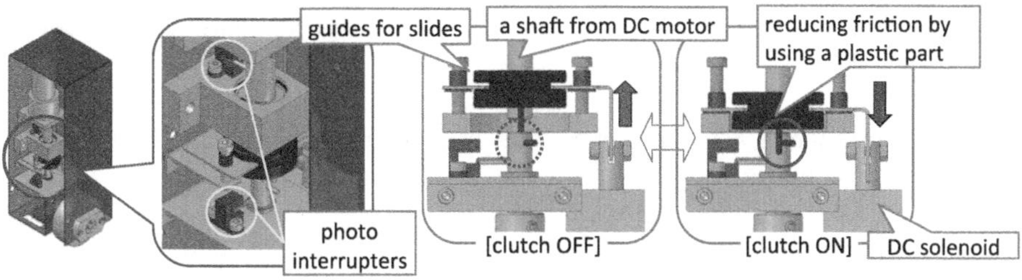

Fig. 5. Detailed description of the clutch mechanism

3.3 Door State Recognition Function by Magnets and Hall Sensors

Recognition of the door state is realized by magnets placed on the floor and hall effect ICs equipped on the down side of the driving unit (Fig. 6). The sensor, DN6852 produced by Panasonic, has binary output according to in- crease/decrease of one way magnetic field. The distance between the sensors and magnets is about 2 [mm]. As shown in Fig. 6, two sensors are equipped side by side. By combining the sensors' outputs, Robo-Door distinguishes four different door state; fully open, fully close, on the magnet's point and the other. 10 × 20 × 1 [mm] neodymium magnets are used in our prototype.

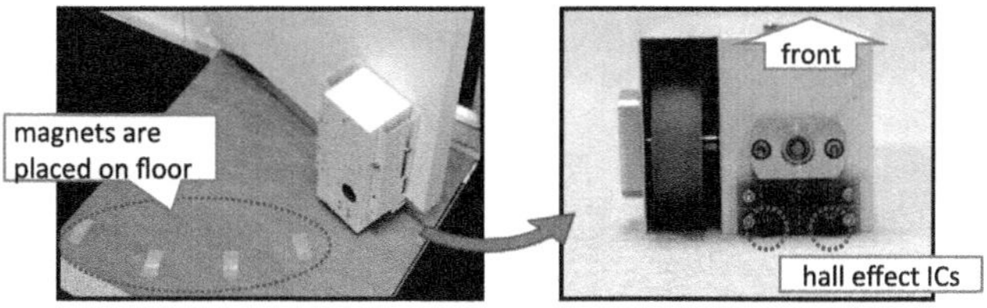

Fig. 6. Magnets and hall-effect ICs for door's position detection

3.4 Easy Installation Function by Segmented Structures

To make installation work as easy as possible, Robo-Door adopts a fixing method without fabrication like punching on a door (Fig. 7, left). Fixing is achieved by (1) clipping the bottom of a door in between the fixing and slider guide units, (2)

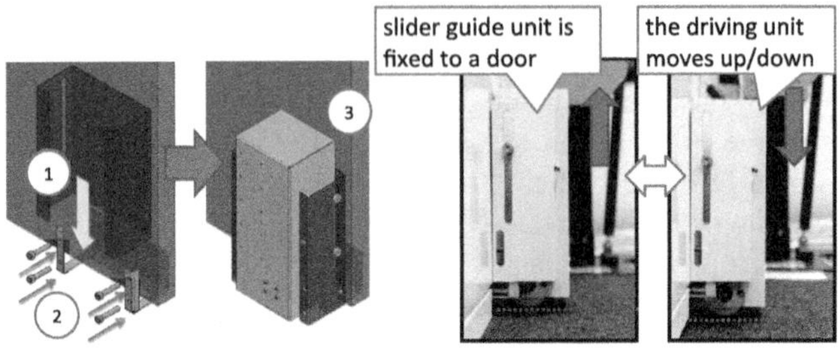

Fig. 7. (Left) Fixing the unit to the door without a punch, (Right) Slide mechanisum for driving force optimization

clamping the slider guide unit against a door and (3) assembling the driving unit on the slider guide unit.

3.5 Driving Force Optimization Function by a Slide Mechanism

As described in section 2.2, the condition of a floor might cause a problem in the case of wheel actuation. Avoiding slip, the driving unit can move up-down along with the channels of the slider guide unit. To get enough driving force, in addition, the driving unit is pulled down to the floor by springs equipped between the slider guide and driving units (Fig. 7, right). This function also provides an advantage that it is needles to adjust the placement appropriately to the gap between a floor and the bottom of a door, though the gap varies according to installation places.

4 Performance Evaluation Experiments

To evaluate the performance of a prototype Robo-Door, two experiments are carried out; (1) examining automatic opening/closing motion of a door and (2) verifying collision detection. The detail of the experiments are described below.

4.1 Automatic Door Operation Experiment

[Condition] The prototype of Robo-Door is equipped to a room door and opens/closes the door according to a command from a wireless communication device (Digi international, XBee). Actuation of the door is tried on three kinds of floor: wood, carpet and cushion floor. In this experiment, the magnets for recognition of door's state are installed only on the wood floor.

[Result] The snapshots of the experiment on the wood floor are shown in Fig. 8 (upper), and the results on the carpet and the cushion floor are depicted in Fig. 8 (lower). As to these three types of floor, Robo-Door actuated the door successfully.

[Discussion] On each type of typical floors, automatic operation of the door by wheel was achieved without problems. Thus, the feasibility of Robo-Door was confirmed. In this experiment, magnets were temporarily fixed with tapes on the floor. The arrangement of the magnets should be modified for real applications.

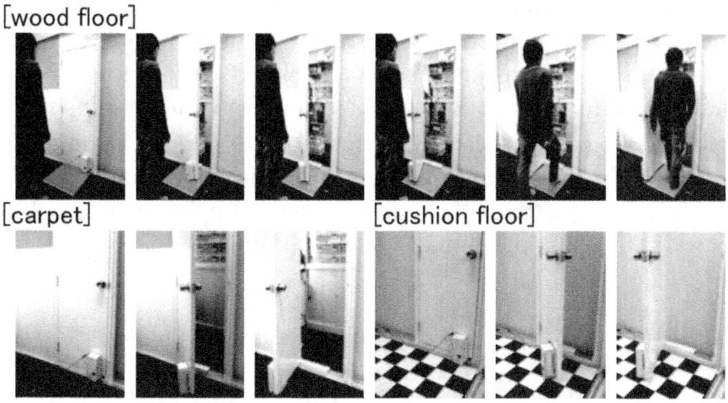

Fig. 8. Sequential snapshots of automatic door operation experiment

4.2 Collision Detection Experiment

[Condition] In this experiment, Robo-Door actuates a door and collides with an object while its operation. A load cell ("LM10KA" produced by KYOWA Sensor System Solutions) and a data logger ("NR-600" produced by KEYENCE) are used to measure the collision force (Fig. 9). Running distances before the collision are 200 [mm] and 400 [mm], and the data is measured three times at each setting.

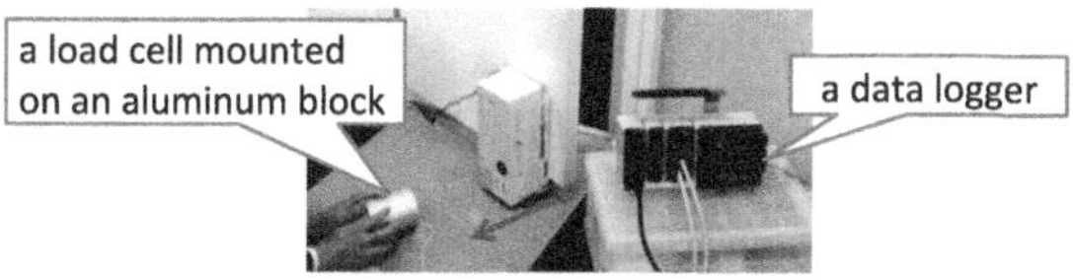

Fig. 9. Snapshot of collision detection experiment

[Result] The results of the collision detection experiment is shown in Fig. 10. The left side of Fig. 10 indicates the maximum applied force and continuous time during which over 10 [N] force was applied in each measurement. The right side of Fig. 10 is sequential force graph of the second trial in distance 400 [mm].

distance	trial	maximum force [N]	applied over 10N [ms]
200 [mm]	1	40.86	111
	2	34.01	86
	3	39.31	72
400 [mm]	1	25.22	350
	2	39.75	442
	3	24.47	684

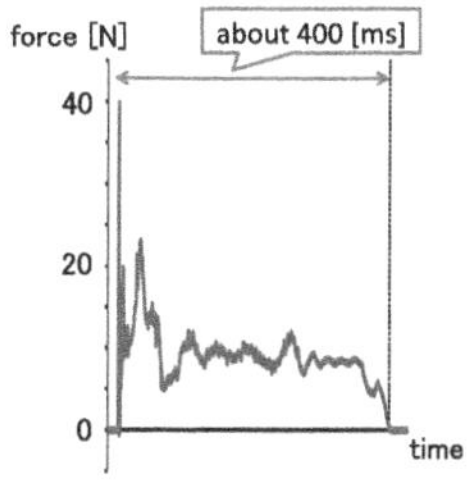

Fig. 10. The experimental result ofcollision detection

[Discussion] The experimental result shows that about 40 [N] force was applied to the object at the moment of impact. It is apparent from the graph, however, that the maximum of applied force was just around a peak. Afterward, lower than 20 [N] was applied continuously for some 100 [ms], and then Robo-Door stopped its motion by detecting collision. An impact energy corresponds to defined by multiplication of a force and its applied time. Therefore, the impact energy by collision is not serious. Consequently, it is demonstrated that collision detection function of Robo-Door using a current sensor has enough performance to ensure safety.

5 Conclusion

In this paper, we develop a device Robo-Door, which opens/closes a door automatically in living spaces. The purpose of Robo-Door is both daily life support for the handicapped and arrangement of intelligent environment for service robots. The main features of Robo-Door are (1) actuation by a wheel, (2) low resistance for manual operation and (3) easy installation into existing environment. It is shown by experiments that Robo-Door achieves opening/closing operation on various kinds of floor and has enough safety against collision with humans and robots.

As a future work, it is urgent to establish the way to arrange magnets properly on a floor for stable recognition of the door state. In addition, Robo-Door now can be equipped only to a hinged door. Therefore, design modification for installing into a slide door is also required.

References

1. Mori, T., Sato, T.: Robotic Room. Robotics and Autonomous Systems 28(2), 141–148 (1999)
2. Youngblood, G.M., et al.: Managing Adaptive Versatile Environments. In: Proc. of 3rd IEEE Int. Conf. on Pervasive Computing and Communications, pp. 351–360 (2005)
3. Helal, S., et al.: The Gator Tech Smart House: a programmable pervasive space. Computer 38(3), 50–60 (2005)
4. Murakami, K., et al.: A structured environment with sensor networks for intelligent robots. IEEE Sensors, 705–708 (2008)
5. Tomokuni, N., et al.: Multi-Functional Active Caster Module for Distributed Actuation Devices. In: Proc. of SICE-ICASE Int. Joint Conference, pp. 2649–2652 (2006)
6. Rusu, R.B., et al.: Laser-based Perception for Door and Handle Identification. In: Proc. of Int. Conf. on Advanced Robotics, pp. 1–8 (2009)
7. Shono, K., et al.: Development of the Indoor Mobile Robot Based on RECS - Oepening And Closing a Door And Charge. In: Proc. of JSPE Spring Meeting, vol. I35, pp. 831–832 (2004)
8. DORMA GmbH, CD80, http://www.dorma.com
9. I.S.T Corp., Kaiheikun3, http://www.kaiheikun.com

Automatic Service Composition with Heterogeneous Service-Oriented Architectures

José M. Reyes Álamo, Hen-I Yang, Johnny Wong, and Carl K. Chang

Department of Computer Science, Iowa State University
Ames, IA, USA
{jmreyes,hiyang,wong,chang}@cs.iastate.edu

Abstract. Service-Oriented Architecture is widely used to program pervasive spaces such as Smart Homes because of its capabilities to handle dynamic and heterogeneous environments. It is often the case that the services required are designed and implemented using different SOAs, such as OSGi and Web Services. Most of the current composition frameworks take a two-tier approach: those services following the same SOA can take advantage of service composition and runtime substitutions, while interactions between services of different SOAs require hardcoded service invocations that do not really provide full advantage of SOA. Some SOAs do not support features such as on-the-fly compositions or a searchable service directory. In this paper, we present a framework to compose and orchestrate services from different SOA implementations and provide the missing functionalities to support composition of heterogeneous SOAs. We present a case study and the performance analysis of the study to demonstrate the feasibility of our framework.

Keywords: Web Services, Service Composition, OSGi, SOA, BPEL.

1 Introduction

A service is defined as an autonomous, loosely coupled, platform independent entity that can be described, published, discovered, and invoked. It can be an atomic service performing a simple computation or a set of services that when combined perform a complex computation [1]. Service-Oriented Computing (SOC) is a programming paradigm where applications are created by having different services interacting in a logical way. Instead of depending on a single component as in the case of stand-alone applications, several orchestrated services in SOC provide the desired functionality. A fundamental characteristic of SOC is the separation of the service implementation from the service specification. Several Service-Oriented Architectures (SOAs) have been proposed for this purpose, which define the specification of services and the protocol to interact with the actual services. SOAs are designed to be loosely coupled and theoretically, any service should be able to collaborate with other services via compatible interfaces. However, in practice it is difficult for services implemented under different SOAs to interact.

Most of the research in SOA has focused on Web Services (WS). As a result, technologies and protocols for WS are well defined and studied. There exists other SOAs

Y. Lee et al. (Eds.): ICOST 2010, LNCS 6159, pp. 9–16, 2010.

whose properties make them more suitable for certain applications such as OSGi, JINI, and UPnP. To comprise the full potential of SOC, we would like to be able to create composite services that are not dependent on a particular SOA. We believe that an SOA standard should be able to accommodate and utilize different services, regardless of the particular languages, platforms, and architectures they are based on. We conjecture that doing so will improve the availability and diversity of the potential applications. This will also increase the number of services to choose from as well as the quality of the composite service. Universal composition of heterogeneous services can also influences performance as we can choose the services that perform better not limiting ourselves to a particular SOA. It can also improve reliability, as a set of services might provide the same functionality but are implemented using different SOAs. If one of the services fails, the framework can select another and still be able to execute our application.

We aim at providing an efficient solution especially useful for Smart Home environments that considers the uses and properties of services. Having an approach to compose, add, remove, start, and stop these services as needed and selecting the SOA that maximizes performance is a primary motivation for this work. A scenario suitable for this kind of applications is the Smart Home environment. A Smart Home is a residential establishment equipped with sensors, actuators, and other technology to help the resident performing activities of daily living. Smart Homes are especially useful for the elderly and persons with special needs. Over the years, researchers have studied a vast number of devices and development approaches for Smart Homes. A service-oriented approach as a solution for the challenges of developing Smart Homes that satisfies the user requirements seems the most plausible. Therefore, we would like to improve Smart Home applications and move a step closer to a comprehensive solution.

In this paper, we explore the different strategies used by the research community to compose services of different SOAs. We present a composition framework that relies on services from different SOAs. We provide a working example of an actual application that combines heterogeneous services, and contrast our framework with other people's work. The rest of the paper is organized as follows: Section 2 presents related work; Section 3 discusses the importance of heterogeneous SOAs composite services; Section 4 outlines the composition framework; Section 5 describes our case study; Section 6 details the performance evaluation; Section 7 is the conclusions and future work.

2 Related Work

Several research works have presented strategies for automatically composing OSGi services. In [2] the authors present a framework to achieve spontaneous compositions of OSGi services. It provides functionality to handle availability of services, links to connect to the services and matching criteria for selecting the best available service. In [3] the authors use the Business Processing Execution Language (BPEL), which is a WS language, to describe the workflow of a composition. They provide a framework that extends OSGi by allowing it to interpret BPEL files, locate the services, and create the composite service. Their framework focuses on composing OSGi services only. The authors in [4] present a strategy for automatically composing OSGi services by first converting them to WS and then use WS composition techniques. Our work is different, in that we want to use different services in their original architecture without the need of converting them.

Other researchers have focused on the problem of composing heterogeneous SOAs such as OSGi services and WS. In [5] the authors support BPEL for workflow description and allow composite services to use OSGi services and WS. In their work, they add a set of custom tags to the BPEL file. These tags specify service type and binding information. These approaches are different from ours as we automatically gather this information from a service repository without extra tags. Therefore, the BPEL file needed in our framework is simpler, less verbose and represents a more interoperable solution. As there is no need to provide details about a service in the workflow specification file, this allows our framework to be extendable to other SOAs. A similar approach is followed by technologies such as the Service Composite Architecture (SCA) [5] found in frameworks such as Apache Tuscany [6], Fabric3 [7] and the Newton Framework [8]. The basic unit in SCA is a component, which is a service developed using any accepted SOA such as OSGi, WS, and Spring. SCA offers a framework where developers can create composites using services with heterogeneous implementations. They rely on annotation and a special XML language to define the components and composites. The problem with SCA is that the tags and annotations have to be included in the source code of the service so the framework can understand it. This limits the services that can be used to only those developed under a SCA infrastructure. In our work, we use the services in their original implementation, allowing us to reuse services already available.

3 Heterogeneous Service Composition

There is still a great need for a SOA-independent solution for service composition. The foundation of the SOA is the separation of the specification of a service from its implementation. Platform and language independence is one of the main features of SOA. However, in real life implementations it is difficult to integrate services of different SOAs. As described in the related work, some researchers have focused on automatically composing OSGi services while others attempted to combine technologies like OSGi and WS. Our work moves one-step closer towards the goal of having a platform, language, and SOA independent solution.

We present a framework for creating composite services that is extendable to accept services in different SOAs. Our solution consists of a framework capable of automatically composing OSGi services extended to include WS. In order to combine both types of services we carefully investigate different SOAs, especially WS compositions. We evaluate and integrate several existing WS protocols and technologies to accommodate for a heterogeneous set of services from different SOAs. We also examine the OSGi framework [9] that has been the subject of research for many years, it is standardized, and it has several open-source and commercial implementations available. We notice that certain very desirable features for smart home environments of the

OSGi framework are not available for WS. These features include security, dynamic installation and removal of bundles, automatic package resolution, as well as a set of essential services provided by the standard like the HTTP server and log service.

During the design and development of our framework for automatic composition of heterogeneous services we have addressed several technical challenges. One of the challenges is to ensure full support of each of the SOAs to allow seamless invocation of services. Another challenge is regarding to the lack of support for automatically creating composite services in some SOAs. We create the necessary tools to support these missing but necessary functionalities. The end-result is a composition framework that supports seamless integration of heterogeneous SOAs, both OSGi services and WS. This allows transparent heterogeneous service composition using OSGi bundles or WS without the need to modify them, as contrasts to previous approaches that rely on tags, annotations, or transformations of services.

4 Composition Framework

We describe how our composition framework operates in the following: First, we provide a BPEL file with the description of the composite service workflow because it is based on XML, is widely supported in the industry and the research community as well as it has become the de-facto standard for WS compositions. After invoking the composition framework with a BPEL file as input, the framework performs a syntax check. If the check finds no errors, the framework parses the BPEL file and extracts the composite service information. Using the information, it locates the candidate services in a service repository that stores information for both WS and OSGi. Once the framework gathers the services' binding information it proceeds with the actual

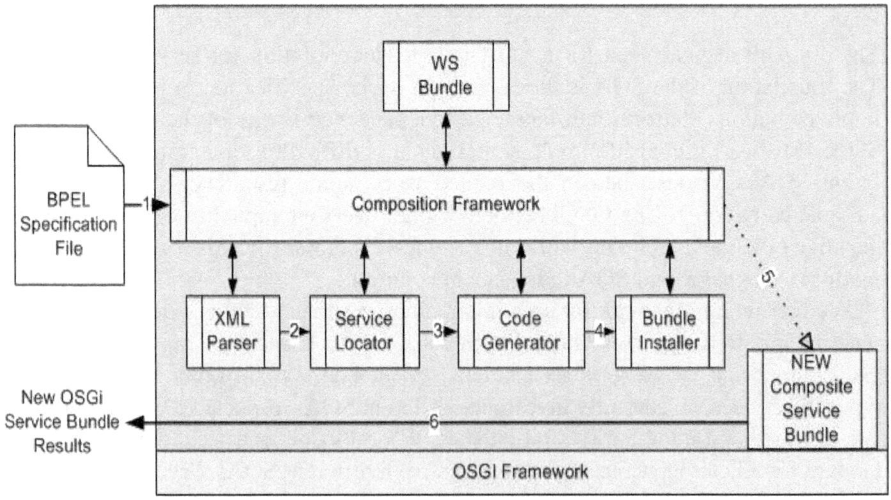

Fig. 1. BPEL2OSGi Composition Framework Architecture

creation of the composite service. After that, it translates the orchestration logic into executable Java program. Since the implementation of the composed service is an OSGi bundle, the framework creates the remaining components such as the service interface, the activator class, and the manifest file and includes the service references. These files are then automatically compiled, packaged into a jar file, and installed into the OSGi framework. If the service is error free it will run after a few instants otherwise, it will throw exceptions and display error messages. All these steps are automatic and transparent to the user. Figure 1 depicts a graphical representation of this framework. Because our composition framework takes as input a BPEL file and produces an OSGi bundle, we call our framework BPEL2OSGi.

5 Case Study (MISS)

We demonstrate the feasibility of our composition framework with a case study where we provide a BPEL file, create the composite service, install, and execute it. The case study is an implementation of the Medicine Information Support System (MISS) [10] that helps patients with the management of their prescriptions. It integrates the doctor, the pharmacy, and the smart home, allowing subsystems to share information with each other and uses a trusted third party to check for conflicts. Its main purpose is to increase safety by checking for conflicts among new prescription and previous medicines, health conditions and foods. By checking new prescription data with the patient's local record at each subsystem, MISS detects all possible paths of conflicts.

The workflow of MISS can be described as follows: at the doctor's subsystem, the doctor enters the new prescription's data and checks for conflicts with previous prescriptions using a trusted third party [11]. If no conflict found, MISS uses a secure communication channel to forward the prescription data to the pharmacy. At the pharmacy subsystem, MISS checks for conflicts using the patient's local pharmacy record. If no conflicts found, MISS uses a secure communication channel to forward the prescription data to the Smart Home subsystem. At the Smart Home, MISS checks for conflicts using the patient's local Smart Home record of medications, foods, and conditions.

Figure 2 shows a BPEL diagram of the workflow of MISS. This figure shows specifically the interaction between the pharmacy and the Smart Home subsystem. The process execution starts at the main node followed by the Receive Input operation, which is the default BPEL operation indicating the beginning of the execution. After that, we call a series of services. First, the Invoke RFID Service for reading the RFID tags of the medicine used by the Invoke Pharmacy Server to query the prescription information. Then we assign data to several variables and call the Invoke MCD Service [11] that checks for conflicts among the new prescription and with previous medicines and food items at home. Depending whether there is a conflict we invoke the Invoke Speech Server and Invoke Notification Service with the corresponding message. If no conflict is found the new prescription data is stored into the Smart Home subsystem by the Invoke Medicine SH Server service.

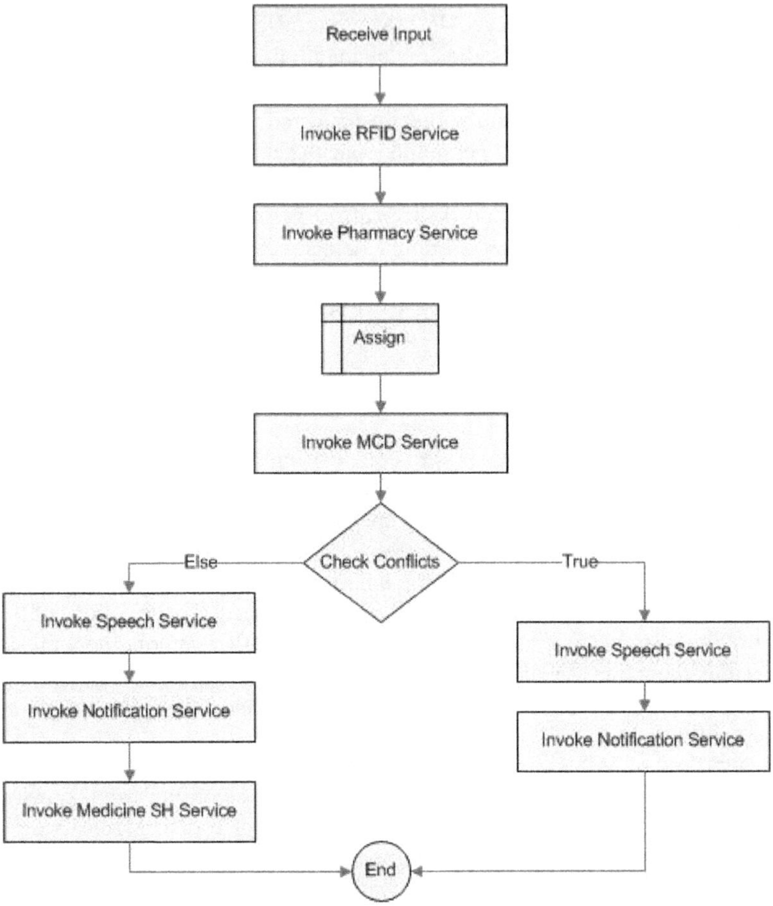

Fig. 2. BPEL Diagram of MISS

6 Evaluation

We study the performance of our composition framework by measuring the time it takes to create a composite service, how much overhead it adds and compare it to current compositions approaches. We compare the execution time of composite services using a single SOA against those using heterogeneous SOAs. In our experiments, we create a composite service that only uses OSGi services (MISS_OSGI), another that only uses WS (MISS_WS), and a third that uses a combination of both (MISS_BPEL). The overhead for parsing the XML file, locating the services, and creating the composite service is about the same in all cases. Our hypothesis is that MISS_OSGi will perform better, followed by MISS_BPEL and MISS_WS will have the worst performance. We base our hypothesis in the fact that OSGi services are local and their communication protocol is faster, while WS use HTTP that is a slower protocol. We observe a significant difference in the execution time of the composite service. Figure 3 shows the result of our experiments after we execute the three types of composite services at least 100 times and we measure the execution time.

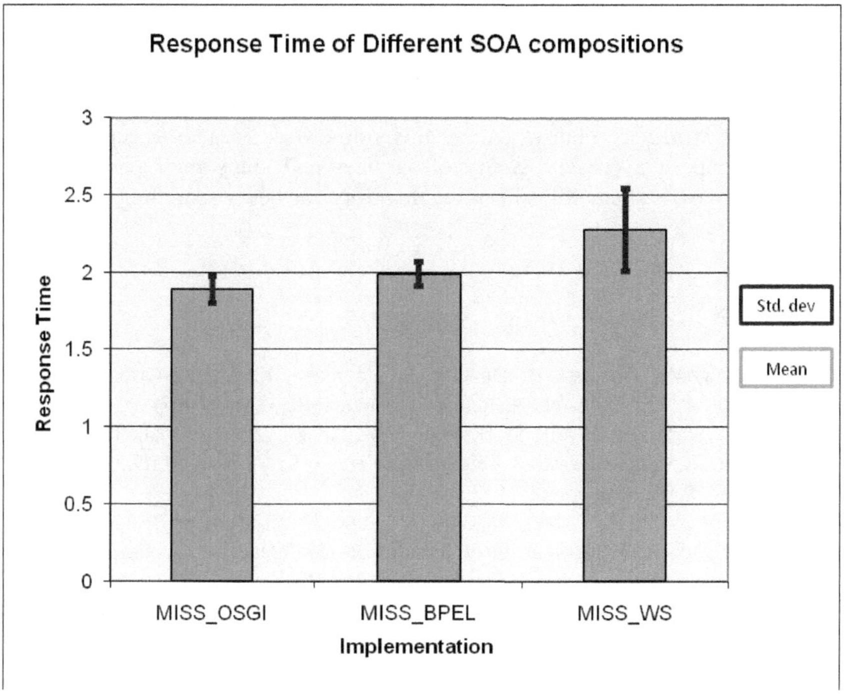

Fig. 3. Execution time of each implementation. The black line (left) indicates the minimum and maximum. The red line (right) indicates the standard deviation.

Our result supports our hypothesis as the MISS_OSGi had the best performance, closely followed by MISS_BPEL and the composition with the worst execution time is MISS_WS. Nevertheless, the time difference among them is in the worst case 0.3848 or less than half a second. This amount of time for this particular application is acceptable and observed by a human being, it is almost unnoticeable. The fact that WS are the slower but are the most popular and widely used, gives us an upper bound on the time that is acceptable for these applications. Another positive result is that we reduce the execution time of the worst case by using heterogeneous services. It is a great advantage the fact that we can choose different implementations of services providing the same functionality. Figure 3 also shows that the MISS_BPEL has the smallest standard deviation (and variance) of all three, making the execution and communication time more consistent and predictable.

7 Conclusions and Future Work

Service-Oriented Computing has been widely used in pervasive spaces such as Smart Homes. However, we would like to compose services from different SOAs. We present a framework that actually makes the automatic composition of heterogeneous services possible, requiring minimum intervention from the user. The framework provides automatic, on-the-fly compositions, a searchable service directory, and supports different SOAs like OSGi and WS.

We present a case study in which we compare the performance of the composite service created by the framework with composite services created manually. The analysis shows that the performance is acceptable sitting between the best case and the worst-case scenarios with the advantages that the framework offers.

For future work, we plan to extend this framework by adding support for other SOAs to compose a greater variety of services and study their performance. We also want to have a standardized service directory for better searching and binding to services.

References

1. Papazoglou, M., Traverso, P., Dustdar, S., Leymann, F.: Service-Oriented Computing: State of the Art and Research Challenges. Computer 40, 38–45 (2007)
2. Wood, A., Stankovic, J., Virone, G., Selavo, L., He, Z., Cao, Q., Doan, T., Wu, Y., Fang, L., Stoleru, R.: Context-aware wireless sensor networks for assisted living and residential monitoring. IEEE Network 22, 26–33 (2008)
3. Redondo, R., Vilas, A., Cabrer, M., Arias, J., Lopez, M.: Enhancing Residential Gateways: OSGi Services Composition. In: International Conference on Consumer Electronics, ICCE 2007, Digest of Technical Papers, pp. 1–2 (2007)
4. Anke, J., Sell, C.: Seamless Integration of Distributed OSGi Bundles into Enterprise Processes using BPEL, Bern, Schweiz
5. Lee, C., Ko, S., Kim, E., Lee, W.: Enriching OSGi Service Composition with Web Services. IEICE Transactions 92-D, 1177–1180 (2009)
6. Apache Tuscany, `http://tuscany.apache.org/` (March 23, 2010)
7. Fabric3 - Open Source SCA, `http://www.fabric3.org/` (March 23, 2010)
8. Newton Framework, `http://newton.codecauldron.org/site/index.html` (March 23, 2010)
9. Marples, D., Kriens, P.: The Open Services Gateway Initiative: an introductory overview. IEEE Communications Magazine 39, 110–114 (2001)
10. Reyes Álamo, J.M., Wong, J., Babbitt, R., Chang, C.: MISS: Medicine Information Support System in the Smart Home Environment. In: Helal, S., Mitra, S., Wong, J., Chang, C.K., Mokhtari, M. (eds.) ICOST 2008. LNCS, vol. 5120, pp. 185–199. Springer, Heidelberg (2008)
11. Reyes Álamo, J.M., Yang, H., Wong, J., Babbitt, R., Chang, C.: Support for Medication Safety and Compliance in Smart Home Environments. International Journal of Advanced Pervasive and Ubiquitous Computing 1, 42–60

A Flexible Privacy and Trust Based Context-Aware Secure Framework

Pierre E. Abi-Char, Abdallah Mhamed, Bachar El-Hassan, and Mounir Mokhtari

Laboratory of Reseaux et Service De Telecommunication (RST),
Telecom SudParis (ex. INT), 9 Rue Charles Fourier, Evry, France
{Pierre.abi_char,abdallah.mhamed,mounir.mokhtari}@it-sudparis.eu,
Bachar_elhassan@ul.edu.lb

Abstract. Ubiquitous and pervasive technologies contribute significantly to the quality of life of dependent people by providing personalized services in context aware environments. The deployment of these services within indoor and outdoor environments still require security, privacy and trust issues for dependent persons. Considering the strong links between these three issues, our challenging task was to integrate them in a common and flexible framework using contextual information. In this paper, we propose a security framework that integrates context awareness to perform authentication and access control in a very flexible and scalable model while ensuring both privacy and trust. The framework focuses on the authentication of users who request access to the resources of smart environment system through static devices (i.e. smart card, RFID, etc.), or dynamic devices (i.e. PDA, mobile phones, etc.).

Keywords: Context-Aware, Authentication, Access Control, Smart Spaces, Privacy Control, Trust Management, Risk Assessment.

1 Introduction

The growing evolution of Information and Communication Technology (ICT) systems towards more pervasive and ubiquitous infrastructures contribute significantly to the deployment of services anywhere, at anytime and for anyone. To provide personalized services in such infrastructures, we should consider security, privacy and trust in both indoor and outdoor pervasive environments.

Basically, the common goal of the three issues (security, privacy and trust) is to prevent threats which can affect any information, stored, used or communicated in smart environments. Since this information can be hold by both software and hardware components and can be associated to the user, to computer devices, to network protocols or to assistive devices, its protection techniques fall into one or several of these three issues. This is the reason why it is usually difficult to consider each of these issues individually [1].

Security describes all the techniques used to secure both communications channels and required data. If we consider the protection of information storage and transport, security controls who may access, use or modify context information. Considering the

Y. Lee et al. (Eds.): ICOST 2010, LNCS 6159, pp. 17–23, 2010.

protection of user's personal information, there is a growing concerns about privacy and trustworthiness of such environments and the data they hold. Privacy is the ability to keep user's personal information confidential by whether, when, and to whom information is to be released. Trust is the ability to evaluate the confidence level related to the information issued by the involved entities (users, devices, platform).

As the main objective of our work is dedicated to dependant users (aging, disabled people), the basic user related security services on which we focused our contribution are authentication and control access.

The rest of this paper is as follows. Section 2 provides some background and a summary regarding relevant related work. Our proposed agent framework its process description and implementation are introduced in section 3 and 4 respectively. Finally, section 5 conclude our paper by giving some future directions.

2 Background and Related Work

Firstly, we briefly introduce and discuss some main concepts and key ideas that justify the great necessity of a novel scheme and constitute our background thought and design of our proposed framework.

Context-Awareness: is an emerging computing paradigm that tries to exploit information about the context of its users to provide new or improved services. A context is commonly defined as any information that can be used to characterize the situation of an entity. An entity is a person, place, or object that is considered relevant to the interaction between a user and an application. Generally, the context includes user's location, environmental information (temperature, loudness, and brightness), terminal attributes, and network status (QoS), etc.

Authentication and Access Control: Authentication systems are used for security purposes to verify the authenticity of communicating parties or entities during a transaction. Most traditional identity based authentication methods are not efficient in pervasive environments: either, they do not scale in distributed environments, with hundreds or thousands of embedded devices, or they are inconvenient for users roaming between various living spaces. As authentication requirements differ greatly among different spaces, applications and contexts, a context-aware authentication and access control should be provided using a new approach: (1) Collect and recognize the user's current context, and (2) Generate and control a secure user environment based on the current context.

Privacy Effects: Addressing user privacy is somehow contradictory with user authentication because the act of authentication often involves some disclosure or confirmation of personal information. When designing an authentication system or developing control access policies, we should have a well-defined purposes of the process and ways that the contextual data are collected, shared among active entities, or manipulated by information owners.

Secondly, we briefly highlight the investigated research work related to attribute-based authentication, privacy, and trust.

Authors, in [2], have defined a model that uses contextual attributes to achieve an approach to authentication that is better suited for dynamic, mobile computing environments. They examined the use of trusted platforms to provide assurances for these contextual attributes. Although authors claimed that their model provides a seamless and flexible user experience that can protect privacy and reduce administrative overhead, it does not provides trust and reasoning and there no mention about how to protect privacy (i.e, user, attributes, and data privacy). Marc Langheinrich [3] introduces a privacy awareness system that allows data collectors to both announce and implement data usage policies. The announced data collections of each services and their policies is delegated by a mobile privacy assistant to a personal privacy proxy residing on the platform, which interact with corresponding service proxies and inquires their privacy policies (Privacy Beacon). Corner et al. [4] describe Transient Authentication as a means of authenticating users with devices through a small, short-ranged wireless communications token. This research is limited to the use of location-based context (i.e., proximity) as an attribute in authentication. A similar approach is taken by Glynos et al. [5] where they combined traditional authentication with a limited set of contextual information used to identify users. Other similar approaches were taken by [6] where they also have used a limited set of attributes to perform authentication process. However, we have presented a more generic approach that allows any attributes to be used for authentication. Creese et al. [7] present a general overview of security requirements for authentication in pervasive computing and discuss how traditional authentication does not fit these requirements. Although they discuss authentication of entities using attributes, they did not present a framework for authentication as we have done. In [8], Authors present a service provision mechanism which can enable effective service provision based on semantic similarity measure with the combination of user profiles and situation context in WLAN enabled environment. The paper suggests the combination of user profiles and contextual information to provide a more pervasive service experience in smart assistive environments with mobile device. Behzad et al. [9] propose a framework to construct a context-aware authentication system. Although the framework is flexible and privacy preserving, it is not context-aware user authentication and does not support user trust-worthiness evaluation neither user role assignment. Moreover, the framework is designed to be applicable to Ad-Hoc network, does not provide users a way to control attributes, and not suitable for static environments where users may be holding RFID tags only. In [10], authors propose an authentication scheme for a mobile ubiquitous environment, in which the trustworthiness of a user's device is authenticated anonymously to a remote Service Provider (verifier), during the service discovery process. However, the scheme does not provide support for contextual information, and does not support fuzzy private matching.

3 Toward a New Solution

Here, we briefly outline our proposed authentication-based privacy enhancing infrastructure. Our framework is based on a privacy control layer, a context-aware authentication broker, a context-aware Access Control broker and the use of attributes-based private set intersection and trust evaluation engines. Our framework is a layered architecture that discriminates service providers (context consumers), privacy control process, authentication process, access control process, service receivers (context producers) and the borders that separate these layers. The figure below (Figure 1) shows the process of granting access to resources with the help of user and attributes. Attributes can contain identity and other contextual information (i.e user's profile).

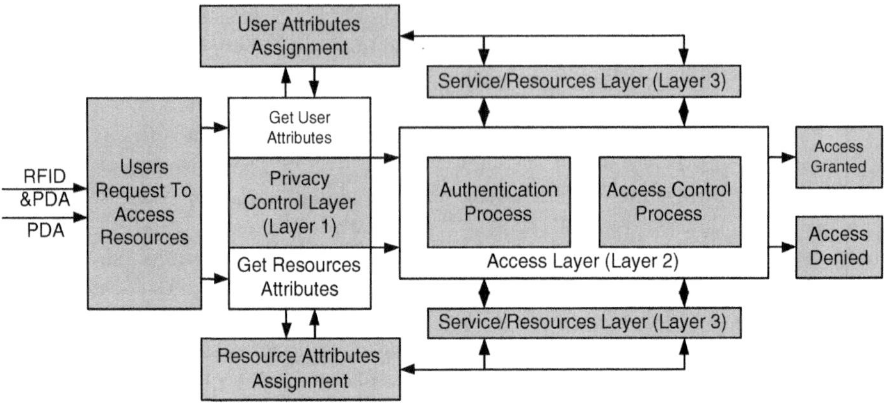

Fig. 1. Context-Aware Framework

In our framework [11], [12], we design an integration scenario where mobile subjects (i.e users) carrying embedded devices (i.e., smart phones, PDA, etc.) receive pervasive services according to their identity and real-time context information environments. Moreover, users with Special needs will have a Body network sensor (BN S) woven into their coat, not visible, which reveal data to the context-awareness system. The cornerstone of our framework is the flexibility to provide authentication and access control for independent and dependent (With a special need) people both at context level and where privacy is preserved. Moreover, our framework provides a distributed infrastructure that allows the tracking of the context in a real-time manner. A high-level overview of these logical components and how they interact is given in following figure 2

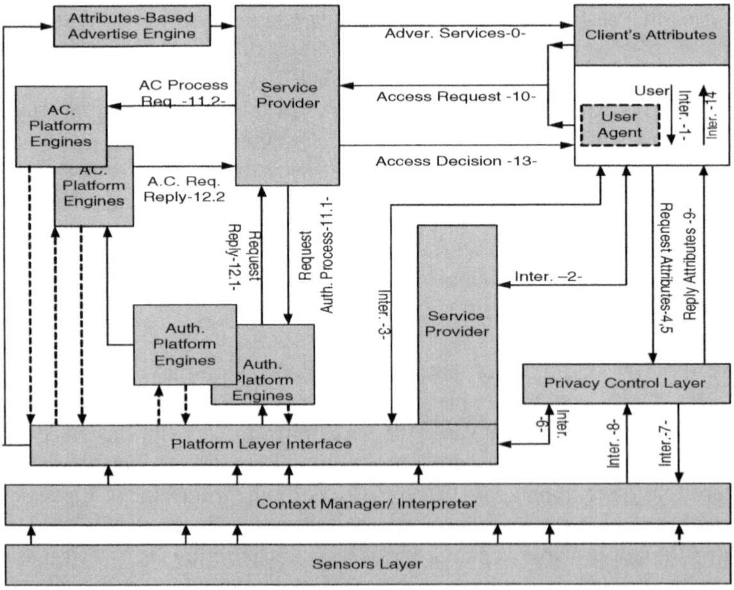

Fig. 2. A High-Level View

3.1 Framework Interaction

In the following, we will give a summary of the interaction [11] that takes place when a user wants to invoke a context-aware service. We consider these interactions occur after the user has received the advertisement message and want to invoke a service. Figure 2 shows the following interaction steps We consider these interactions occur after the user has received the advertisement message and want to invoke a service. These interactions are as follow:

1: The user tells the user agent what context-aware service it should invoke.

2: The user agent obtains the privacy policy of the context-aware service.

3: The user agent compares the policy to the user's preferences, and if the policy is acceptable, it registers the user's context-dependent preferences in the platform.

4 & 5: The user agent invokes the context-aware service through the privacy control layer and requests the service's contextual information.

6: The privacy control layer checks whether the user about whom the context-aware service is requesting information has registered context-dependent preferences, and evaluates these preferences.

7: If the context-dependent preferences are satisfied, the privacy layer passes the request for the contextual information to the context interpreter.

8. The context interpreter processes the request and returns the requested information to the privacy layer.

9. The privacy layer returns the contextual information to the user agent.

10. The user agent packages all the needed data that fulfill the access request and sends the data package to the access server.

11. The access server processes the data package and forwards each, the authentication process and the access layer, the corresponding set of data.

12. The authentication and access control brokers evaluate the data through their built-in engines and reply with a relevant access request decision to the access server.

13. The access server evaluates the access request decisions and returns the final request decision to the user agent.

14. The user agent evaluates the request decision and displays the context-aware service's result to the user.

4 Framework Implementation

The following section details the implementation phases that were done. For our different set of experiments, we generated a series of access request using different set of rules, roles, complex policies and modules including trust engine, contextual information rules, etc. The framework presented has been integrated in the Eclipse platform. In our implementation, policies are defined through the eXtensible Markup Language (XML). XML provides an efficient structure for storing the policy that is generated and enforced by our security services. The experiments were conducted on a cluster of workstations using dual-2.20GHZ Intel processors, running windows XP Professional. Figure 3 represents the user's service selecting process. Depending on the user based contextual information, the access server will select the corresponding context based services and deliver them to the user. In our following example, these corresponding services are services S0, S1 and S3.

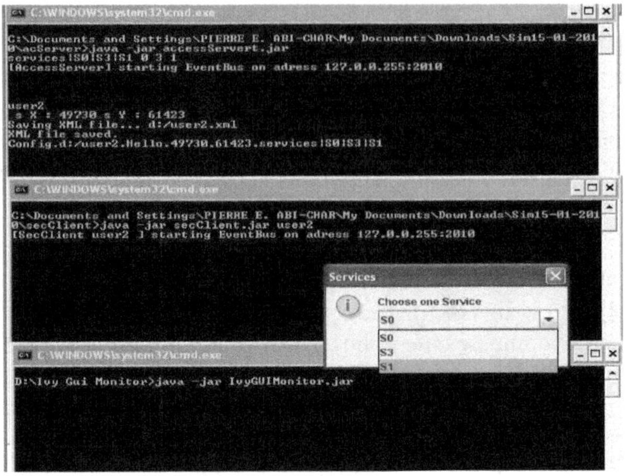

Fig. 3. User Selection Service

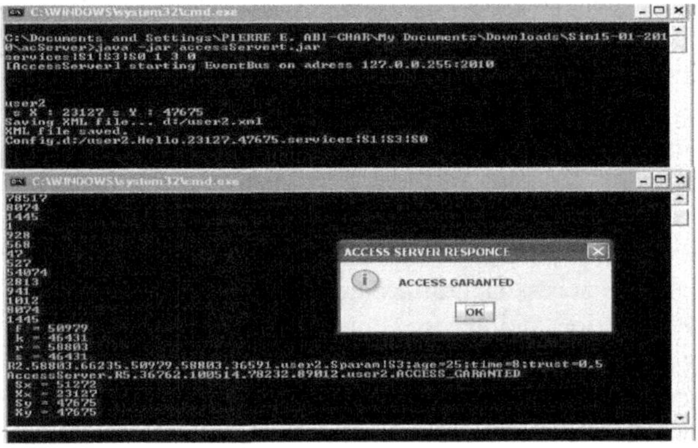

Fig. 4. User Access Granted-1-

Figure 3 illustrates a user with the option of selecting a service from the available context-based services. In our case, the user has the ability to select a service form these three services. As illustration, the user select the service namely S3.

Figure 4 shows that the user has been granted access the service. As demonstration, the user's contextual information fulfill the service's access requirements and therefore the user will be allowed to access the server.

5 Conclusion

In this paper, we have proposed a flexible and scalable dynamic context aware authentication framework for pervasive environments. The design of our framework is built on a robust attribute-based authentication scheme and support a privacy control and trust management tools in order to provide access controls for personalized services. This framework was implemented within the service delivery platform at

Handicom lab of Telecom SudParis and the prototype is currently under deployment to perform real world experimentation. Moreover, the deployment of this framework is under study to experiment it using RFID tags for users in indoor spaces. Future work consist to deeply investigate contextual parameters which will allow us to refine and adapt the privacy and trust models to user profile of dependant people.

References

1. Mhamed, A.: Safety, Security, Privacy and Trust in Smart Environements. In: Helal, A., Mokhtari, M., Abdulrazak, B. (eds.) The Engineering Handbook on Smart Technology for Aging, Disability and Independence. Computer Engineering Series. John Wiley & Sons, Chichester (2007), ISBN 0471711551
2. Covington, J.M., Sastry, M., Manohar, D.J.: Attribute-Based Authentication Model for Dynamic Mobile Environments. In: Clark, J.A., Paige, R.F., Polack, F.A.C., Brooke, P.J. (eds.) SPC 2006. LNCS, vol. 3934, pp. 227–242. Springer, Heidelberg (2006)
3. Marc, L.: A Privacy Awareness System for Ubiquitous Computing Environments. In: Borriello, G., Holmquist, L.E. (eds.) UbiComp 2002. LNCS, vol. 2498, pp. 237–245. Springer, Heidelberg (2002)
4. Corner, M.D., Noble, B.D.: Protecting Applications with Transient Authentication. In: Proceeding of the First International Conference on Mobile Systems, Applications and Services, pp. 57–70 (2003)
5. Glynos, D., Kotzanikolaou, P., Douligeris, C.: Preventing Impersonation Attacks in MANET with Multi-Factor Authentication. In: Proceeding of the Third International Symposium on Modeling and Optimization in Mobile Ad-hoc, and Wireless Networks, pp. 59–64 (2005)
6. Jakob, B., Rasmus, K., Michael, P.: Context-aware user authentication: Supporting proximity-based login in pervasive computing. In: Dey, A.K., Schmidt, A., McCarthy, J.F. (eds.) UbiComp 2003. LNCS, vol. 2864, pp. 107–123. Springer, Heidelberg (2003)
7. Creese, S.J., Goldsmith, M.H., Zakiuddin, B.R.: Authentication in Pervasive Computing. In: Proceeding of the First International Conference on Security in Pervasive Computing, SPC (2003)
8. Qin, W., Daqing, Z., Mounir, M., Yuanchun, S., Kejun, D.: Combining User Profiles and Situation Context for Spontaneous Service Provision in Smart Assistive Environments. In: Proceeding of the 5th International Conference on Ubiquitous Intelligence and Computing, pp. 187–200 (2008)
9. Behzad, M., Ali, M., Ahmed, K.: A Framework for Context-Aware Authentication. In: Proceeding of 2008 IET 4th International Conference on Intelligent Environments, pp. 1–8 (2008)
10. Adrian, L., Chris, M.J.: Ninja: Non Identity Based, Privacy Preserving Authentication for Ubiquitous Environments. In: Krumm, J., Abowd, G.D., Seneviratne, A., Strang, T. (eds.) UbiComp 2007. LNCS, vol. 4717, pp. 73–90. Springer, Heidelberg (2007)
11. Abi-Char, P., Mhamed, A., El-Hassan, B., Mokhtari, M.: A Dynamic Trust- Based Context-Aware Authentication Framework With Privacy Preserving. Proceeding of International Journal of Computer and Network Security, IJCNS 2 (accepted) (to appear)
12. Abi-Char, P., Mhamed, A., El-Hassan, B., Mokhtari, M.: Secure Authenticated and Key Agreement Protocols with Access Control for Mobile Environments. Proceeding of International Journal of Computer Science and Information Security, IJCSIS 6(2), 170–183 (2009) (Best Paper Award)

Security, Privacy, and Dependability in Smart Homes: A Pattern Catalog Approach

Pierre Busnel and Sylvain Giroux

University of Sherbrooke, DOMUS lab, Sherbrooke
J1K 2R1, QC, Canada
{Pierre.Busnel,Sylvain.Giroux}@USherbrooke.ca

Abstract. Security, privacy and dependability are crucial issues if one wants to build a real smart home. First, in addition to established home security requirements, smart home adoption requires to solve brand-new security vulnerabilities deriving from the automated facets of smart homes. Thereafter, pervasive computing and ambient intelligence allow to collect a lot of information, to analyze it to derive new facts, and make them explicit. Finally, systems that are usually safe and dependable can fail when their behavior is becoming controlled as the result of complex interactions between many intertwined information systems. Unfortunately, application developers in smart home environments are usually neither security experts, nor familiar with ethical and legal requirements related to privacy. Security patterns can help to anticipate, overcome, and document systematically these difficult issues in building pervasive information systems in smart homes for cognitively impaired people. In this paper, we illustrate how security patterns can be extended and applied to Smart Home to foster autonomy of elderly or cognitively impaired people, then, we sketch the structure of the catalog which will be populated with a few patterns.

Keywords: Security patterns, ubiquitous computing, health care, smart home, cognitively impaired people.

1 Introduction

Occidental countries are facing great challenges from a population of elders increasing rapidly while the birth rate cannot sustain it. According to U.S. Census Bureau estimations, there were more than 36 million people that are aged 65 and over in 2003, and this population is projected to increase to 72 million in 2030 [1]. Thus, it is easy to forecast an increase of health injuries related to normal and pathological aging that will lead toward loss of autonomy and greater fragility, which result in a reduction of quality of life. People may need continuous supervision when either injured, sick, cognitively impaired, elderly, or fragile. If resources are not adapted at home, then people are more often transferred to a hospital setting. Thanks to ubiquitous and pervasive computing, Smart Homes (SH) can interact with residents to foster their autonomy and to provide for health monitoring [2].

Nonetheless, security, privacy and dependability are crucial issues to build a real SH. They must be equipped with privileged, secure, and dependable ambient

Y. Lee et al. (Eds.): ICOST 2010, LNCS 6159, pp. 24–31, 2010.

information systems. This implies that traditional information systems must be adapted to ambient intelligence (AmI) specific requirements. First, in addition to established home security requirements, SH adoption requires to solve brand-new security vulnerabilities deriving from the automated facets of SH. For instance, a thief can intrude into a SH sensor network to learn about one's habits and be aware precisely when he is home, when he is not and for how much time. Second pervasive computing and ambient intelligence allow to collect a lot of information, to analyze it to derive new facts, and to make them explicit. Before the rise, in everyday life, of pervasive and connected systems, such information was latent or hidden. Indeed, pervasiveness will take place in everyday life transactions where technical systems are not involved at all like, for instance, taking a bath[1] or social relationship[2] [14]. Finally, systems that are usually safe and dependable, such as heating systems, can fail when their behavior is becoming controlled as the result of complex interactions between many intertwined information systems, e.g. user interfaces to set the temperature, ecological control systems for saving energy, electricity company controlling the overall demand in the city, etc.

Unfortunately, application developers in SH environments are usually neither security experts, nor familiar with ethical and legal requirements related to privacy. Security[3] patterns can help to anticipate, overcome, and document systematically these difficult issues in building pervasive information systems in smart homes for cognitively impaired people. They can enable SH to meet the required security, privacy, and dependability. A security pattern describes a particular recurring security issue that arises in specific contexts, and presents a well-proven generic solution for it. Several security patterns have already been written to assist developers to select and deploy security solutions in their applications. However, elements used to describe them and assist developers in their choice does not take into account the particular infrastructure of SH and the cognitive impairments of their residents.

In this paper, we show how security patterns can be extended and applied to SH to foster autonomy of elderly or cognitively impaired people. First, a simple case study is used to illustrate where security, privacy and dependability issues can arise in a smart home with health related services (§2). Then, an overview of security patterns is presented (§3). The current description of their structure is too generic to catch the peculiarities of smart homes. Thus, it is extended with facets specific to smart homes, health services, and cognitively impaired people. Once the description of security patterns is well extended, the structure of the catalog is sketched and populated with a few patterns (§4).

---

[1] While you are on the way home, Smart Hydro can prepare your bath according to your preferences and inform you on your cell phone. http://www.ihouse.com.br/ and http://gadgets.softpedia.com/gadgets/Household-and-Office/The-Smart-Hydro--Intelligent--Bath-Tub-994.html

[2] When a friend is visiting you, what will happen if a note appears on your TV screen saying you rated his wife as boring on one of your preferred social network...

[3] For convenience, in the rest of the paper the term "security" encompasses information systems security, privacy and dependability.

2 Case Study

Smart homes in a medical context raise difficult and complex security issues; often, programmers are not able to cope with these specific issues. Security patterns can then become an invaluable help. This section presents a case study involving a patient in his smart home, his physician, his daughter, and a health-monitoring center that allow us to pinpoint security requirements in smart homes. First, the profiles of the actors involved are sketched (§2.1). Then, a scenario about monitoring an elder is cut into small scenes, each one illustrating a specific security issue (§2.2).

2.1 Actors

The case study involves the following actors: the patient Bob, his smart home, his daughter Rachel, the doctor Andrew, and the Monitoring and Emergency Response Center systems (MERC) as shown in Fig. 1.

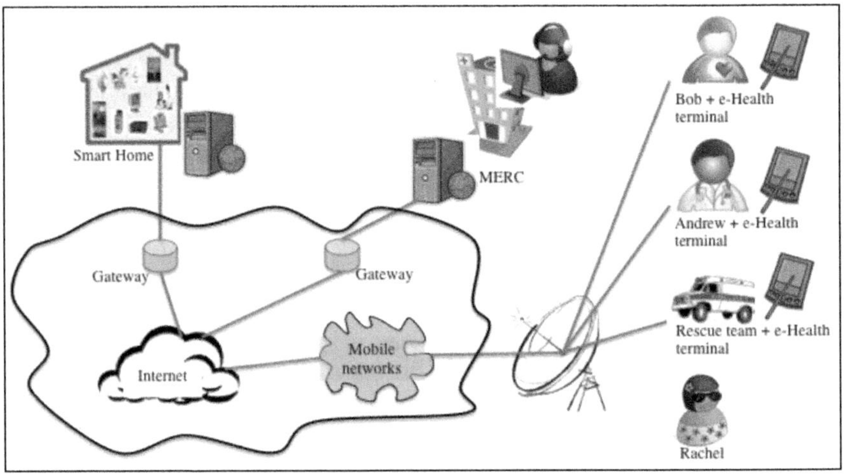

Fig. 1. Actors involved in the case study

- *Bob* is a 70-year-old widowed man. Six months ago, he had a Cerebral Vascular Accident (CVA). Bob spent 4 months at the hospital after his accident. Since he still suffers from various troubles, his health status needs to be monitored daily. Before leaving hospital, he subscribed to a Smart Home (SH) program to get assistance in his daily activities and to make his heart rate monitored continuously.
- The *MERC* receives and handles emergency and assistance requests triggered by monitored patients. It also coordinates the activities of many other actors including doctors and social workers.
- Dr. *Andrew* is a physician working at the MERC. In the case study, Andrew is Bob's personal doctor, who is in charge of Bob's case.
- *Rachel* is Bob's daughter. Since her father's CVA, she often runs his errands and visits him twice a week. Rachel, in contrary to other visitors, is a privileged user and can enter the SH using her RFID tag and password, as approved by her father Bob.

- The *Smart Home* is a conventional apartment equipped with various types of sensors and effectors, to monitor and assist the patient in his Activities of Daily Living (ADL) [3], [4], [5]. Pressure mats, electro-magnetic sensors, infra-red and flow meters in the apartment, are used to recognize activities performed by the patient and prompt him with advices when necessary. *Microphones*, *speakers* and *cameras* are available to facilitate communications between the patient, the medical staff and his family. *RFID tag readers* are available at the Smart Home door for authenticating the access requesters among the medical staff, doctors, family and others during home visits.
- The *SH terminal* combines an interface to interact with the SH server and the MERC server. It displays a calendar accessible through the MERC for adding medical or maintenance visits. It also hosts an ADL assistant [4] and a communication interface with the MERC for emergency request or request for doctor assistance.

2.2 Scenario

The general scenario is exploring the management of security and privacy when people come into Bob's home. This scenario is divided in two main parts. In the first part, the visits of a doctor and a technician are planned and organized by the MERC. In the second part, the focus is put on the access by persons with different status at Bob's home.

According to Bob medical records, the MERC has to schedule weekly medical visits for Bob's check-up. The MERC also schedules regular maintenance visits for sensors check-up. So each week, a medical visit is assigned to an available doctor, and events detailing the arrival time of the doctor and his identity are added to Bob's calendar by the MERC. Therefore, Bob is always warned in advance and aware of these planned visits. Accordingly, when Dr. Andrew is assigned to visit Bob this week, Bob has to allow and acknowledge the visit thanks to his electronic calendar. The same procedure is used for the maintenance visit.

Next the scenario is divided into three small scenes that highlight security and safety issues that need to be solved when Bob receives visitors. The first scene corresponds to the medical visit at Bob's home. This visit involves known participants and is scheduled beforehand (Fig. 2). Then, in Scene 2, an unexpected visitor comes in while the doctor and Bob are watching private medical data (Fig. 3), and, finally, Scene 3 describes an emergency situation when nobody, except Bob, is at home and someone has to get in (Fig. 4).

- **Scene 1: the doctor visit (Fig.2)**

  When Dr. Andrew arrives at the SH's door, the door bell rings as the RFID tag carried on his badge gets scanned and analyzed by the SH. At the same time, the outdoor webcam takes a picture of Dr. Andrew. Bob, notified by the doorbell, sees on his screen both the picture taken outside and the one corresponding to Dr. Andrew's identification badge and the MERC, and unlocks the door from his terminal. Then, the doctor logs in to access the medical record of Bob (1). The MERC retrieves the record, sends it to the SH and it is displayed on the TV screen (2). When Rachel arrives at the door, her authentication RFID tag is read and, since she has special access right, the door automatically unlocks and grants her access inside. Since confidential data are displayed on the TV screen and a new person is in the living room (3), the system immediately hides these data (4). Then, Andrew has to log in again to get access to the data (5).

Scene 1 and 2 illustrate security and privacy issues related to providing access inside the SH and to sensible data involving a mix of devices (RFID tag reader, camera, movement detectors, TV screen…) and information (photo, RFID tag number…), authorization policies and procedures (login and password, explicit authorization…).

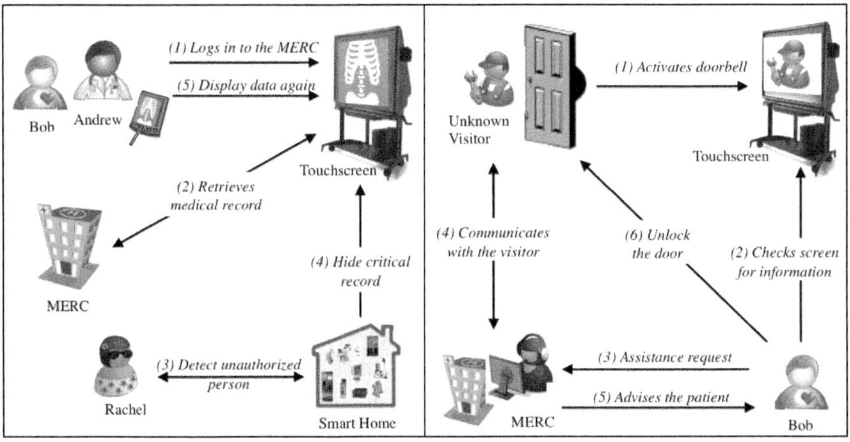

Fig. 2. Scene 1 – the doctor visit (left side) and scene 2 – the unknown visitor (right side)

- **Scene 2: the unknown visitor (Fig. 2)**
  Bob is in the living room when the doorbell rings (1). An unknown visitor picture appears on the screen situated next to him (2). Bob does not recognize this visitor and even after talking to him through the interphone, hesitates to open the door. He finally decides to ask assistance to the MERC (3) which communicates with the visitor (4) in order to advise Bob to grant access or not (5). Since the MERC advises Bob to grant access to the visitor, he unlocks the door (6).
- **Scene 3: the assistance request (Fig. 3)**
  Bob's is at home when he suddenly feels giddy and uses his e-health terminal to send an emergency request (1). The MERC forwards the assistance request to an available doctor (2). The doctor consults the medical record and the medical data recently collected by the SH sensors and sends a report to the MERC saying that an emergency team must be sent to help Bob (3). Thanks to the localization service, the MERC localizes Bob in his home. The localization service was granted special

and temporary access rights to sensors data stocked in Bob's home server (4). The MERC sends an emergency intervention request to the rescue team (5). While the rescue team is on its way to the SH's door, the MERC grants temporary access to the SH's door to the members of the rescue team, in order to let them enter into Bob's home (6). This scene is treated more extensively in [6].

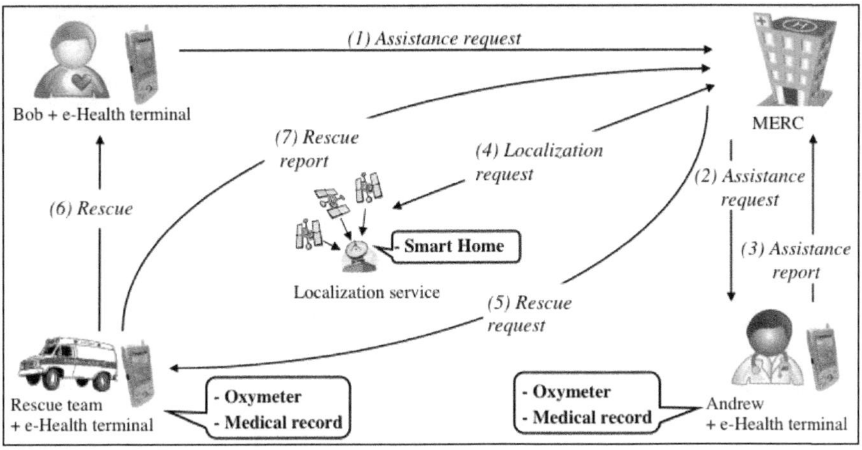

Fig. 3. Scene 3 – the assistance request

3 An Overview of Security Patterns

The pattern approach has been adopted into software engineering as a method for object-based reuse [8]. Design patterns capture recurring solutions to common problems in software design. The following items describe a design pattern: *name*, *intent*, *alias*, *motivation*, *applicability*, *structure*, *participants*, *collaborations*, and *consequences*. Given the success of the Gang of Four in eliciting and organizing expert knowledge in object-oriented programming, a similar methodology was applied to security issues. Schumacher [9] applied the pattern approach to security problems by proposing a set of security patterns for the development process. Yoder and Barcalow [10] proposed architectural patterns that can be applied when introducing security into an application. Fernandez and Pan [11] described patterns for the most common security models, such as *Authorization*, *Role-Based Access Control*, and *Multilevel Security*.

One of the main limitations of these proposals is that they neither capture explicitly the very nature of SH and pervasive systems, nor they take into account specific issues related to resident, for instance cognitive deficits. For instance, Table 1 presents an eXtensible Access Control Markup Language (XACML) based pattern that tries to make these peculiar requirements more explicit.

Table 1. XACML based access control pattern to enforce confidentiality

Pattern name	XACML based access control pattern
Context	While confidentiality is enforced at the hospital to access medical information, such data need to be accessible outside with the same level of confidentiality. During home visits at the patient's smart home, medical staff needs to access the medical record and display it on the living room screen. The data displayed must only to be seen by the patient and the medical staff.
Legal issue	Medical data are confidential
Ethical issue	Not available
Problem	With the presence of others actors and family members having privileged access to the smart home, confidentiality while displaying medical data during a home visit is at risk.
Solution	The smart home sensors are used to identify any incoming visitors by using RFID badge at the main door of the apartment and using an XACML policy enforced both at the smart home and the MERC side.
Smart Home infrastructure requirements	An RFID reader must be deployed at the entrance of the door and connected to the smart home events server.

4 Towards a Catalog of Patterns

Without a general classification scheme, design patterns would just have become a long list difficult to search in and understand. The beauty of the Gang of Four solution is that they also provide a general organization scheme to better understand, search and use design patterns. This organization takes the form of a classification table ordered into class and instance patterns on the rows side and creation, structure, and behavior aspects on the column side. Also, a graph shows the interrelations between patterns use. Then, a catalog of patterns becomes more than a collection of patterns and can offer guidance to select and use patterns. It is a tool for both patterns writers to organize their solutions and developers to find the adequate patterns to apply. Catalogs of patterns in domains such as code design [8] and security [9], [12], [13], already exist. However, no one is dedicated to Smart Homes.

We are currently working on such a catalog. This catalog of security patterns will assist SH developers to choose a security solutions adapted to their needs and their context of utilization. In our context, several elements such as the sensors network, the use of mobile devices, the participation of healthcare workers and the cognitive troubles of SH residents are taken into account in order to explicit the consequences of the possible security solutions.

5 Conclusion and Future Work

This paper presented, by using a simple use case, the necessity to create security pattern and to structure them in a catalog dedicated to Smart Homes, in order to assist SH developers in the integration of security solutions in their application. Up to now, two patterns have been written and successfully implemented in remote healthcare prototype [6], [7]. Many patterns are on their way to a complete description. Future works will focus on the validation of new elements composing security patterns in the context of smart homes and on writing new security patterns in order to populate the catalog.

References

1. He, W., et al.: 65+ in the U.S.: Current Population Reports, pp. 23–209. U.S. Bureau of the Census, Washington (2005)
2. Jorge, J.: Adaptive tools for the elderly new devices to cope with age induced cognitive disabilities. In: Proceedings of the 2001 WUAUC, pp. 66–70 (2001)
3. Pigot, H., Mayers, A., Giroux, S.: The intelligent habitat and everyday life activity support. In: Proceedings of the 5th International Conference on Simulations in Biomedicine, Slovenia, pp. 507–516 (2003)
4. Bauchet, J., Vergnes, D., Giroux, S., Pigot, H.: A pervasive cognitive assistant for smart homes. In: Proceedings of the 2006 ICADI, USA, p. 228 (2006)
5. Bauchet, J., Mayers, A.: A modelisation of ADLs in its environment for cognitive assistance. In: Proceedings of the 2005 ICOST, Canada, pp. 221–228 (2005)
6. Busnel, P., El Khoury, P., Giroux, S., Li, K.: Achieving Socio-Technical Confidentiality using Security Pattern in Smart Homes. In: 3rd International Symposium on Smart Home (SH 2008), China (2008)
7. El Khoury, P., Busnel, P., Giroux, S., Li, K.: Enforcing Security in Smart Homes using Security Patterns. International Journal of Smart Home (IJSH) 3(2) (2009)
8. Gamma, E., Helm, R., Johnson, R., Vlissides, J.: Design patterns: Elements of Reusable Object-Oriented Software. Addison-Wesley Professional, Reading (1994)
9. Schumacher, M.: Security Engineering with Patterns: Origins, Theoretical Models, and New Applications. LNCS, vol. 2754. Springer, Heidelberg (2003)
10. Yoder, J., Barcalow, J.: Architectural Patterns for Enabling Application Security. In: Conference on Pattern Languages of Programs (1997)
11. Fernandez, E., Pan, R.: A Pattern Language for Security Models. In: Conference on Pattern Languages of Programs (2001)
12. Schumacher, M., Roedig, U.: Security Engineering with Patterns. In: Conference on Pattern Languages of Programs, USA (2001)
13. Kienzle, D., Elder, M., Tyree, D., Edwards-Hewitt, J.: Security Patterns Template and Tutorial (2002), `http://www.securitypatterns.com/documents.html`
14. Everyware: The Dawning Age of Ubiquitous Computing, 272 p. Peachpit Press Publications, Berkeley (2006)

A Taxonomy Driven Approach towards Evaluating Pervasive Computing System

Bessam Abdualrazak[1], Yasir Malik[1], and Hen-I Yang[2]

[1] University of Sherbrook, DOUMS Lab, Dept. Informatique, 2500 Boulevard de Universite, Sherbrooke, Canada
[2] Iowa State University, Department of Computer Science, USA
{bessam.abdulrazak,yasir.malik}@usherbrooke.ca, heny@isu.edu

Abstract. This paper presents taxonomical classification of pervasive computing system that allows characterizing the system and helps to identify most defining performance parameters for evaluation. Tremendous efforts have been put in the related research, but there is no standard or commonly accepted model to benchmark systems and to identify direction for future research. We survey various systems published in the literature and identify their distinctive features to construct a classification scheme, and the outcome is the taxonomy of pervasive computing systems that allows us to devise strategy on how to evaluate a wide variety of these systems.

Keywords: Pervasive Computing, Taxonomy, Evaluation, Standardization, Parameters, Classification, validation.

1 Introduction

Today pervasive computing is shifting the computing paradigm toward everywhere computing. The emergence covers distributed and mobile computing, sensor networks, human computer interaction and artificial intelligence under umbrella of pervasive computing. Nearly two decades since Weiser's vision [23] was introduced, very few practical and promising systems have been deployed, and even fewer actually generated significant impact and received acceptance. As the technology is improving there is a great need of standard acceptance model to position pervasive computing systems and define directions for future research.

Researchers around the globe use evaluation techniques to benchmark their proposed work, similarly evaluation techniques are currently being used on pervasive computing and subsequently published in literature [4, 5, 9, and 19]. However, since there is no standard evaluation model, it is difficult to agree performance results presented in literature. Evaluation of pervasive computing has struggled due to the complexity, openness and diversity of technology, as a result new assessment and evaluation techniques are required to set standards. In our effort to create a comprehensive evaluation framework for pervasive computing systems, we found that it will be very effective to first categorize the systems based on some criteria and define key parameters to evaluate the systems.

Y. Lee et al. (Eds.): ICOST 2010, LNCS 6159, pp. 32–42, 2010.

In this paper, we present the taxonomy as our first step towards designing the evaluation framework for pervasive computing system. We studied different aspects of pervasive computing and classified them into different categories. Within each aspect, we identify key parameters that can be characterized and measured. We believe this taxonomy driven approach will help in evaluating the system in term architecture, enabling technologies and application domain.

The rest of the paper is organized as follows. In section 2, we present a brief summary of all surveyed paper focusing on pervasive computing evaluation and few taxonomical classifications. In section 3, we present our taxonomy for classifying the pervasive computing system along with the key parameters. Finally in section 4, we summarized the paper and discuss about future work.

2 Related Work

Several models and schemes have been presented to evaluate and benchmark pervasive computing system. In section, we review some presentative works that address different evaluation challenges present in the domain. Gabriele suggested that traditional performance approaches are no longer applicable for pervasive computing environments due to their high QoS requirements, proactive performance tuning activities and interdependencies between user behavior and system [17]. Similarly Scott and Jennifer studied three case studies and suggested some major challenges like applicability of metrics, scale, ambiguity and unobtrusiveness for evaluation [6].

Scholtz and Consolvo presented a ubiquitous computing evaluation areas framework [9]. The goal of this framework was to develop consensus among research community for evaluating and positioning pervasive computing systems. Mark and Chris presented a comparison of quantitative and qualitative evaluation strategies and suggested a hybrid evaluation framework [5]. Jennifer and Scott suggested using unobtrusive methods to gather data by combining quantitative and qualitative methods [19]. John et al suggested selecting the metrics from scenarios that are driven by real problems rather than by the technology [4].

On the other hand, Anand Ranganathan et al divided the pervasive computing framework roughly into three layers (system support, application programming support, and end-user interface) and suggested evaluating metrics respectively [22]. Laurent and colleagues proposed a generic framework for mobility modeling in dynamic networks and argue that in future their framework can change the way for dynamic and behavior depended technology evaluation [7]. Andrea et al presented automated methods that inputs UML model of application and gives complete extended queuing network model as an output that can be evaluated with any evaluation tool [10]. Kay proposed a mathematical predictive model based on user's perception of usefulness, ease of use, social influence, trustworthiness and integration to evaluate user acceptance in pervasive computing environments [8]. Ali and colleagues presented a privacy model based on user control over private information, expressiveness of privacy policies and unobtrusiveness of privacy mechanisms [11]. Stephen introduces the Place Lab a living laboratory to study and evaluate the ubiquitous technologies in home settings [15].

The aforementioned evaluation methods are quite limited and only focused on specific areas. Our study shows that pervasive systems are highly diverse in areas such as software architecture, enabling technologies and application domain, thus it is very difficult to establish a generic and comprehensive performance evaluation framework for pervasive computing systems. Based on our observation, we conclude that as a first step toward evaluating pervasive computing system, it is necessary to examine the common characteristics and differences that separate them apart.

Taxonomy of pervasive computing systems allows us to characterize the systems and helps to identify the most defining performance parameters for evaluation. There is quite limited research on the classification of pervasive computing due to the heterogeneity of various technologies. Jeon and colleagues presented the taxonomy of ubiquitous applications and suggested the three main criteria's i.e. (subject, time and place) to classify ubiquitous applications [16]. Similarly Kista and Rajiv presented taxonomy of mobile and pervasive computing applications [12], Dennis and colleagues presented taxonomy of ubiquitous computing environments [18], Joanna and colleagues presented taxonomy of pervasive healthcare system [21], and Modahl and colleagues presented the taxonomy for a ubiquitous computing software stack called UbiqStack [20]. All these taxonomies and classification mentioned here are limited to specific domains and do not cover the complete system.

3 Taxonomy of Pervasive Computing System

After a careful study of various systems presented in literature, we analyze the distinctive features and bring together the most suitable classification. This taxonomy is by no means complete, but merely reflects on the classification scheme that best suited for the purpose of effective performance evaluations.

Based on analysis of distinctive feature of pervasive system, we have chosen seven criteria's that would exhibit vastly different characteristics and can generate the most compelling categories. The diversity of pervasive computing prevents the use of well-formed hieratical classification scheme. We take a different perspective and identify criteria's that define major divisions in operational paradigm. We first identified the differentiating parameters that can be used to categorize pervasive systems. Once the criteria and their differentiating parameters are identified, we define the categories and identify the key aspects and parameters.

Each system to be evaluated can be categorized based on one of the seven different criteria (as defined later in different subsections), and it will fall into one of the categories each time a different criterion is applied. The candidate parameters of interest for each system could be the union of the common parameters, the differentiating parameters and the key parameters associated with the category. Since there are multiple criteria employed in the taxonomy, any system can belong to multiple categories. Therefore, the set of categories the system belongs to can be used to define its character. For instance, a smart house would be considered as a centralized, assistive system that works within a single house.

The taxonomy is designed to give researchers a reference when deciding which parameters are most relevant to a particular pervasive computing system. The key aspects and parameters associated with each category are not the only parameters of interests. The specified parameters are identified that are of particular interest to each category but do not provide an exclusive list of every parameter to be evaluated.

There are common parameters that are of interest for all systems such as throughput, response time, and user acceptance. The taxonomy clarified the scope, commonalities and range of diversity of pervasive computing systems. It also generates a reference and provides guidance when researchers and implementers wish to evaluate and benchmark different systems. In next section, we present the detail description of our seven criteria presented in taxonomy.

3.1 Criteria 1: Architecture

Architecture describes the conceptual design and functional structure of all hardware and software components in pervasive systems. It provides the blueprint and operational manual during development and deployment of pervasive system. We have divided the architectural characteristics of pervasive computing system in to two major sub categories (Infrastructure and Design). Following we present the details and key evaluation parameters associated with each category.

3.1.1 Infrastructure

As one of the primary characteristic of pervasive systems is communication and computing capabilities that are integrated into environment with the possibility for a system to provide all the services from personal to global scale. We categorize systems according to the distribution of data and control, mobility of users and devices, infrastructural support of the network and the geographic span. We identify the following differentiating parameters: architectural characteristics at the system level, node-level characteristics, communication performance & cost and economical considerations that allow us to distinguish one system from another based on their differences in the network infrastructure and geographic span. Following, we define the categories under this criterion, and identify the key aspects and parameters.

CATEGORY: Network
Sub-Type: Centralized
Key Aspect:
- Resource Usage

Key Parameters:
- Software footprint
- Data storage scheme
- Scalability

Type: Distributed
Subtype: Stationary
Key aspect:
- Deployment
- Safety

Key parameters:
- Maintainability
- Security & privacy

Subtype: Grid
Key aspect:
- Resource Usage
- Safety

Key parameters:
- Process Management
- Data Management
- Data storage scheme
- Security & privacy

Subtype: Mobile (Infrastructure)
Key aspect:
- Resource Usage
- invisibility

Key parameters:
- Software footprint
- Power profile
- Data storage & manipulation
- Reliability & fault-tolerance
- Node-level characteristics & privacy

Subtype: Mobile (AdHoc)
Key aspect:
- Speed & Efficiency
- Resource Usage

- Safety
- Deployment
- Compatibility
- Invisibility

Key parameters:
- Communication performance & cost
- Data storage scheme
- Software footprint
- Node-level characteristics
- Security and privacy

CATEGORY: Geographic Span

Type: Personal-Range

Key Aspect:
- Resource Usage
- Usability
- Invisibility

Key Parameters:
- Software footprint
- Power profile
- Data storage & manipulation
- Acceptance
- Node-level characteristics

Type: Local-Range

Key Aspect:
- Safety
- Deployment

Key Parameters:
- Reliability & fault-tolerance
- Security & privacy
- Scalability

Type: Wide-range

Key Aspect:
- Resource Usage
- Deployment
- Compatibility

Key parameters:
- Power profile
- Data storage scheme
- Node-level characteristics
- Adaptability ,maintainability and self-organization

3.1.2 Design

The vision of pervasive computing is to provide user with access to computational environment anywhere anytime [23]. Thus the goal of pervasive computing system is to design software architectures that support multiple application and services in pervasive environment. The diverse nature of pervasive computing has made it difficult for software designers to adapt one common model that can meet all the requirements of pervasive computing. The major challenges that make the software design difficult are ability of software architectures to support interoperability due to various network technologies and implementations, need of user and service mobility [3]. After a careful review of different software architectures, we have identified the key differentiating parameters *(coordination, coupling, versatility and generation)* that can help to classify different software architectures used for pervasive computing. Following are the categories and the key aspect along with key parameters.

CATEGORY : Application based architecture

Key Aspects
- Modularity
- Software dynamic
- Design

Key Parameter
- Coupling And Cohesion
- Dependency between application
- Interpretability

CATEGORY : Component Oriented architecture

Key Aspects
- Modularity
- Software dynamic
- Management
- Design

- **Key Parameters**
- Component compilation
- Orchestration
- Coupling And Cohesion

CATEGORY : Service Oriented architecture

- **Key Aspects**
- Modularity
- Compatibility
- Management
- Software Dynamic
- Design

- **Key Parameters**
- Orchestration
- Runtime service generation
- Coupling And Cohesion
- Scalability
- Interoperability

CATEGORY : Agent Oriented architecture

- **Key Aspects**
- Management
- Design

- **Key Parameter**
- Choreography
- Embedded intelligence
- Autonomy
- Interpretability

3.2 Criteria 2: Application Purpose

The services and functionalities that pervasive computing systems are designed to provide are extremely diverse. The requirements and emphasis on various performance parameters are heavily dependent on their primary purposes. For example assistive services allow users to enhance and expand their communication, learning, participation, well-being, quality of life and achieve great levels of independence [21, 14]. We have define some key differentiating parameters like quality of context, reliability, fault tolerance, security, privacy and effectiveness that can be use to categories the pervasive computing applications. After analyzing the pervasive application presented in literature, we define the key differentiating parameters and categories according to their purposes. Following, we present key aspects and parameters that define each category.

CATEGORY
Assurance

Key Aspect
- Safety
- Sentience

Key Parameter
- Reliability & fault-tolerance
- Security & privacy
- Quality of Context

CATEGORY
Assistive

Key Aspect
- Usability
- Safety
- Invisibility

Key Parameter
- Reliability & fault-tolerance
- Node-level characteristics
- Security & privacy
- Modality and Effectiveness

CATEGORY
Return on Investment

Key Aspect
- Speed
- Efficiency

Key Parameter
- System performance
- Comm. performance & cost
- Economical considerations
- Data storage scheme
- Learning ability
- Efficiency

CATEGORY
Experience enhancement

Key Aspect
- Sentience
- Usability

Key Parameter
- Context characteristics
- Explicitness
- Learning ability
- Satisfaction

CATEGORY
Exploration

Key Aspect
- Sentience
- Deployment

Key Parameter
- Quality of context
- Maintainability

3.3 Criteria 3: Autonomicity

Pervasive computing systems are distributed, heterogeneous, and dynamic. Unlike computers as traditionally defined, these systems have more and diversified software and hardware components, thus making manual management and development is much more expensive. Automaticity is an aspect that describes how a pervasive computing system is initialized, how it evolves automatically to accommodate faults and failures, adjusting to users requirements, integrating new resources, and how it can identify and fend off the potential attacks. The differentiating parameter of this criterion includes the report process of new or changed requirements, number of people involved in making required changes, and level of integration between business and programmed logic. Following, we define the categories and key aspects and parameters.

CATEGORY: Static

Key Aspect
- Speed & Efficiency
- Safety

Key Parameter
- Computational performance
- I/O performance
- Reliability & Fault-tolerance

CATEGORY: Dynamic

Subtype: Self-Learning

Key Aspect
- Sentience
- Usability

Key Parameter
- Quality of context
- Knowledge representation scheme
- Error
- Learning ability
- Explicitness

Subtype: Re-Programmable

Key Aspect
- Programmability
- Deployment
- Compatibility

Key Parameter
- Ease of programming
- Maintainability
- Service & application
- Extensibility
- Backward compatibility

Subtype: Re-Configurable

Key Aspect
- Usability

Key Parameter
- Adaptability
- Ease of programming
- Self optimization

3.4 Criteria 4: Integration

Pervasive computing systems by its nature require integration of many different subsystems with very different characteristics. These subsystems include computational facilities, communication devices, mechanical or chemical sensors and actuators, smart appliances, and existing control systems. Plenty of research efforts have been spent on solving various integration issues, and different implementers have tried on different approaches. Based on the approach taken, systems usually exhibit different architectures and therefore present vastly different characteristics. After careful study of different system integration presented in literature and our own experience in building smart spaces [1,2,13], we define some differentiating parameters like maintainability, standardization, reliability, fault-tolerance, security, privacy, architectural characteristics and scalability that can be use to categories the system based on their integration methods.

CATEGORY: AdHoc Integration
Key Aspect
- Method

Key Parameter
- Designated Black-box

CATEGORY: Universal Interface
Key Aspect
- Method

Key Parameter
- Analyze data flow
- Analyze pattern
- Analyze content in pipeline

CATEGORY: Plug-In
Key Aspect
- Method

Key Parameter
- Analyze and check the performance of utilities provided in middleware.
- Pattern and efficiency of integration between application components and middleware.

3.5 Criteria 5: Interaction

In pervasive computing system, human-computer interaction and machine to machine interaction are the important components and they are becoming highly dynamic and implanted in environment. A system should adapt the interaction and presentation using various components available for interfacing based on behavior sensing, service mobility and events happening in the environment. We identify presentation as the key differentiating parameter (i.e. human to machine and machine to machines) that helps us to categorize and classify the interaction in pervasive systems. Following we define the categories under this criteria and key aspects and parameters.

CATEGORY: Human to Machine
Key Aspect
- Human Capabilities
- Preferences

Key Parameter
- Perceptual, cognitive, motor
- Interface designs
- Interaction Mode (audio, video, tangible)

CATEGORY: Machine to Machine
Key Aspect
- Interoperability

Key Parameter
- Communication protocols
- Platforms
- Computational capacities

3.6 Criteria 6: Intelligence

Pervasive computing environments are embedded with computing based devices that have ability to learn from user behaviors, their needs and preferences to adapt the environment accordingly. Ambient intelligence techniques allow these devices to help people when performing their daily living activities reactively or proactively. In our observation, we found that there are two kinds of environments, one that interacts and responds to the user behavior and preferences according to changes in user's context and behavior. The second environment is the one which personalized according to the user preferences set in his/her context (profile), and doesn't respond and adapt when the user's context or behaviors are changed. For example when a person enters to a smart room the system recognizes and personalized the environment according to his/her profile but if the person behavior is change the environment don't adapt that change. Following, we present the key aspects and parameters.

Key Aspect
- Context awareness

Key Parameter
- Quality of context
- Learning
- Reasoning

3.7 Criteria 7: Service Availability

The goal of pervasive computing system is to provide its user with rich set of services that are embedded in the user's physical environment and integrated seamlessly with their everyday tasks. Unlike services that are provided by internet, pervasive computing services are invisible, intelligent and invoked automatically depend on the events happening in the environment, user context or conditions that satisfy their invocation. The quality of pervasive service can be evaluated in many aspects, the key differentiating parameter that can help to categorize these services is its ubiquity. We categorize the pervasive service based on the definition of pervasive computing (i.e. any where any time). Following, we define the category under this criterion, and identify the key aspects and parameters.

CATEGORY: Any where Any -Time

Key Aspect
- Discovery
- Location
- Adaptation
- Availability
- Mobility

Key Parameter
- Discovery Protocol
- Service deployment
- Service composition
- Execution
- Resource availability

4 Conclusion and Future Work

There is an inherent difficulty when evaluating pervasive computing systems because of their complexity, openness and diversity of technology, therefore new standards for assessment and evaluation techniques are required. Our survey suggests that it would be extremely difficult to devise a single evaluation framework that is applicable to all systems. Instead, by first categorizing the pervasive computing system based on their distinctive features, we have established the taxonomy of pervasive computing systems. In association with each criterion, the differentiating parameters are identified to categorize various systems. Within each category, we further define their key aspects and parameters so the evaluation and comparison can be performed under a standardized and meaningful context with proper perspectives. We are currently working on a common set of scenarios that can categorize and generate the checklist to design evaluation framework that can help researcher to compare their work among other competing systems, position their work and drive future research directions. We hope that as the research community continues to move forward and new systems come into life, the taxonomy can be adjusted and expanded.

References

1. Abdulrazak, B., et al.: Integration of home networking in a smart environment dedicated to people with disabilities. In: Proceeding IEEE International Conference on Information & Communication Technologies: From Theory to Application. IEEE, Los Alamitos (2004)
2. Abdulrazak, B., Helal, S.: Enabling a Plug-and-play integration of smart environments. In: Proceedings of the second International Conference on Information & Communication Technologies: from Theory to Application, pp. 820–825. IEEE, Los Alamitos (2006)
3. Andre da Costa, C., et al.: Toward a general software infrastructure for ubiquitous computing. IEEE Pervasive Computing 7(1), 64–73 (2008)
4. Barton, J., Pierce, J.: Finding the right nails: Scenarios for evaluating pervasive systems. In: Common Models and Patterns for Pervasive Computing Workshop (2007)
5. Burnett, M., Rainsford, C.: A hybrid evaluation approach for ubiquitous computing environments. In: Workshop: Evaluation Methodologies for Ubiquitous Computing (2005)
6. Carter, S., Manko, J.: Challenges for Ubicomp evaluation. Technical report ucb-csd-04-1331, Computer Science Division. University of California, Berkeley (2004)
7. Ciarletta, L., et al.: Towards standards for Pervasive computing evaluation: using the multimodel and multi-agent paradigms for mobility. Technical report, INRIA - LORIA (2008)
8. Connelly, K.: On developing a technology acceptance model for pervasive computing. In: Proceedings of Ubiquitous System Evaluation (USE) - a workshop at the Ninth International Conference on Ubiquitous Computing, Austria (2007)
9. Consolvo, S., Scholtz, J.: Toward a framework for evaluating ubiquitous computing applications. IEEE Pervasive Computing 3(2), 82–88 (2004)
10. D'Ambrogio, A., Iazeolla, G.: Performance model building of pervasive computing. In: FIRB-PERF 2005: Proceedings of the 2005 Workshop on Techniques, Methodologies and Tools for Performance Evaluation of Complex Systems, Washington, DC, USA, p. 44. IEEE, Los Alamitos (2005)
11. Dehghantanha, A., et al.: UPEM: User-centered privacy evaluation model in pervasive computing systems. Ubiquitous Computing and Communication Journal 4(4) (2009)
12. Dombroviak, K., Ramnath, R.: A taxonomy of mobile and pervasive applications. In: SAC Proceedings of the ACM symposium on Applied computing, USA, pp. 1609–1615. ACM, New York (2007)
13. Giroux, S., Pigot, H. (eds.): From Smart Home to Smart Care. Assitive Technology Research series. IOS Press, Amsterdam (2005)
14. Helal, S., Mokhtari, M., Abulrazak, B.: The Engineering Handbook on Smart Technology for Aging, Disability and Independence. John Wiley and Sons, Chichester (2007)
15. Intille, S., et al.: A living laboratory for the design and evaluation of ubiquitous computing technologies. In: Extended Abstracts of the 2005 Conference on Human Factors in Computing Systems, pp. 1941–1944. ACM Press, New York (2005)
16. Jeon, N., Leem, C., Kim, M., Shin, H.: A taxonomy of ubiquitous computing applications. Wirel. Pers. Commun. 43(4), 1229–1239 (2007)
17. Kotsis, G.: Performance management in ubiquitous computing environments. In: Proceedings of the 15th International Conference on Computer Communication (2002)
18. Lupiana, D., et al.: Taxonomy for ubiquitous computing environments. In: First International Conference on Networked Digital Technologies, July 2009, pp. 469–475 (2009)
19. Manko, J., Carter, S.: Crossing qualitative and quantitative evaluation in the domain of ubiquitous computing. In: CHI 2005 Workshop on Usage Analysis: Combining Logging and Qualitative Methods, Portland (2005)

20. Modahl, M., et al.: Ubiqstack: A taxonomy for a ubiquitous computing software stack. Personal and Ubiquitous Computing 10(1), 21–27 (2006)
21. Muras, J., Cahill, V., Stokes, E.: A taxonomy of pervasive healthcare systems. In: Pervasive Health Conference and Workshops, pp. 1–10 (2006)
22. Ranganathan, A., et al.: Towards a pervasive computing benchmark. In: PerCom Workshops, pp. 194–198 (2005)
23. Weiser, M.: The computer for the 21st century. Scientific American 265(3), 66–75 (1991)

A Robotic System for Home Security Enhancement

Andreas Gregoriades[1], Samuel Obadan[1], Harris Michail[2], Vicky Papadopoulou[1], and Despina Michael[3]

[1] European University Cyprus, Cyprus
{samice2k,a.gregoriades,v.papadopoulou}@euc.ac.cy
[2] University of Patras, Greece
michail@ece.upatras.gr
[3] University of Nicosia, Cyprus
michael.d@unic.ac.cy

Abstract. Central to smart home security is the need for adequate surrounding awareness. Security systems have been designed for remote exploration and control, however, these still lack the simplicity needed by elderly and disabled. The majority of elderly people find the control of such systems laborious. This highlights the need for usable designs that take into consideration the cognitive limitations of this category of people. This paper contributes towards this problem through the introduction of a novel vehicular Remote Exploration Surveillance Robot (RESBot), capable of monitoring in real time the environment in response to events. The interaction with the system is achieved through natural language commands and hence, provides improved usability over traditional approaches. Results from the experimental usability evaluation of the RESBot system revealed considerable improvement over conventional home security systems.

Keywords: Human-robot interaction, Situation awareness, Home security, Teleoperation.

1 Introduction

The worldwide population of elderly people is growing rapidly and in the coming decades the proportion of old people will change significantly. This demographic shift will create a huge increase in demand for domestic home security technologies. Smart homes have been credited with saving the lives of many elderly, disabled and senior citizens [5]. The first generations of home security systems are mainly using CCTV cameras. However, these provide limited flexibility in maintaining sufficient situation awareness [7]. Plus, these systems are controlled using keyboard and joystick that hence pose cognitive strain on elderly users. According to [18] CCTV is ineffective for day-to-day safety and security. Specifically, CCTV cameras could be badly placed, broken, dirty, or with insufficient lighting and this limits their overall effectiveness and efficiency. When CCTV is used for command and control, safety operators performance is hampered by the large number of information sources, and inefficient audio communication channels. This suggests that CCTV for crime

Y. Lee et al. (Eds.): ICOST 2010, LNCS 6159, pp. 43–52, 2010.

prevention can only be effective as part of an overall set of measures and procedures designed to deal with specific problems. When it comes to elderly, the use of CCTV is inappropriate for all of the above reasons along with the fact that elderly are characterized by limited attentional resources that in effect constrain their capabilities. For elderly and disabled people to maintain adequate situation awareness it is important to provide them with only the salient cues from the environmental context. Too much or too little information may have the opposite effect with regards to situation awareness. Therefore, central to smart homes is the need for technologies that sufficiently address these requirements. Prerequisite for adequate situation assessment is effective interaction with the technology. Despite their success stories, smart homes have their limitations. It has been reported that smart home technology will be helpful only if it's tailored to meet individual needs [2]. This currently poses a problem as many of the interface control console designed do not take into consideration non-functional limitations associated with the elderly. In the same vein, there is a fundamental problem in making IT system user friendly for the elderly and disabled [11,12]. This work is motivated by the need to improve the safety living conditions of elderly/disabled by addressing two important factors that interest this category of people, namely, usability and cost. The former prerequisites usable interfaces designed that improve users' task performance through reduced cognitive effort. This requirement strive engineers in investigations for best fit between man and machine by considering the constraints and capabilities of elderly people. The later factor we address through a simple generic robotic platform.

Given that elderly and disabled are characterized by reduced memory and attention, the home security system proposed in this study uses an interaction metaphor that minimizes user effort and improves situation awareness. To that end, we adopted a human-centered approach for the human-robot interaction through simple natural language instructions. The underlying technology of the interaction metaphor is a mobile phone. The ubiquitous property and low weight of mobile phones overcomes fundamental problem during interaction. The proposed implementation utilizes a vehicular robotic surveillance system capable of indoor/outdoor remote observation in response to natural language commands. This constitutes an improvement over traditional approaches to home security management, characterized by dexterous manipulation of joy stick and keyboard interfaces that obstruct the users from the primary task. The research question that we address in this work is: "Does voice activated robotic surveillance system provides improved situation awareness for elderly/disabled compared to existing home security systems?"

The paper is organized as follows. Next section covers the literature on developments of human centered robotics especially in smart home security technologies. Following this is a detailed breakdown of the 'RESBot' architecture, design methodology and software implementation. Next, follows a usability evaluation of the proposed system and an interpretation of the results. The paper concludes with future directions.

2 Literature Review

The last 10 years witnessed robots becoming increasingly common in non-industrial applications, such as homes, hospitals, and service areas. These robots are often referred to as "human-centred" or "human-friendly" robotic systems due to the way the robot interfaces with the human users [15,9]. This close interaction can include contact-free sharing of a common workspace or direct physical human-machine contact. Contrasts to industrial robots where specific tasks are performed repetitively, human-centred robots are implemented on a totally different set of requirement [11]. These include: safety, flexibility, mechanical compliance, gentleness, and adaptability towards user, ease of use, communicative skills, and sometimes possession of humanoid appearance and behaviour. According to Heinzmann and Zelinsky [12] human centred robotics should have natural communication channels that involve not only language but also facial gestures and expressions along with providing high level of functionality and pleasure. Some successful human-centred robotic implementations include: Rhino the museum tour guide robot that was assigned tasks via internet teleoperation technique [14]. Among their other roles, robotic systems have been designed to aid home, industrial and business security. An example of robot security management system is the Mobile Detection Assessment and Response System (MDARS) [19] deployed by the department of defense. MDARS simultaneously control multiple autonomous robots that provide automated intrusion detection and warehouse inventory assessment. Similarly, robots are becoming popular in home security and telecare [1-4]. Telecare is defined as the use of a combination of communications technology and sensing technologies to provide a means of manually or automatically signaling a local need to a remote service centre, which can then deliver or arrange an appropriate care response to the telecare service user. AVENUE is an example telecare robot [16]. However, current telecare and home security robots require dexterous manipulations [10] and hence, failed to take into consideration the human-requirements of elderly and disabled. Efforts have been reported that aim in easing the complexity of the interaction between elderly users and the robot. Phonebot, is an example that uses cell phone communication between user and robot [7]. Phonebot responds to calls via, a ring detector circuit, which establishes a connection between the user and the robot. The main limitation of Phonebot is the lack of a voice activated control mechanism and this creates a communication overload that obstructs the user from achieving his/her goals [25]. This one of the limitations we address in this research.

An additional issue that has emerged in the field of human-robot usability is the notion of enjoyment during interaction as reported by [17]. Specifically, [17] identified that there is high correlation between enjoyment and intention to use of a robotic system in a usability analysis conducted with elderly people. This indicates the need for enjoyment to be part of robot design. This constitutes another motivating factor of the research conducted and described in here.

3 The Remote Exploration Surveillance Robotic System (RESBot)

RESBot is a roving maneuverable vehicular surveillance system, which projects in real time contextual information of the environment for enhanced situation awareness of elderly and disabled people. The RESBot is a voice activated control mechanism that enables remote command and control for home security purposes. The main components of the system are classified in user and robot side as depicted in figure 1 and described below:

- User interface component
- Communicator
- Autonomous obstacle avoidance component
- Onboard contextual assessor.
- Actuators

User interaction and navigation is achieved through a voice recognition component. This can be trained in any language of choice and provides natural means for interacting with the system. This is of major importance to elderly and disabled people that are characterized by low cognitive and motor capabilities. Through this technology, we built a robotic system by incorporating existing technology into a unified robotic surveillance system.

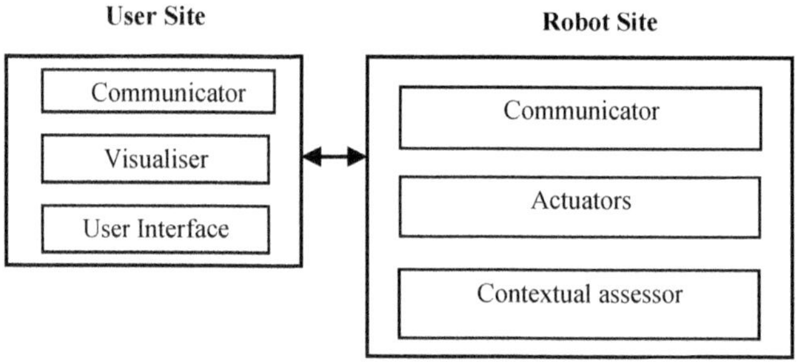

Fig. 1. RESBot architectural components

The robot's on-board controlled camera provides 360 degrees visual coverage and thereby provides its users with the necessary contextual cues for improved situation awareness. For brevity, the user is capable of interacting with the robotic system using voice commands over GSM mobile phone. The visual feedback display enables the user to carry out real time surveillance of a remote environment and as such support users' contextual awareness. The scope of this work concentrates on vehicle teleoperation that enable remote task execution.

The other main component of the actuator sub-system is the autonomous obstacle detection and avoidance system that provide effortless navigation of the robot. Finally, the automatic intrusion detection component provides real time recognition through a motion sensor that also supports user's situation awareness. This component is responsible for the automatic orientation of the camera and notification of the user of an intrusion event. An overview of the communication mechanism between user-side and robot-side is presented in Figure 2.

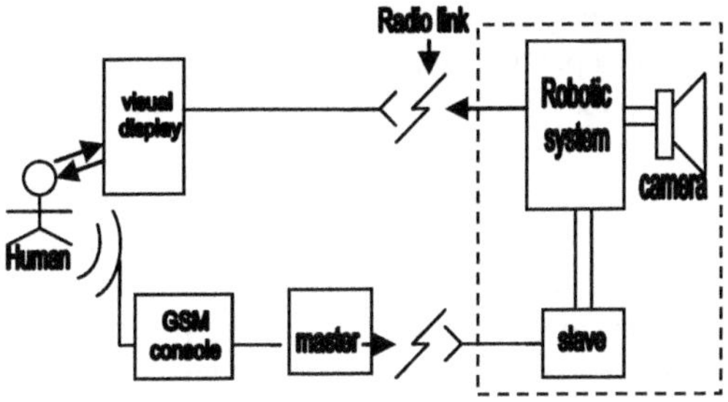

Fig. 2. Outline of client-robot communication architecture

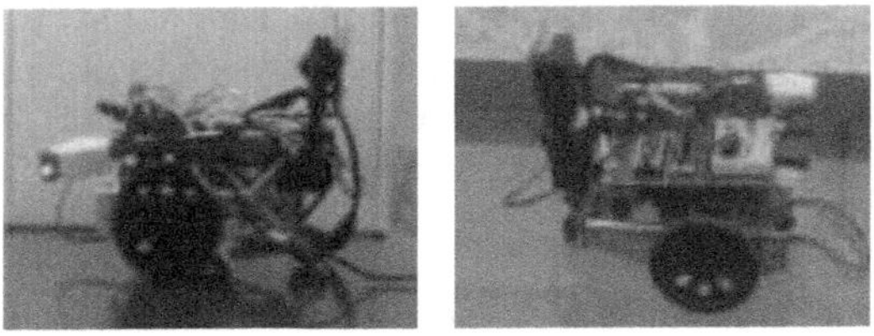

Fig. 3. The RESBot implementation

4 Design and Implementation of RESBot

The RESBot is a novel implementation of a voice activated robotic system leveraging the use of modern GSM technology. The parallax Board of education (BOE) was used as the platform for its development. The robot is a small, skid-steered wheeled vehicle capable of limited outdoor/indoor work. The robot is equipped with a ring of infrared proximity sensors, power monitoring, and voice recognition decoder. An onboard pinhole camera provides forward video. Digital/Analogue transmitters are used for video and data communication. An on-board micro-controller processor performs navigation and obstacle avoidance.

The communication between the user and the robot is achieved through GSM digital transmission. GSM digital signals can pass through an arbitrary number of regenerators with no loss in signal and thus travel long distances with no information loss [8]. Users perceive situational cues from the environment through the onboard video feedback and accordingly respond to them by engage the robot in a voice command. The command and control mechanism is based on a user-centred interface design methodology in which visual displays provide information for decision-making and control [9]. Through this we achieve easy robot-user interaction for adequate contextual awareness [10]. A wireless video camera is used to enhance motion planning. An onboard infra-red sensor provides situational cues that are analyses by the central system and subsequently inform the user through an automatic events generation.

The user can request status updated by invoking the robot at any time. The voice recognition decoder is responsible for recognizing the user input and accordingly converting this into an instruction for the robot's actuators. This component can be trained to recognize up to 40 instructions. After training, the user can instruct the robot using the specified language corpus. During training the user can validate the system's knowledge by repeating a trained word into the microphone. During the validation of this component, the index of the corresponding human instruction was displayed on a digital display. This helped to verify that the right instructions are associated with the right indexes. Output from the voice recognition circuit is fed into the robot's microcontroller for navigation. To achieve a more robust interaction between user and the robot, words with the same meaning were associated with the same action in the language corpus. Central to the robot is the microcontroller that processes human instructions for command and control. This component is responsible for the rotation of the on board camera during surveillance mode. Recognition of an event raises an alert to the user that accordingly navigates the robot and orients the camera. The robot is also equipped with an obstacle detection and avoidance algorithm that enables its autonomous navigation. To achieve this feature, three infrared sensors are used. Intrusion detection is achieved through an on board motion detector sensor. For the rotation of the camera and the wheeling of the robot sstandard and rotational servos are used. Figure 3 depicts the implemented RESBoat system.

5 Usability Evaluation of the RESBot

Core to the success of the proposed home security system is adequate usability, given that the indented users have special needs and attentional constraints. Therefore, it was essential to primarily understand prospective users' relevant skills and mental models and accordingly develop evaluation criteria. However, robotics systems differ significantly from desktop user interfaces and hence, the use of empirically defined set of heuristics such as Nielsen are not suitable. To that end, it was decided to use an experimental usability evaluation approach in controlled settings. Typical HCI evaluations use efficiency, effectiveness, learnability and user satisfaction as evaluation metrics. Efficiency is a measure of performance time; effectiveness is a measure of task performance; learnability is a measure of how easy is to learn a system by a novice user and satisfaction a measure of pleasure. Learnability is considered as a key indicator for usability in human-robot interaction with elderly and disabled since it significantly affect system acceptance. Learnability incorporates several principles like familiarity, consistency, generalizability, predictability, and simplicity. These four measures were deemed appropriate for the experimental evaluation of the RESBot system and its comparison against the most popular home security system, namely CCTV.

To benchmark the proposed system against available low budget home security systems such as CCTV, we opted for a comparative study using two groups of participants. Each group was composed of 10 participants of age 60 and over. Throughout the study, CCTV and RESBot systems were referred to as System A and B respectively. Prior to the experiment each participant had to complete a consent form. Participants of each group were given instructions and demonstration on how to use each system through example scenarios. During training, participants were encouraged to ask questions. The evaluations involved two experiments using system A and B accordingly. The scenario of each experiment, involved participants independently investigating an alarm caused by a human intruder. The experiments took place in the participants' homes and a TV was used for video feedback. For system A, a static camera was mounted in the participant's garden. The CCTV camera was also equipped with a motion sensor that raised an alarm whenever it sensed motion within the covered area.

The first experiment was conducted with the use of the CCTV system and group A. The evaluation scenario required users to locate the hiding position of an intruder that was allowed to move around at will. In this experiment, it was assumed that intruder was not aware of the position of the CCTV camera. During the experiment, participants were asked to locate the intruder and specify his hiding position. The second experiment was conducted with the use of the RESBot system and group B. This group did not participate in the first experiment. Prior to the use of the RESBot system, participants were expected to train its instructions corpus. During this experiment, the RESBot was placed in the surroundings of each participant's home and the goal was to locate an intruder. Participants were informed of the intrusion through the system alarm. The manipulation of the RESBot was performed with the aid of a mobile console using voice commands. Visual feedback from the robot was projected on the TV. In both experiment the scenario was terminated with the recognition of the intruder's position.

Throughout the experiments, participants' actions and mistakes were recorded by the researchers along with their tasks and task's completion times. To assess users' situation awareness, we opted for the SAGAT approach described by Endsley[6]. Hense, during the scenarios, participants were asked to designate at different intervals, where they though the intruder was located. The actual and perceived location of the intruder enables the quantification of their situation awareness, that in turn guided their consequent actions/instructions with the system. With the completion of both experiments, each participant was asked to complete a questionnaire. This included constructs relating users' perceptions of: ease of use, usefulness, attitudes, and intention to use of the system. In addition, behavioral information regarding satisfaction and user experience with both systems, were also collected. Each participant's response was associated with a unique identification number to avoid bias during data analysis.

The evaluation of the two systems' was based on the level of user-acceptance, the assessment of which was based on the Technology Acceptance Model (TAM) [17]. TAM has been successfully used to study user's acceptance of IT systems using quantifications of users attitude that define the positive or negative feelings toward the IT system. In its most basic form it states that perceived usefulness and perceived ease of use determine the behavioral intention to use a system that can predict actual use. Specifically:

- *Perceived ease of use* (P1): defines as the degree to which an individual believes that learning to use a technology will require little effort. The participants' perceptions that system (A or B) was easy to use were captured with 12, five-point Likert-scale questions.
- *Perceived usefulness* (P2): examines individual believes that use of the technology will improve performance. The participants' perceptions of systems' usefulness were captured in 8, five-point Likert-scale questions

- *Attitude* (P3): feeling or emotion about using the technology. The participants' attitudes towards using the system (A or B) were assessed using 5, five-point Likert-type questions.
- *Intention to use* (P4): the likelihood that an individual will use the technology in the future. The participants' intention to use each system was assessed using 4 five-point Likert-type questions.

Questionnaires were used as the main instrument for measuring these influences. Each component of the TAM model was expressed in a number of questions. Items of the instrument that measured the same influence were grouped together to form generic constructs. In addition to the core TAM constructs, an extra set of questions regarding user satisfaction were also incorporated in the research instrument.

5.1 Analysis and Results

Data collected from the experiments was analyzed using the statistical package SPSS. Comparative analysis between the two systems was performed using a 2-tailed t-test for each of the constructs of TAM. Since we have no strong prior theory to suggest any relationship between the TAM components of system A and B, we opted for the 2-tailed t-test. The analysis performed a paired samples t-test to check the difference between the scores in each dimension. The difference between the two paired mean scores for TAM constructs ranged from P1-P4. P1 compared perceived usefulness of the two systems. P2 compared perceived ease of use, while P3 and P4 attitude towards use and intention to use respectively.

The collated results of table 1 highlight that for each of the TAM constructs, the mean scores between systems A and B differ significantly. The output begins with the means and standard deviations for the two systems. The "Mean Difference" statistic indicates the magnitude of the difference between means. When combined with the confidence interval for the difference, this information explains the importance of the results. In particular, perceived usefulness of system B is significantly higher than system A. Similarly, perceived ease of use, attitude and intention to use is significantly higher for system B. The 2-tailed test indicates that the difference between the two systems is significant and the results are not due to chance. This is identified from the significance value which is less than .05 and means that the variability in the performance of the two systems is not the same and the scores in the one system vary much more than the scores in the second system. The negative sign on t value designates that system B which is the RESBot outperforms system A in mean values.

The results shows that the robotic system provides better usability and control over the CCTV system by better addressing the needs and capabilities of the elderly and disabled.

Table 1. Paired sample t-test

Pair	Mean	Std Dev	t	df	Sig
P1	-12.800	2.616	-15.472	9	.000
P2	-12.600	5.037	-7.909	9	.000
P3	-12.100	2.282	-16.762	9	.000
P4	-3.700	2.057	-5.687	9	.000

Additional data regarding the usability of the robotic system revealed that 90% of participants could use and interpret the feedback from the visual display with ease. Moreover, 90% of participants feel that the alarm produced by the system is suitable for attracting attention. Overall, the results yielded from the experiments demonstrated that:

- 80% of participants were able to navigate the robot with the voice recognition system.
- 70% of the participants spotted the intruders' changing position faster with the RESBot than the CCTV.
- Participants were not able to get the system to respond to the 'survey' and 'hold-on' commands using RESBot. Nevertheless, the other commands were sufficient for effective navigational surveillance.
- 90% of participants found customizing the commands with easy to remember words in their preferred language very satisfying
- Throughout the experiment 20% of participants complained about issuing a command more than once over the control console, for the robotic response.
- 100% of the participants were satisfied with the latency (reaction time) between a recognized command and robotic response.
- 90% of the participants agreed they had an enjoyable, engaging and satisfying experience using the RESBot.
- 80% of participants managed to locate the intruder in less time using the RESBot.
- 70% of participants had better situation awareness with the RESBot.

6 Conclusion/Future Direction

As smart homes implementation gradually become widely adapted due to increasing aging population [13], the need for improving the safety living conditions of the elderly/disabled increases along with it. Similarly, there is a stressing need for usable human-robot interface designs that meet the needs and constraints of elderly and disabled [6]. In this research, we demonstrate the implementation of a vehicular robotic surveillance system (RESBot) capable of remote surveillance of the environment in response to natural language commands. This is an improvement over keyboard and joystick controls and hence, provides a more usable communication metaphor between elderly users and robotic systems. The study also highlighted an important issue in the literature by examining the effects of robotic systems operated by elderly people for enhanced home security through improved contextual awareness. The current research results provide key information to educators and commercial industries in providing a more robust security implementation of smart homes.

Future direction will be geared towards incorporating audio processing capabilities to address the needs of users with speech impediment. A possible implementation could also be the combination of visual and voice interface in a single control console such as PDAs.

References

1. Kinsella, A.: Home telecare in the United States. J. Telemed. Telecare 4, 195–200 (1998)
2. Doughty, K., Cameron, K., Garner, P.: Three generations of telecare of the elderly. J. Telemed Telecare 2, 71–80 (1996)
3. Ruggiero, C., Sacile, R., Giacomini, M.: Home telecare. J. Telemed. Telecare 5, 11–17 (1999)
4. Stoecke, J., Lorch, S.: Why go see the doctor? Care goes from office to home as technology divorces function from geography. International Journal Technology Assessment in Health Care 13, 537–546 (1997)
5. Cheek, P.: Aging Well With Smart Technology. Nursing Administration Quarterly 29(4), 329–338 (2005)
6. Endsley, M.R.: Design and evaluation for situation awareness enhancement. In: Proc. Human Factors Society 32nd Annual Meeting, Santa Monica, CA (1988)
7. Sobh, T., Mihali, R., Gosine, G., Batra, P., Singh, A., Pathak, S., Vitulskis, T.: Web-Controlled Devices and Manipulation: Case Studies. In: Remote Learning for Automation and Robotics, World Automation Congress (2002)
8. Fong, T.: Collaborative Control: A Robot-Centric Model for Vehicle Teleoperation. The Robotics Institute Carnegie Mellon University Pittsburgh, Pennsylvania (1998)
9. Newman, W., Lamming, M.: Interactive System Design. Addison-Wesley, Reading (1995)
10. Riener, R., Lünenburger, L., Nat, R., Colombo, G.: PhD Human-centered robotics applied to gait training and assessment. Journal of rehabilitation research and development 43(5), 679–694 (2006)
11. Zinn, M., Roth, B., Khatib, O., Salisbury, J.K.: A new actuation approach for human friendly robot design. Int. J. Robot Res. 3(4-5), 379–398 (2004)
12. Heinzmann, J., Zelinsky, J.: A safe-control paradigm for human-robot interaction. J. Intell. Robot Syst. 25(4), 295–310 (1999)
13. Toprani, K.: Smart houses become reality. The Triangle Online (2004)
14. Burgard, W., Thrun, S., fox, D., Cremers, A.B., Harnel, D., Lakemeyer, G., Schulz, D., Steiner, W.: Experiences with an interactive museum tour-guide robot. Artificial Intelligence 114(1-2), 1–53 (1999)
15. Dehuai, Z., Cunxi, X., Xuemei, L.: Design and Implementation of a security and patrol robot system. In: IEEE International Conference on Mechatronics and Automation (2005)
16. Allen, P., Stamos, I., Gueorguiev, A., Gold, E., Blaer, P.: AVENUE: Automated site modeling in urban environments. In: Proceedings of 3rd Conference on Digital Imaging and Modeling in Quebec City, Canada
17. Heerink, M., Kröse, B., Wielinga, B., Evers, V.: Enjoyment, Intention to Use And Actual Use of a Conversational Robot by Elderly People. Hogeschool van Amsterdam, Instituut voor Information Engineering Almere, Netherlands year (2007)
18. Sasse, M.: Not seeing the crime from the cameras? Communications of the ACM 53(2) (2010)
19. Everett, H.R., Gage, D.W., Gilbreath, G.A., Laird, R.T., Smurlo, R.P.: Real-world issues in warehouse navigation RDT&E Division. In: Naval Command Control and Ocean Surveillance Center, San Diego (1994)

Why Is My Home Not Smart?

Patrick Holroyd, Phil Watten, and Paul Newbury

University of Sussex
School of Informatics, Falmer, Brighton, BN1 9QJ, UK
{p.holroyd,p.l.watten,p.newbury}@sussex.ac.uk
http://www.sussex.ac.uk

Abstract. Although the idea of the smart home has been around for over three decades the smart technology that enables it has yet to reach the mass market. Spending on smart technology is expected to rise, but it is still negligible when compared to overall spending on consumer electronics. This paper examines the benefits of the smart home, peoples attitude towards them and smart technologies and the possible reasons for lack of interest and adoption of such technologies.

Keywords: smart home, smart technology, benefits, attitude, interest.

1 Introduction

The term smart home was coined by the National Association of Home Builders (NAHB) in the early 1980s after it set up a group to push for the adoption of smart technologies in the design of new homes [1]. Since then, there has been limited research into the area with the majority of this focused on the development of example smart houses showcasing the possibilities this type of technology could bring. However, this research, along with the efforts of the NAHB and others, has yet to deliver the smart home life envisioned by many during the late 20th and early 21st century. Most of the western world is still living in homes more similar to their grandparent rather than those conceived by the early smart home pioneers. This paper examines the benefits of the smart home, such as support for the elderly and energy saving, people's attitude towards them and smart technologies and the possible reasons for lack of interest and adoption of such technologies.

A smart home is a domestic residence that incorporates common devices to control features of the home. The most basic feature of a smart home is the ability to control devices remotely or automatically [2]. Originally this may have been limited to switching the heating or lighting on or off, but as technology has improved almost any device can now be controlled remotely or automatically. Smart homes are now capable of incorporating large amounts of computing power to monitor the activities of its occupants and anticipate their wants and needs. They can provide users with complex customisation options to allow them to tailor their environment to precise requirements [3].

At the turn of the century the advent of high speed broadband (ADSL, cable etc.) and the always connected quality of this type of technology gave rise an to explosion

Y. Lee et al. (Eds.): ICOST 2010, LNCS 6159, pp. 53–59, 2010.

in home networking. With broadband companies giving away wireless router technology more people than ever are being exposed to the possibilities a connected home can bring. A report by Continental Automated Buildings Association Connected Home Research Council in 2008 [4] found that approximately nine-tenths of Americans have access to broadband Internet and approximately two-fifths have a home network. With access to high speed broadband people are downloading more data than ever before and are consuming vast amounts of content. A smart home used to be regarded as home where devices could be controlled or monitored remotely or automatically, but they are now regarded as technology rich multimedia environments. Only 10 years ago, the thought of remotely setting your living room personal video recorder (PVR) on the move then watching the program back in the bedroom was nearly impossible. Now using a home network you can connected to your PVR using a mobile phone then watch back the show in the bedroom using your laptop [5].

2 Benefits

Although the benefits for smart homes are numerous they can be divided into four distinct categories, these being:

- Energy saving
- Support for elderly or disabled
- Security and safety
- User convenience

User convenience is an area that has long been associated with smart technology, energy saving and support for the elderly or disabled have been more recently explored and, due to the global warming and an aging population, both of which are today very much in vogue. Each of these categories are briefly discussed below.

2.1 Energy Saving

The need to significantly reduce carbon emissions is arguably todays greatest challenge. Energy efficient smart technology can be utilised within the home to offer the user a host of energy saving ideas. The installation of smart meters, promised by many governments, will allow a whole host of energy saving techniques to be implemented within the home. Those who generate their own energy will be able to sell it back to the energy grid. Smart meters will allow feedback of energy consumption to easily be delivered to the user. Wood et al. [6] explores the idea of using energy feedback displays to inform user of the amount of energy being used by the various devices currently active within the home. With these displays motivation techniques can be used to encourage a reduction in energy usage. Darby [7] investigates the use of a TV or PC to deliver information back to the user showing them their historic consumption, daily costs and comparisons with other homes. Other systems such as smart heating systems and smart lighting systems (the idea of a single off button for the home, which will turn off all but essential items) are being explored and researched.

2.2 Support for the Elderly or Disabled

Kidd et al. describe The Aware Home, developed by Georgia Institute of Technology, which "focuses on the computing needs of people within their everyday lives, specifically, the part of their life not centred around work or the office" [8]. Kidd et al. identify support for the elderly as a specific application for smart homes. With a baby boom generation fast approaching retirement age, smart homes could provide them with cheap affordable home support and health care advice. Governments are beginning to see smart home technology as a viable option in reducing the financial burden of supporting this generation through their retirement. Raad et al. have developed a sensor-based system which utilises telecommunication technologies to provide a cost-effective telehealth system for the elderly and disabled [9]. The aim of this system is to "provide a continuous communication link between patients and caregivers and allow physicians to offer help when needed". This type of system could allow the elderly to stay within their own home while providing them with essential care at an affordable cost.

2.3 Security and Safety

Security and safety are important issues for many people. A study by Min-Soo et al. [10] found that nearly 43% of the elderly respondents were worried about the event of an accident involving gas and approximately 22% were "anxious that outsiders would suddenly invade their home" [10]. Smart home technology offers many benefits for preventing accidents and reducing security fears. IP bases security cameras are commonly used as a home security feature. These types of cameras can be controlled from remote locations by sending control commands allowing users to view their home from the office or on their mobile phone while out. Security aware smart systems are a more advanced security feature. This type of system can monitor occupants in the home, learn daily routines and use a whole host of sensing technology to analyse and flag potential security risks to the user.

2.4 User Convenience

The Gator Tech Smart House [11] showcases many convenience smart home technologies. The first generation of ubiquitous environments were generally closed off systems unable to adapt to the newly developed technology. This problem meant that once a home was considered complete it became very difficult to install new devices or systems within that home. The house tries to address this limitation by developing "programmable ubiquitous spaces in which a smart space exists as both a runtime environment and a software library". Although the home is specially designed for the elderly and disabled with an overall goal of creating assistive environments it demonstrates the type of convenience technologies which could be common place in the average home. The house boasts an impressive array of smart devices that are connected to the homes network and are designed to monitor all aspects of daily life. Example of these devices includes a smart mailbox, capable of sensing when the post arrives, and a smart front door complete with RFID tag for keyless entry. The smart bathroom is capable of detecting low toilet paper, toilet flushes, occupants cleanliness as well as regulating the shower water temperature. Along with a whole host of other devices, the home is capable of sensing itself and the resident so it can, for example, replenish stocks when necessary or automatically controlling the home entertainment system depending on your location. The benefit of all these technology would be similar to the adoption home appliances during the 1940-1950s. It would begin to free people from the last remaining mundane aspects of running a modern home.

3 Attitudes

3.1 Mass Market

Although many academic and industrial research institutions have conducted research into smart homes and their potential there is distinctly less investigation into what a consumers attitudes and needs are regarding smart home technology. In order to understand peoples attitude towards smart homes we must first look at their attitudes to previous new technology and consumer products. Pragnell et al. have tried to assess the smart home market potential with a report published by the John Rowntree Foundation [12]. Pragnell et al. describes the S-curve of new technology adoption which is "characterised by slow take-up in the early years followed by a more rapid increase in adoption which moves the product into the mass market". Fig 1 shows an example of this type of curve showing that as time goes on more households adopt the new technology. It is worth noting that different technologies follow different S-curve shapes, some rapidly making it to mass market, some more slowly. This can be affected by a number of key factors:

- Economic
- Social
- Consumer
- Technological
- Global/political

Pragnell et al. go on to describe the demand for smart homes and groups society into three categories:

- The interested - Generally aged between 15-34; technophiles with home entertainment systems, PCs, Internet access and higher income
- The ambivalent - Marginally more likely to be older and on medium/low incomes
- The uninterested - Generally aged 55 and over; technophobes with no PCs, internet access or home entertainment systems

It is perhaps unsurprising that the younger more technology aware section of society is the most interested in the smart home concept. However even in the younger generation this interest does not translate to a wiliness to invest in smart home consumables. An ON World report [13] predicts that by 2012 the smart home market will be worth $2.8 billion. According to an iSuppli estimate the worldwide consumer electronics OEM revenue in 2010 will rise to $317.3 billion [14]. This means that the smart home market represents less than 0.1% of overall spending on consumer electronics. The 21st century question that faces the smart home industry is not what is possible with the smart technology, but what is preventing the technology being

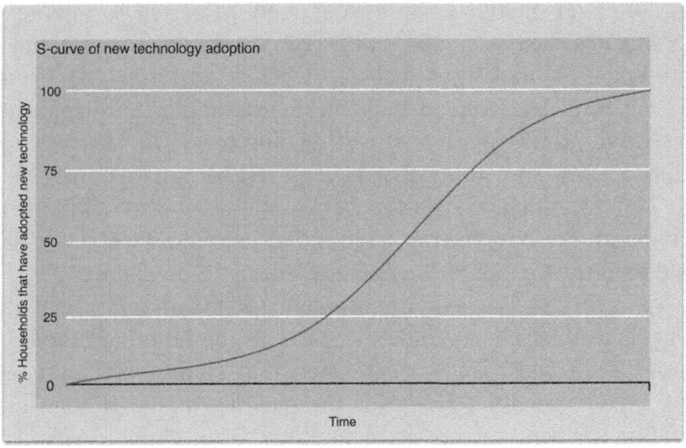

Fig. 1. S-curve of new technology adoption

adopted by the average consumer. With over three decades of development people are still unwilling to invest.

3.2 Problems with Adoption

The problem of adoption cannot be pinned on one overridding smart home feature but with hosts a problems. These can be boiled down into 4 key areas:

- Retrofitting
- Usability - lack of killer feature
- Cost
- Interoperability

By retrofitting a standard home into a smart home you are adding new technology without making any major alteration to the existing home. At present the technology for a smart home is usually installed during construction of the building or during a major renovation. Expensive cabling, planning and simulation is undertaken to ensure that bespoke designed systems and devices are connected together [2] [15]. An individual rarely undertakes this type of building work and therefore the technology is almost never found in older buildings. Construction companies are also unlikely to budget for unnecessary building costs in all but luxury domestic buildings therefore many new builds are still constructed without the ability to even accommodate new smart technology. The potential for a smart home retrofit has improved with the development of wireless network devices and power line smart transceivers such as the ZigBee Alliance [16] and LonWorks [17] platform respectively. These types of technologies are useful for sending small amounts of control data between devices but unable to cope with the high data rates of multimedia applications.

The usability of a smart home defines the way an end user will interact with various smart devices and system preferences. It has until recently been largely overlooked but it is something which is of huge importance. If a user finds a system too complicated or unintuitive they will simply not use it. Jeong at el demonstrates this point when they researched the smart home interface preferences between U.S and

Korean users. Jeong at el found the "respondents preferred to interact with a smart home using a physical device (a computer, cell phone, or remote control) rather than through communication modalities such as speech or gesture" [18]. From the result of the survey Jeong at el recommend that interfaces should be adapted to a particular culture and go on to propose culture-specific guidelines. The lack of one clear benefit or killer feature is also something that is required for smart homes to penetrate the mass market. This recent success of the Apple iPhone, with the killer mobile internet browsing feature, shows how having an intuitive user interface alongside a killer feature can create a product people want and are willing to pay money for.

The issue of cost has long been a problem for smart home manufacturers. The problem being that either all non smart devices in the home are replaced along with expensive installation and cabling cost mean that smart homes are generally only available to societies wealthy. However the success of the iPhone has shown that people are willing to spend money on technology. The iPhone is relativity expensive, especially compared to other phones, which are given away free. Where the iPhone differs is that Apple took a modular approach to each aspect of the device ensuring that each feature of the phone was not only up-to date but also that it didnt confuse the user [19]. If a similar approach was taken to smart home design users may be more willing to invest in the technology.

It is not only the interface which may confuse the user or stop them investing but the lack of interoperability. Although various smart home control protocols exist (e.g. X10, Lonworks [17] and KNX [20]) there still exist problems when different devices are connected together. The movement towards universal connectivity rather than individual designed and controlled smart devices can only work when manufactures use open and common standards. This would allow users to bundle together different products bought at different times allowing them to invest slowly in various smart technologies safe in the knowledge that the next product they buy will still connect with existing purchases.

4 Conclusion

Why is my home not smart? Although smart homes and smart technology has been available for some time it has yet to enter the mass market. The main reason for this is the complex installation and user interface, which have long been associated with smart homes. This twinned with lack of interoperability has prevented adoption of this type of technology to all but the wealthy and technophile. The issue of retrofitting could become less of problem if manufacturers use open standards that utilise the wireless and power line transceiver technologies such as Zigbee and KNX.

The commitment by many governments to install smart energy meters into homes nationwide may have the desired effect of kick starting the smart home revolution. The reduction in green house gases may also be a catalyst for this revolution as energy production moves towards micro generation whereby people use their smart energy meter to sell power back to the grid. This, however, will not happen until smart technology systems and smart homes in general become more user friendly with each area having a killer feature which can be used as a main selling point. More research needs to be conducted into what the user really wants from a smart home and how this is best delivered in an intuitive, easy to use manner. The benefits of smart home are vast and we are only beginning to understand how this will affect future generations. By researching smart home interfaces and interoperability, this revolution may happen faster than ever before.

References

1. Harper, R.: Inside the smart home. Springer, Heidelberg (2003)
2. Cook, D., Das, S.K.: Smart environments. John Wiley Sons, Inc., Hoboken (2005)
3. Ricquebourg, V., Menga, D., Durand, D., Marhic, B., Delahoche, L., Loge, C.: The Smart Home Concept: our immediate future. In: 2006 1ST IEEE International Conference on E-Learning in Industrial Electronics, pp. 23–28 (2006)
4. 2008 State of The Connected Home Market Study Executive Summary. Continental Automated Buildings Association Connected Home Research Council (2008)
5. Kamel, I., Akinlar, C., El-Sayed, H.: QoS guarantee for multimedia traffic in smart homes. Multimedia Tools and Applications 47, 87–103
6. Wood, G., Newborough, M.: Energy-use information transfer for intelligent homes: Enabling energy conservation with central and local displays. Energy and Buildings 39, 495–503 (2007)
7. Darby, S.: The Effectiveness of Feedback on Energy Consumption. In: A., F.a.R. (ed.) Department for Environment. Environmental Change Institute, University of Oxford (2006)
8. Kidd, C.D., Orr, R., Abowd, G.D., Atkeson, C.G., Essa, I.A., MacIntyre, B., Mynatt, E.D., Starner, T., Newstetter, W.: The Aware Home: A Living Laboratory for Ubiquitous Computing Research. In: Proceedings of the Second International Workshop on Cooperative Buildings, Integrating Information, Organization, and Architecture. Springer, Heidelberg (1999)
9. Raad, M., Yang, L.: A ubiquitous smart home for elderly. Information Systems Frontiers 11, 529–536 (2009)
10. Min-Soo, K., Kyung Mi, K., Hee-Cheol, K.: A questionnaire study for the design of smart home for the elderly. In: 8th International Conference on e-Health Networking, Applications and Services, HEALTHCOM 2006, pp. 265–268 (2006)
11. Helal, S., Mann, W., El-Zabadani, H., King, J., Kaddoura, Y., Jansen, E.: The Gator Tech Smart House: a programmable pervasive space. Computer 38, 50–60 (2005)
12. Pragnell, M., Spence, L., Moore, R.: The market potential for Smart Homes. Joseph Rowntree Foundation. York Publishing Services Ltd., England (2000)
13. Gurganious, D., Hatler, M., Ritter, M.: WSN for Smart Home: A Market Dynamics Report. ON World, San Diego, California (2008)
14. Deffree, S.: Revenue gain expected in 2010 consumer electronics market. Electronic News (10616624) 56, 3 (2010)
15. Hamdhaidari, M.: High LevelModelling And Simulation of Pervasive Multimedia Systems and Environments Informatics. University of Sussex, Brighton (2009)
16. Alliance, Z.: Zigbee Alliance, vol. 03/03/2010 (2010)
17. Echelon: Lonworks 2.0, vol. 03/03/2010 (2010)
18. Jeong, K.-A., Proctor, R.W., Salvendy, G.: A Survey of Smart Home Interface Preferences for U.S. and Korean Users. Human Factors and Ergonomics Society Annual Meeting Proceedings 53, 541–545 (2009)
19. Eye phone. The Economist. The Economist Newspaper Limited, London (2007)
20. KNX: KNX Standard, vol. 2010, KNX (2009)

Augmented Photoframe for Interactive Smart Space

Koen De Voegt, Mohamed Ali Feki, Laurence Claeys, Johan Criel, Pascal Zontrop, Marc Godon, Marc Roelands, Marjan Geerts, and Lieven Trappeniers

Alcatel-lucent, Bell Labs, Belgium
Coopernicuslaan 50, Antwerp 2018
Koen.De_Voegt@alcatel-lucent.com

Abstract. Existing "photoframes" are single application closed proprietary systems. In this paper, we will outline the possibilities that emerge when we expose the control API of the digital "photoframe" to the local network. The "photoframe" is connected to an execution environment that aggregates intelligence in the smart space. We will describe briefly the Execution environment functionalities and then focus on the new interaction with the "photoframe" this enables. We will report our experience to proof that usage of a "photoframe" in this fashion creates real added value for elderly users in an assisted living environment.

Keywords: Photoframe, smart space, assistive living.

1 Introduction

Smart spaces can be used for elder people and those with disabilities, providing safe and secure environments. It allows the user to control many features or automate these features. The user can also be monitored by the Smart Home system to ensure their safety, and alert people in case of difficulties.

Several worldwide projects have been developed recently on smart spaces which leaded to multiple experimental houses generally dedicated to dependent people (aging and people with disabilities). The most well-known works today are:

- The Gator Tech Smart House: The University of Florida's Mobile and Pervasive Computing Laboratory is developing programmable pervasive spaces in which a smart space exists as both a runtime environment and a software library. Service discovery and gateway protocols automatically integrate system components using generic middle-ware that maintains a service definition for each sensor and actuator in the space. Programmers assemble services into composite applications, which third parties can easily implement or extend. [1]

- The PlaceLab MIT: The PlaceLab is a highly instrumented, apartment-scale, shared research facility where new technologies and design concepts can be tested and evaluated in the context of everyday living. Not a prototype and not a demonstration environment, the PlaceLab allows researchers to collect fine-grained human behavior and environmental data, and to systematically test and evaluate strategies and technologies for the home in a natural setting with volunteer occupants. The PlaceLab

Y. Lee et al. (Eds.): ICOST 2010, LNCS 6159, pp. 60–66, 2010.

is capable of accommodating multiple and simultaneous experiments proposed by academic researchers and MIT industrial collaborators. It is particularly useful for hypothesis testing and for generating pilot data prior to longer-term studies. [2]

- The Aware Home research Initiative: Georgia tech: The Aware Home Research Initiative (RHRI) at the Georgia Institute of Technology should response following questions: "Is it possible to create a home environment that is aware of its occupant's whereabouts and activities? If we build such a home, how can it provide services to its residents that enhance their quality of life or help them to maintain independence as they age? The Aware Home Research Initiative (AHRI) is an interdisciplinary research endeavor at Georgia Tech aimed at addressing the fundamental technical, design, and social challenges presented by such questions." [3]

- Intel research: Aging-in-Place: Advanced Smart-Home Systems: In collaboration with Intel Research Seattle, the Proactive Health team is building an advanced smart-home system to help those like Carl and Thelma deal with Alzheimer's. Researchers are integrating four main technology areas into a prototyping environment to be tested in the homes of patients: sensor networks, home networks, activity tracking, and ambient displays. [4]

Moreover, some industrials are making their own business model to commercialize in a short term such smart home like Panasonic in Japan, IBM United States, etc. Theses research works are mainly focusing on home environment to assist elderly. Our work is in line with them, augmenting the smart space with a distributed digital photoframe, we allow the photoframe to grow beyond its pure ambient functionalities and enriches the way people interact with them. (E. g: showing instructions how to brush teeth …).

In this paper we will first analyze existing photoframe concepts and devices, then outline the software and hardware architecture of new assistive interaction methodology, using our photoframe integrated in the smart space.

2 The Photoframe in the Market

In this paragraph we refer to a number of state of the art photoframes currently on the market or soon to be released. Some photoframes do have a notion of communication built in, but often this is very limited.

In [5], the Isabella Products' Vizit has a GSM/GPRS module built in. This photoframe will be able to receive media through MMS, email or the web. A service will also be provided to share photos straight from the frame itself. Connection will require a monthly fee to the service provider [6]. A similar technology, Pandigital's Photo Mail LED frame [7], the difference lays in the way the connection costs are paid for. This frame comes bundled with 500 photo downloads. And you will be able to buy extra download bundles when you need them. Some devices are by no means just a photoframe, e.g. the D-Link's Xtreme N DIR-685 [8], is a wired/wireless LAN router, a NAS and a photoframe. So it's at least a very well connected photoframe. In contradiction to the previous examples this device uses a wired Internet connection. Photo sharing through specialized on-line photo-sharing tools like Facebook or Flickr is also supported by this device. [9]

Previous examples represent a powerful digital photoframe in term of stand-alone capabilities, however we found it is impossible to make the photoframe react to or interact with events in its environment. Our prototype is not intended as a stand alone consumer appliance, but to integrate in an end-users smart home. In this sense it is part of the Casensa project on which we will elaborate more in the following sections.

3 Research Methodology: The Photoframe in the Smart Space

3.1 Casensa Concept and Implementation

Current smart homes mostly allow users to change the home's behaviour by letting them configure predefined behaviors (see figure 1), profiles or settings. For a true personalized behaviour of the environment, a more programmatic approach is needed; requiring technical skills that even go beyond that of professional caregivers. In contrast to this, Casensa allows elderly to define their own so-called smart objects, starting from pictures they took in their home. By tagging and making semantic links to existing concepts, they can further redefine them; specify how they interrelate and which behavior is expected from them. By means of easy & collaborative definition of layered ontological concepts and rules, the Casensa system allows users to specify the smart home's behavior in terms of their own smart objects while at the same time it allows to translate these semantic specifications to low-level execution platforms.

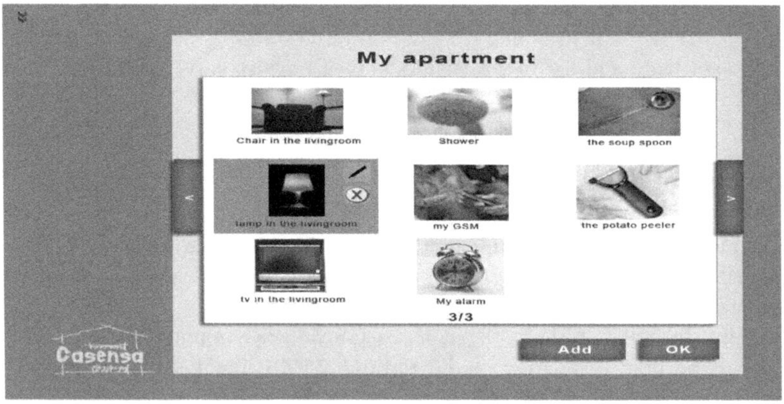

Fig. 1. Casensa creation environment

3.2 Photoframe Design and Implementation

For the creation of our prototype we choose the java programming language. The audio and video player part is built using the jVLC libraries. In this fashion we were able to seamlessly embed a VLC client in our application. The photo viewing part uses java's built in photo handling capabilities. To expose our API to the local network we use the Apache CXF libraries. Using this technique we make a Java servlet that we can deploy to an application server. For compilation and code dependency management we used Maven. Maven also allows us to easily combine compilation and deployment to the jetty web-server. As we where involved in a larger project aimed at less technically skilled people we had to keep the number of options limited. The options where also kept very simple straight forward.

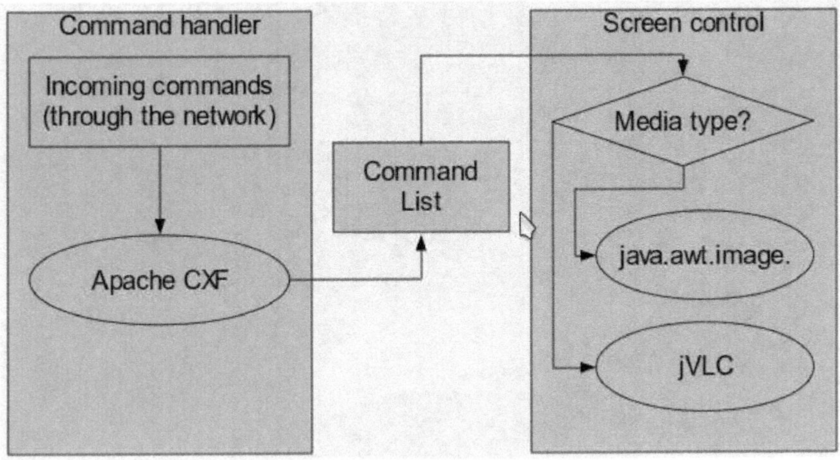

Fig. 2. Photoframe architecture

To make sure our application would not miss any incoming commands we choose a structure using two threads. The first thread is intended to continuously listen to all incoming commands. The second one will actually process these commands and thus control the screen. For simplicity, we limited our implementation to only "showSlideshow" and "videoPlayer" commands. The strength of this photoframe is derived from its integration in a smart environment.

4 Experimentation

4.1 Prototype Testbed Description

The testing environment is an apartment that is established with smart objects (like an alarm clock equipped with a sensor) in the living room, in the bedroom and in the kitchen. The Casensa board, with five NFC readers built in, (see Figure 3) was mounted to the wall of the kitchen on eye level. The Casensa card box with magnetic cards was located in the kitchen most of the time. It could be taken to the Casensa touch screen with single NFC reader and printer, which was located in the bedroom.

A set of sensors are embedded in the test environment and connected to the sensor gateway. We used sensorML language [10] for data processing and a subscription/polling mechanism for reasoning and semantic retrieval. For instance, we installed a pressure sensor to detect when someone is standing in front of the kitchen

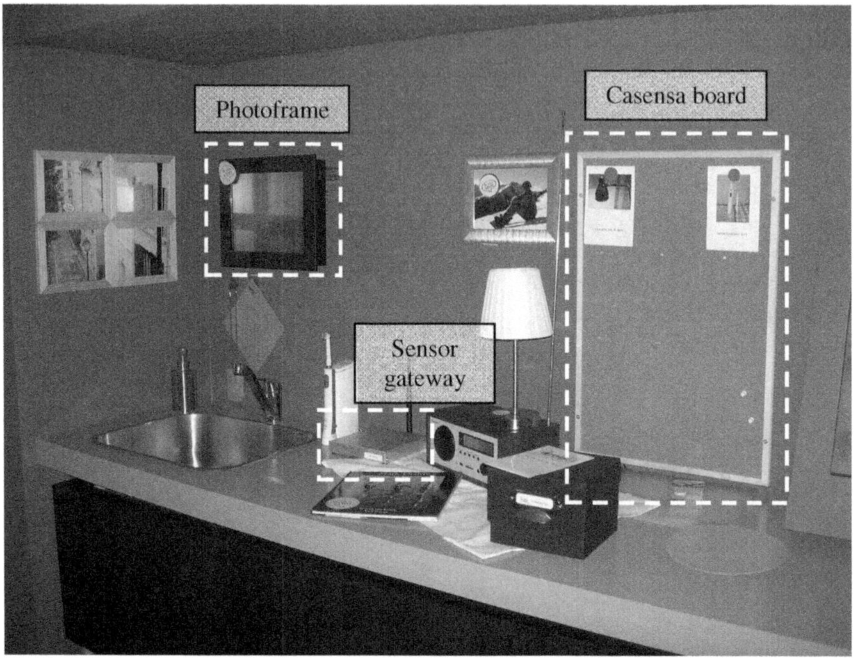

Fig. 3. Smart space demonstrator

sink; we tried out a set of RF distance (contact) sensors for device status retrieval (e.g. door, brush). For a general description of our smart space (Casensa) technology please see [11].

4.2 Examples of Assisting Interaction Based Photoframe

In this section we list a few of the use cases we demonstrated to our users during a field trial. Beyond the traditional functionalities of a digital photoframe (show locally stored picture), we implemented a set of new use cases driven by a user research study analysis For more details about the user research please see our previous publication [12].

The first use case is built to enable elderly to show their family photos. Indeed, a collection of family photos can be given to an elderly or not technically skilled person in the form of a NFC-card. The photo collection has been previously attached by a caregiver or family member to this card. Simply placing the card on the magnetic Casensa board will show the pictures on their photoframe. This is a far simpler and more tangible way of interaction especially for the non-digitally native (Figure 4).

Similar to the previous case, cards can be made to represent the favorite TV-soap of the elderly. When the card is attached to the Casensa board the soap is show on the photoframe when the new episode starts. The user then has the option to keep on following the show on the photoframe or just sit down relax and turn on the TV.

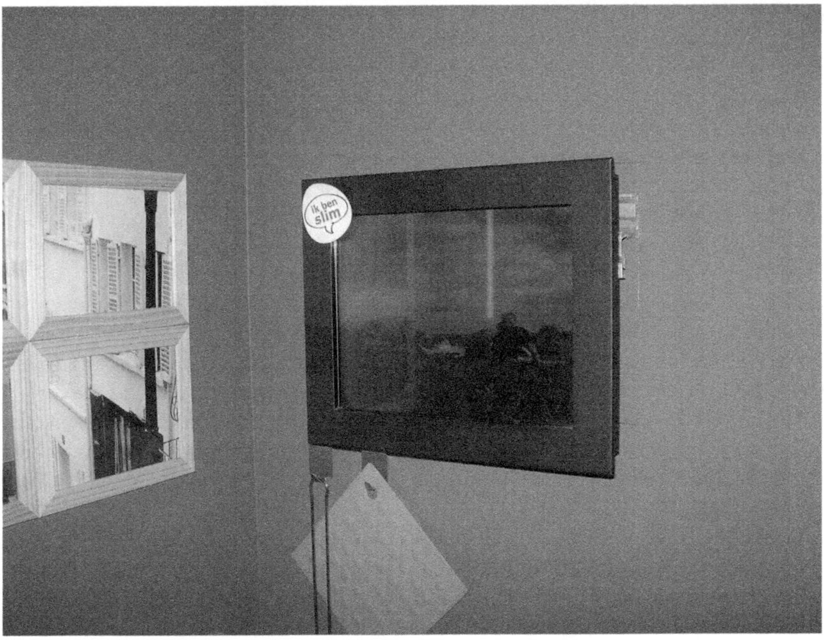

Fig. 4. Photoframe showing family pictures

To assist elderly users suffering from mild-dementia, we implemented several specific use cases among them we will describe the brush teeth and wash hand use cases. In fact, when a demented patient picks up his toothbrush, instructions on how to brush her tooth are shown on the photoframe. In addition, when she steps on a pressure sensor near her sink, she is reminded to wash her hands by showing a video on the photoframe with instructions.

5 Conclusion

In this paper, we described a new connected photoframe we integrate into a smart space and outlined the opportunity to augment current assistive services. We have shown the value added in a concrete use cases and explained the software architectures and the integration (photoframe-smart space) details.

We are planning to make a more stable photoframe version and expand its functionalities in an urban environment with public services.

References

1. Helal, S.: Programming Pervasive Spaces. IEEE Pervasive Computing 4(1), 84–87 (2005)
2. Intille, S.S., Larson, K., Beaudin, J.S., Nawyn, J., Munguia Tapia, E., Kaushik, P.: A living, laboratory for the design and evaluation of ubiquitous computing interfaces. In: Extended Abstracts of the 2005 Conference on Human Factors in Computing Systems. ACM Press, New York (2005)

3. http://awarehome.imtc.gatech.edu/
4. http://www.intel.com/healthcare/hri/pdf/proactive_health.pdf
5. http://www.engadget.com/2009/11/05/isabella-products-vizit-first-2-way-touchscreen-photo-frame-he/
6. http://www.engadget.com/2009/01/10/isabella-products-intros-cellular-connected-vizit-photo-frame/
7. http://www.engadget.com/2010/01/07/pandigitals-atandt-lovin-photo-mail-led-frame-hands-on/
8. http://www.engadget.com/2009/07/02/d-links-xtreme-n-dir-685-storage-router-hands-on-and-impression/
9. http://www.computerizedspirit.com/2010-02-26/internet/d-links-dir-685-xtreme-n-storage-router
10. http://vast.uah.edu/downloads/sensorML/v1.0/specification/07-000_SensorML_Implementation_Specification.pdf
11. Marjan, G., Laurence, C., Johan, C., Pascal, Z., Marc, De Voegt, K., Trappeniers, L., Dieryckx, L., Verschatse, A., Deboutte, P.: Seniors Re-engineering Context-aware Applications, The Casensa Research process. In: Proceeding of AmI 2009, Salzburg, November 18-21 (2009)
12. Geerts, M., Criel, J., Claeys, L., Godon, M. (Alcatel-Lucent Bell Labs, Antwerp, Belgium), Dieryckx, L., Deboutte, P. (In-HAM, Gits, Belgium): Let the Seniors Hack! Finding daily life practices and hacks of elderly using cultural probes. In: Workshop Capturing Ambient Assisted Living Needs, Ambient Intelligence Conference 2008, Nurnberg, Germany (2008)

Unobtrusive Sleep Posture Detection for Elder-Care in Smart Home

Hongbo Ni[1,2], Bessam Abdulrazak[2], Daqing Zhang[3], and Shu Wu[2]

[1] School of Computer Science, Northwestern Polytechnic University, China
nihb@nwpu.edu.cn
[2] Department of Computer, University of Sherbrooke, Canada
{Bessam.Abdulrazak,shu.wu}@usherbrooke.ca
[3] Handicom Lab, Institut Telecom SudParis, France
Daqing.Zhang@it-sudparis.eu

Abstract. Quality of sleep is an important attribute of an elder's health state and its assessment is still a huge issue. The sleep posture is a significant feature to evaluate the quality of sleep, and how to detect elder's sleep posture is a key challenge in elder-care community. This paper proposes an unobtrusive sleep postures detection solution and introduces pressure sensor matrix to monitor the elder's sleep posture in bed. Based on the proposed sleep detection system, the processing methods of experimental data and the classification approaches for sleep posture detection are also discussed.

1 Introduction

Sleep is essential to people's physical health and emotional well-being, and most people will spend one-third of lives in bed. But, in fact, complaints of sleep difficulty are common among the elder. In an aging study of over 9000 subjects aged 65 and older, more than 50% of older adults reported frequent trouble falling asleep, difficult waking or waking too early, or needing to nap and not feeling rested [1].

Sleep disorders are under-recognized public health problems that have a cumulative effect on elders' physical and mental health, and usually put the older adult at greater risk for decreased physical functioning, problems with memory, increased risk of falls and mortality. Meanwhile, sleep disorders in the elder almost involve abnormal behaviors in the bed, which are also an important marker associated with health-related diseases, including congestive heart failure, cancer, nocturia, shortness of breath due to chronic obstructive pulmonary disease, neurological deficits related to cerebrovascular accidents, and Parkinson's disease [2].

As the proportion of aged people in the population increases, a simple and minimally invasive detecting the sleep behaviors in the bed should be developed to maintain the elders' health. Unfortunately, there are no convenient, unobtrusive and accurate ways to obtain elder's body behaviors during sleep outside of a clinic.

This paper will meet the challenge from monitoring the elder's sleep behaviors using a novel and unobtrusive approach. Body movement is generally considered to be an important index in the analysis of sleep behavior shifts in sleep physiology [3].

Y. Lee et al. (Eds.): ICOST 2010, LNCS 6159, pp. 67–75, 2010.

The term 'body movements' can be described by body postures changing to/from a lying position, to turn from side to side, and to reposition the body while in bed. In the literature to analyze the distribution of behaviors during sleep [4], body movements were classified as minor movements (actogram signal or head leads artifact), major movements (actogram signal plus head leads artifact). Major movements usually are associated with changes in body posture, involving the head, arms, torso rotations, any combination of upper and lower limbs, and any combination of limbs and torso rotations. So, given a time interval, the body movement can been detected by the sleep posture. In this paper, we will concentrate on the three typical normal sleep postures, including left-lateral sleep (LLS), right-lateral sleep (RLS) and supine sleep (SS), and these postures will be detected by a matrix of pellicle pressure sensors deployed in the bed. By detecting the sleep postures, the authors try to recognize the elder's sleep behaviors in bed in a non-invasive means.

The key contributions in this paper include: i) Introducing pressure sensors into sleep detection; ii) Presenting the detailed design of sleep detection system; and iii) Proposing a sleep postures detection approaches based on pressure data.

The rest of this paper is organized as follows: section 2 summarizes the related work in sleep detection; in section 3, we describe the design of sleep detection system with pellicle pressure sensors; section 4 presents the experimental method for sleep posture detection; section 5 proposes the experiments analysis and performance evaluation; finally section 6 presents the conclusion of this paper.

2 Related Work

Many sleep sensing approaches have been proposed for assessment of body behaviors in bed, in this section, we will describe some of the representative work on continuous sensing of body behaviors (movements) in bed.

The assessment of sleep-related motor disturbances is traditionally performed by overnight polysomnograph (PSG) to continuously record oractigraphy[5]. Although polysomnography, which includes EEG measurement, is a widely used and reliable method, the technique is rather complicated and both subject and examiner are seriously restricted [6]. With actigraphy, activity monitors are attached to a person's wrist or lower extremity [7] to assess nocturnal activity. It is commonly used for long-term assessment and medical and behavior therapy in conditions such as insomnia and periodic limb movements during sleep (PLMS) [8]. Most of the actigraph models used in sleep studies can determine sleep and wake periods from the level of activity of the patient, but their algorithms only provide accurate sleep/wake periods if the patient provides bedtimes and get up times.

Besides, accelerometers and RFID can also be used to assess movement in bed [9], but they also place a burden on the subject because the patient has to wear them all the time.

Another important approach in this field is to assess sleep behaviors in bed in a continuous and unobtrusive way by instrumenting the bed itself. Tamura et al. [10] proposed a bed temperature measurement system for detection of body movement. The system detects torso and leg movements by placing arrays of 15 thermistors under the waist and under the legs. The system only reports the frequency of movements and time in bed, and does not classify the type of movement. Several authors [11] have employed the static charge sensitive bed (SCSB) for monitoring of motor activity. The SCSB is composed of two metal plates with a wooden plate in the middle that must be placed under a special foam plastic mattress, which will be difficult to bulid. Van der Loos also proposed a sensing system called SleepSmart, composed of a mattress pad with 54 force sensitive resistors and 54 resistive temperature devices, to estimate body center of mass and index of restlessness [12]. The system does not report the frequency and type of movements, and this large-size equipment is difficult to set up and can only be used in specific laboratories. Other sensing techniques, such as optical fibers and conductive fibers have also been used for monitoring body movement in bed. Tamura proposed a body movement monitoring system using optical fibers [13]. Kimura designed an unobtrusive vital signs detection system, which uses conductive fiber sensors to detect body position, respiration, and heart rate [14]. Technologically, the fiber sensors can be incorporated in a conventional bed sheet, but obviously it will be costly and not applicable for home use. The use of load cells is another approach to detect body movements in bed [15], in which load cells is placed at each corner of a bed. The detection of movements is based on short-term analysis of the mean-square differences of the load cell signals, and not applicable for specific sleep postures detecting.

As mentioned above, the previous solutions are not applicable for sleep detection in home in a non-invasive way, and this paper proposes an unobtrusive sleep posture detection system for elder-care, which is relatively cheap and easy to deploy in a common bed without any special alteration.

3 System Development

In this section, we will discuss our sleep detection system (SDS) in two aspects. On the one hand, we will address the framework and main components of SDS; on the other hand, we will also describe the FFS Matrix deployment.

3.1 The Framework of SDS

To date, we have implemented SDS in the first step, and the goal of SDS is to develop a low-cost, multi-sensor, modular, unobtrusive sleep sensing platform that accurately infer the sleep posture, discover the sleep pattern and provide personalized suggestions in future. The framework of SDS can be seen in Fig.1, and there are four levels in it, including physical sense level, data acquisition level, posture detection level, and service provision level.

Physical Sense: The level consists of a matrix of 32 pressure sensors and a Driving Power Unit (DPU) to sense the body pressure. In SDS, we chose a novel type of pressure sensor named FlexiForce. The Flexiforce sensor (FFS) is ultra-thin, low-cost and flexible. FFS is resistive-based technology and will produce an analog signal. FFS acts as a variable resistor in an electrical circuit. When the sensor is unloaded, its resistance is very high (greater than 5 Meg-ohm); when a force is applied to the sensor, the resistance decreases. To trigger the FFS-Matrix, we applied a direct-current low-voltage driving power unit (DPU). For ensuring the scalability of FFS, we customized a multi-channel port for DPU, and it can support 80 FFSs.

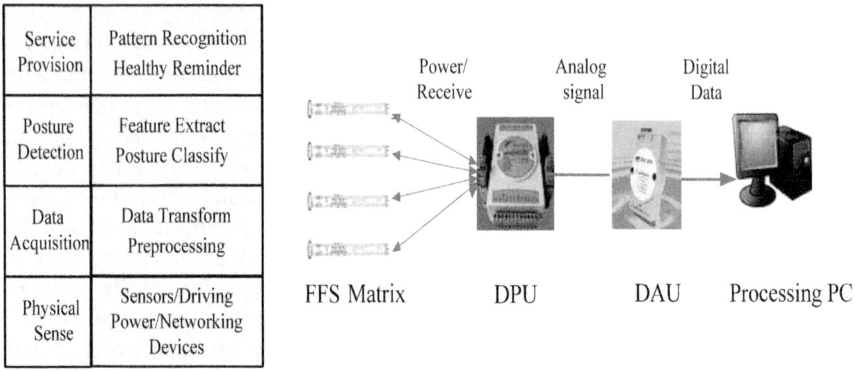

Fig. 1. The framework and main components of SDS

Data Acquisition: This level includes a Data Acquisition Unit (DAU) to process the analog signal. As seen in Fig. 1, DPU power the FFS-Matrix and transmits the analog signals as current, and then the DAU receives and transform these signals into digital data. Concurrently, DAU will also connect with the Processing PC with the Standard MODBUS RTU protocol, and its output is a digitized data that is correlated to the applied pressure but is not an absolute measure of pressure.

Posture Detection: This level is modularized software residing in the Processing PC, including three parts: the receiving module is a soft port to receive real-time digitized data from the DAU; the forwarding module is to input the data into MySQL database for permanent storage and also feed the raw data into posture detection module, which is finally to preprocess the received data and analysis the elder's sleep posture using classification algorithms.

Service Provision: Based on the sleep postures and their duration, we can infer the elderly user's sleep pattern, and evaluate the quality of sleep. On the one hand, the important healthy information will be fed back to the elder and his caregiver; on the other hand, the preferred sleep posture is usually recommended according to the elder's own disease [17], for example, an elder with coronary heart disease is generally suggested a right-lateral sleep posture, thus SDS will also provide necessary reminder to the elder when the sleep pattern is improper for his health. This part is under developing and we will report our progress in future.

3.2 Sensors Deployment

Besides the framework of SDS, we must meet the challenge of sensors deployment. Based on the investigation, we choose FFS to monitor the elder's sleep pressure in bed, which is 203mm long, 14 mm wide, and 0.208 mm thick, with 3 male square pins.

As seen in Fig.2, there is an "active sensing area" at the end of the sensor, which is a 9.53mm diameter circle. The application of a force to the active sensing area of the sensor results in a change in the resistance of the sensing element in inverse proportion to the force applied. FFS is constructed of two layers of substrate, such as a polyester film [16]. Meanwhile, known from common sense that the elder's body posture is mainly relied on his trunk, hence the FFS Matrix was deployed as seen in Fig.2, and there are two arrays to monitor the body pressure of back and hip separately. To ensure the accuracy, these two FFS arrays are fixed onto a flexible and rigid pad, and which occupies 2M by 0.75M, with sensor elements spaced 10 CM apart. The pad is placed on the bed under the coverlet and on the top of normal mattress, without any special installation requirement. Please note, this is the first step of our implementation, and the normal width of this material is 0.75M (we have booked a customized king-size pad from the vendor). Moreover, the 10CM-distance between the FFSs is from our trial experiments, which is proper arrangement for detecting an adult's pressure. We will try more experiments and adjust the distance if the solution applied to child-care.

Since FFS is ultra-thin and non-invasive, the elder will not feel any uncomfortable for FFS Matrix and can be easy to accept the unobtrusive monitoring manner. Furthermore, we developed a 48-channel hub-like port to assemble so many wires connecting sensors, which is placed under the bed together with DPU and DAU.

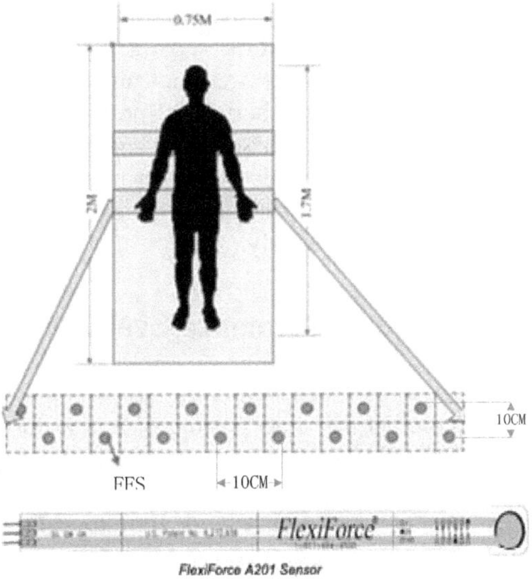

Fig. 2. The deployment of FFS Matrix

4 Data Collection

In this section, we will introduce the approach of collecting data from pressure sensors. In order to verify the usability of SDS, we selected ten students (8 men, 2 women; ages 21 to 26 years) with no mobility problems participated in the study, and especially their body forms are very diverse. Table 1 shows the height, weight, and the mean pressure of each subject. From Fig.3, we can get the first expression of SDS's characteristics, and the approximate curve fitting shows that the mean pressure is nearly proportional to the weight, which is comply with the principle of the FFS, and we would confirm it by a larger data set in future.

Table 1. Height,Weight and Mean Pressure of Subjects

Subject ID	Height (CM)	Weight (KG)	Mean Pressure
1	170	80	293
2	162	53	232
3	174	60	273
4	160	44	221
5	182	70	280
6	165	60	241
7	168	56	242
8	175	59	224

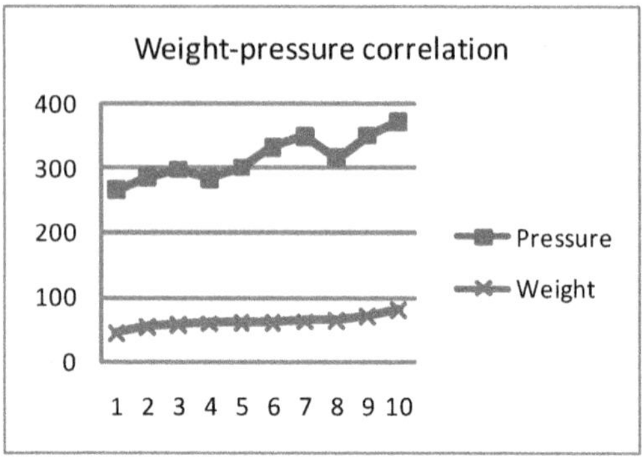

Fig. 3. Qualitative correlation between weight and pressure

The sensors' data were collected from the experiments as follows: every subject slept on the SDS for 15 times in turn, and randomly lied in the left-lateral sleep, right-lateral sleep and supine sleep for 5 times separately. Please note, the subjects' positions and respective gestures for sleep were not restricted, that is, they lied in the bed as they preferred. Although there should be more postures in real world, this paper is to report the primary work of our solution, and we will do more experiments to verify the system in near future. After the experiments, 150 groups of raw data were obtained, and as mentioned in 3.1, the data was sent to the MySQL database and the posture analysis module simultaneously.

5 Posture Detecting and Performance Evaluation

To analyze the experimental data and detect the sleep posture, we implement two classification methods to predict the sleep posture of a new observation based on the training sleep posture data set. The first one is Naïve Bayes. Since Naive Bayes classifier, which is a simple probabilistic classifier based on applying Bayes' theorem with attribute independence assumption has worked quite well in many complex real-world situations, it is implemented on our data set. Meanwhile, since the sleep data set is a high-dimension data set, the different importance of dimensions may impact the result significantly. For this reason, we import the Random Forest method, which has advantage in estimating weight of dimensions and is suitable for high-dimension data set.

Two evaluated validations are involved into the analysis of the experimental results, 10-fold cross-validation and leave-one-out cross validation. In the 10-fold cross-validation, the sleep data set is randomly partitioned into 10 subsamples. In the 10 subsamples, one subsample is retained as the testing data, and the remaining 9 subsamples are used as training data. This cross-validation process is then repeated 10 times with each of the 10 subsamples used once as the test data. The predict accuracies of 10-fold cross-validation in the following tables are the average result of 10 tests from the folds. As the name suggests, leave-one-out involves using a single observation of the sleep data set as the test data, and the remaining observations as the training data. This is repeated such that each observation in the sample is used once as the validation data. The predict accuracy is the average predict result of 150 times tests.

As mentioned in section 4, the data set contains 150 observations belonging to 3 kinds of sleep postures, which are left-lateral sleep, right-lateral sleep and supine sleep. Before the data analysis, we have tried some typical pre-processes on the data set, for example, discretize, normalization, but the classification accuracy of the data set is decreased. Therefore, the classification methods are implemented on the raw data set. The results of two classification methods and two validation processes are list in the table below.

Table 2. Predict Accuracy with Two Cross-Validations

	10-fold		Leave-one-out	
	Naïve Bayes	Rand om	Naïve Bayes	Rand om
LLS	0.620	0.8600	0.6000	0.8800
S	0.660	0.8600	0.6800	0.8800
RLS	0.760	0.8600	0.7800	0.8600
Averag	0.680	**0.8600**	0.6867	**0.8733**

Comparing with 10-fold cross-validation, the leave-one-out cross-validation has more training observations than 10-fold, so the predict accuracy of leave-one-out validation is slightly higher than 10-fold. The Table 2 also shows the Naïve Bayes and Random Forest method both have a little improvement of predict accuracy on the leave-one-out validation test contrasting with the 10-fold.

We analyze the result in the leave-one-out validation. The Table 2 indicates that when we use the Random Forest as the classification method, it provides us almost 90% accuracy to predict the sleep postures, while the Naïve Bayes attains the accuracy about 69%. The Random Forest method performs over Naïve Bayes method in classifying this high-dimension data set. The table 2 also indicates that the Random Forest method is a stable method. Three sleep postures have similar predict accuracies. While in the Naïve Bayes method, left-lateral sleep has the lowest predict accuracy 60%, while the highest predict accuracy is the right-lateral sleep 78%. Compared the results of these two methods, the Random Forest method has higher predict accuracy and attains more stable results than the Naïve Bayes method in our sleeping postures data set.

6 Conclusions and Future Work

This paper proposed an unobtrusive sleep postures detection system based on a kind of ultra-thin pressure sensor matrix. We presented the design of sensors deployment and the implementation of the sleep detection system. Moreover, based on the experiments, we discussed the data analysis and evaluation of the system and the result proved that the proposed solution is a promising way to monitor the elder's sleep posture. In the near future, we will detect more postures to testify the system, and investigate the elder's sleep pattern and complex body movements based on the sleep postures and corresponding duration, and also invite some older adults to evaluate the real benefice of the system.

Acknowledgment. This work is being supported by the Fonds Nature et Technologies, MELS Program, Quebec, Canada, and partially supported by the National High Technology Research and Development Program of China under Grant No. 2009AA011903.

References

[1] Foley, D.J., Monjan, A.A., Brown, S.L., et al.: Sleep complaints among elderly persons: an epidemiologic study of three communities. Sleep 18(6), 425–432 (1995)
[2] Foley, D., Ancoli-Israel, S., Britz, P., Walsh, J.: Sleep disturbances and chronic disease in older adults: results of the 2003 National Sleep Foundation Sleep in America Survey. J. Psychosom Res. 56, 497–502 (2004)
[3] Aaronson, S.T., Rashed, S., Biber, M.P., Hobson, J.A.: Brain state and body posture: a time-lapse video study of sleep. Arch. Gen. Psychiatry 39, 330–335 (1982)
[4] Muzet, A.: Dynamics of Body Movements in Normal Sleep. Presented at Eighth European Congress on Sleep Research, Szeged, Hungary (1986)
[5] Cheng, C.M., Hsu, Y.L., Young, C.M., Wu, C.H.: Development of a portable device for tele-monitoring of snoring and OSAS symptoms. In: Telemed e-Health 2008, vol. 14, pp. 55–68 (2008)
[6] Wilde-Frenz, J., Schulz, H.: Rate and Distribution of Body Movements during Sleep in Humans. Perceptual and Motor Skills 56, 275–283 (1983)
[7] Shneerson, J.M., Smith, I.E.: The Validation of a New Actigraphy System for the Measurement of Period Leg Movements in Sleep. Sleep Medicine 6, 507–513 (2005)
[8] Tryon, W.W.: Issues of Validity in Actigraphic Sleep Assessment. Sleep 27, 158–165 (2004)
[9] Prill, T., Fahrenberg, J.: Simultaneous Assessment of Posture and Limb Movements (e.g., periodicleg movements) with Calibrated Multiple Accelerometry. Physiological Measurement, 47–53 (2007)
[10] Tamura, T., Zhou, J., Mizukami, H., Togawa, T.: A System for Monitoring Temperature Distribution in Bed and Its Application to the Assessment of Body Movement. Physiological Measurements 14, 33–41 (1993)
[11] Rauhala, E., Erkinjuntti, M., Polo, O.: Detection of Periodic Leg Movements with a Static-Charge-Sensitive Bed. Journal of Sleep Research 5, 246–250 (1996)
[12] Van der Loos, H.F.M., Ullrich, N., Kobayashi, H.E.R.: Development of sensate and robotic bed technologies for vital signs monitoring and sleep quality improvement. Autonomous Robots 15(1), 67–79 (2003)
[13] Tamura, T., Nishigaichi, A., Nomura, T.: Monitoring of body movement during sleep in bed. In: Proceedings of the Annual International Conference of the IEEE Engineering in Medicine and Biology Society, pp. 1483–1484 (1992)

[14] Kimura, H., Kobayashi, H., Kawabata, K., Van der Loos, H.F.: Development of an unobtrusive vital signs detection system using conductive fiber sensors. In: Proceedings 2004 IEEE/RSJ International Conference on Intelligent Robots and Systems, pp. 307–312 (2004)

[15] Adami, A.M., Hayes, T.L., Pavel, M., Singer, C.M.: Detection and classification of movements in bed using load cells. In: IEEE 27th Annual International Conference of the Engineering in Medicine and Biology Society, pp. 589–592 (2005)

[16] The website of Tekscan Int., `http://www.tekscan.com/flexiforce/flexiforce.html`

[17] Simonceli, L., Bittar, R.S.M., Greters, M.E.: Posture restrictions do not interfere in the results of canalith repostureing maneuver. Braz. J. Otorhinolaryngol. 71, 55–59 (2005)

Context-Aware Personal Diet Suggestion System

Yu-Chiao Huang[1], Ching-Hu Lu[1], Tsung-Han Yang[1], Li-Chen Fu[1], and Ching-Yao Wang[2]

[1] Department of Computer Science and Information Engineering
National Taiwan University, Taipei, Taiwan
[2] Information and Communication Laboratory
Industrial Technology Research Institute, HsinChu, Taiwan
{b95902066,D93922004,D98922024,lichen}@ntu.edu.tw,
cyw@itri.org.tw

Abstract. Keeping a healthy and balanced diet has long been a critical issue for a person wanting to stay fit and energetic in her/his daily life. We can always turn to a dietitian (or a nutritionist) for professional diet suggestions if necessary. However, we cannot have a dietitian staying with us all the time, which renders daily nutrition control very challenging. Therefore, it is desirable for each individual to receive handy and informative diet suggestions whenever necessary. In this work, we propose a Context-aware Personal Diet Suggestion System (CPDSS) which tries to maximize an aggregated health utility function and provides useful diet suggestions according to some contextual information. In order to increase the practicality of the pro- posed system, we have integrated the CPDSS with an everyday appliance–a smart refrigerator–so that we can readily access the suggestions about one's diet, receive instant context-aware reminders while preparing foods, and keep long-term diet history to extract more useful pat- terns to caregivers to provide suggestions for health improvement.

Keywords: context-awareness, activity level, diet suggestion, smart refrigerator.

1 Introduction

We often have the experience of sitting in front of a menu, unable to decide a meal to order, let alone making a quick and wise purchase of balanced-diet foods from a supermarket. In addition, some factors including personal preference, food intake inhibition, purchase cost of food, advice from professional medic care organization, are all important to our decision making. Apparently, a smart diet-suggestion system that can help us figuring out these problems will be helpful, both for convenience and for improving one's health condition. These suggestions are especially helpful for those who need stricter diet control such as children suffering from Attention Deficit Hyperactivity Disorder (ADHD), or elders suffering from high blood pressure or other chronic diseases.

Most of prior researches [1-5] on diet suggestion primarily focus on proposing some mechanisms, such as Linear Programming (LP), to achieve nutrition or cost optimization. However, some other factors regarding human-related concerns are

Y. Lee et al. (Eds.): ICOST 2010, LNCS 6159, pp. 76–84, 2010.

ignored, and most of these works perform well only when optimizing over cost or nutrition limitation. Reference [6] tries to make use of Case Base Reasoning to implement diet suggestion in hospital to solve those human-involved problem.

Due to the advances in sensing technologies and machine learning, we propose a context-aware Personal Diet Suggestion System (abbreviated CPDSS) to take human-related factors into consideration. The objective of the system, as its name suggests, is to help a user designing his or her individual diet menu based on as many available contexts as possible. The contexts to help optimizing diet suggestion include the nutrient of a food, the diet advisory from specialists, user prior preference, current food stocking, the cost of food, the diet histories of users, and most importantly the activity level inferred from ambient sensors. By correctly inferring the personal activity level, which is estimated based on the performed activities within a specific interval; we can dynamically suggest menus to fulfill nutrition needs from different users based on their unique concerns.

Due to the ever increasing research interest in Smart Home and Tele-healthcare, more and more regular appliances are enhanced by the state-of-the-art ICTs and populated in our daily lives. Some of them [7] aim for personalized healthcare purposes.

One appliance is the so-called smart fridge [8-9], which is often equipped with bar-code scanners or RFID sensors to help residents easily monitor all stocking information like expiration date, nutrient contents, and food quantities via a simple GUI interface. In order to ease information access like most of prior works, this work integrates a smart fridge as the main user interface of the CPDSS. As an enhancement to most of other prior works, our smart fridge is not a stand-alone appliance and it can access and control other appliances via an integration platform in our smart-home system.

2 Context-Aware Personal Diet Suggestion System

2.1 System Overview

Fig. 1 illustrates the proposed CPDSS where an integration platform [10] can integrate all appliances, modules to gather all contexts of interest. The integration platform can provide information for remote access via the Internet (which will be implemented as an information cloud using Apache Hadoop). Due to the integration platform, our diet suggestion modules can be executed on a RFID-equipped smart fridge and interconnect with other components to access various contexts and provide instant control for the purpose of more satisfactory diet recommendation. The sensors deployed in our home environment can be used to extract features for later inference of ADLs (activities of daily living) [11] and the inferred ADLs can be mapped to one's activity level as an important context for diet suggestion. The activity level performed outdoors (such as jogging or walking, etc) can be recorded/estimated by a mobile or a wearable device, and the result stored in the device can be fed into the system once the device can be accessed by the CPDSS.

In order to illustrate the CPDSS, here is a brief scenario to demonstrate the benefits a user can obtain from the proposed CPDSS. Laura is an octogenarian who lives alone and her house has the proposed CPDSS. Since she suffers from some cardiovascular diseases such as high blood pressure, she needs to pay more attention to her diet. Each day when she wakes up, she clicks the touch screen on her smart fridge to get a suggested menu for her breakfast based on her food stocking. Suggested by a doctor, she need to exercise more than one hour every morning and do some chores, which can be correctly detected by the ADL Inference Engine. One day, because of enough exercise in the morning (her activity level is, say, high) and the hot weather, which is a context provided by Other Context Generators, the CPDSS therefore suggests lighter yet higher-calorie food in the menu at noon. The nutrition-aware application can provide a reminder via a speaker connected to the integration platform to inform her for regular replenishment of water or some mineral drink. The system can check food stocking and then automatically send summarized information (including a shopping list) to her families or a healthcare center for future reference. That after- noon, Laura's activity level is low because of her long afternoon break, so the system prepares a menu that suggests a menu with fewer calories and less nutrients replenishment. The system also automatically avoids recommending high-sodium or high-fat recipes according to the suggestion of her dietician. In addition to providing diet suggestions, the CPDSS can provide Laura's diet histories via the information cloud to share or exchange useful information if necessary.

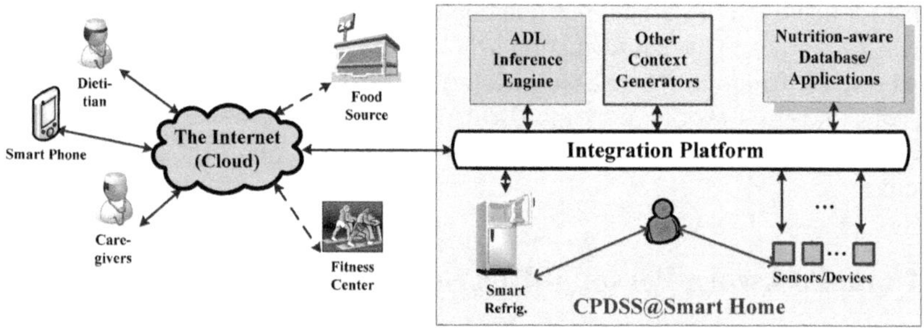

Fig. 1. System Overview

2.2 Problem Formulation

The main objective of CPDSS system is to improve a user's quality of daily living via balanced diet. For easier evaluation of the system, we define one utility for each context to be considered in our system. Therefore, the objective can be formulated as a problem to search food types and their corresponding quantities to maximize a user's aggregated utility, denoted as U, which is the weighted summation of various individual utility functions u.

Before the formulation, we define some notations first. A food f is defined by a nonnegative valued vector describing the nutrition it contains. That is, $f = (n1, n2, \ldots, nk)$, where ni means the ith nutrient that f contains, assuming there are k nutrients at total. In addition, $ni(f)$ denotes the ith nutrient of food f and F is the aggregated set of all foods. With the definition of F, food type T is a subset of F, which contains at least one kind of food. Furthermore, the union of all T is exactly F. From the definition we can infer that any kind of food in F must belongs to at least one food type. For simplicity, we assume there are h food types.

We define a utility function u taking in a food f and linearly mapping it to a real number R. That is, $u(f1) + u(f2) = u(f1 + f2)$ and $u(qf) = qu(f)$. With the individual utility functions, we calculate an aggregated utility U, which is simply the weighted summation of the functions, and all weights are pre-configured. U is the objective function that we wish to optimize. To be more specific, assuming we have a subset F' of F, our objective is to decide a quantity for each food in F', which collectively are denoted as Q. That is, the solution will be consisted of F' and Q, a food list and their corresponding quantities. The above description can be represented by:

$$Q = \langle q_1, q_2, \ldots, q_m \rangle = \underset{\langle q_1, q_2, \ldots, q_m \rangle}{\arg\max} \left[U\left(\sum_{i=1}^{m} q_i f_i\right) \right], \text{ where } |F'| = m \tag{1}$$

If we further factorize the equation, we can get equations (2) and (3)

$$Q = \underset{\langle q_1, q_2, \ldots, q_m \rangle}{\arg\max} \left[U\left(\sum_{i=1}^{m} q_i f_i\right) \right] = \underset{\langle q_1, q_2, \ldots, q_m \rangle}{\arg\max} \left[\sum_{i=1}^{m} q_i U(f_i) \right] \tag{2}$$

$$\Rightarrow Q = \underset{\langle q_1, q_2, \ldots, q_m \rangle}{\arg\max} \left[\sum_{i=1}^{m} q_i \left(\sum_{j=1}^{p} w_j u_j (f_i) \right) \right] \tag{3}$$

where w is a weight for each utility function and there are totally p utility functions. To be more succinct, we define a matrix Ω so that $\Omega ij = ui(fj)$, and a matrix W, which contains p weights of all utility functions. As a result, the desired Q^* is a one by m matrix which satisfies:

$$Q^* = \underset{Q}{\arg\max} \left[(W\Omega) \cdot Q^T \right] \tag{4}$$

Note that the matrix multiplication $W\Omega$ can be pre-computed if F' and W are decided before the optimization. Therefore, the optimization problem is reduced to an m degree linear programming (LP) problem, where ($W\Omega QT$) is exactly the objective function that we want to optimize.

The constraints in the formation of a LP problem regarding diet suggestion are traditionally limited by nutrition and food types. Unlike most of prior works, the CPDSS system first infers one's activity level or other contexts so that the system can use the information as guidance to construct context-related constraints for efficiently searching the optimized solution of equation(4). In our work, each activity has a pre- defined score based on the characteristic of the activity. As a result, an activity level is the average of summarized scores of all performed activities in a time interval. Currently, we define three activity levels including LOW, MEDIUM, and HIGH. We preconfigure the statistics of daily allowance [12] of each nutrient and food type given each activity level so that we can create a lower bound and upper bound for each nutrient and food type. That is, different activity levels will correspond to dif- ferent bounds, leading to different searching space. For example, a user who exercises a lot will definitely require more water and nutrition supply. Mathematically speaking, if a user's activity level is L, and if the upper-bound and lower-bound of the *ith* nu-trient allowance for the user are denoted by ni (L) and ni (L), we can express the nutrient constraints by:

$$\sum_{i=1}^{m} q_i n_j(f_i) \le n_j^+(L) \text{ and } \sum_{i=1}^{m} q_i n_j(f_i) \ge n_j^-(L), \quad for\ j = 1\ to\ k \tag{5}$$

Likewise, we can define *ρi (L)* as the upper-bound of the quantity of the *i* food type under a given activity level *L*, and *ρi (L)* is the lower bound. Then we can have additional 2*h* (*h* is the number of food types) constraints over food quantities:

$$\sum_{f_i \in T_j} q_i \le \rho_j^+(L), \text{ and } \sum_{f_i \in T_j} q_i \ge \rho_j^-(L), \quad for\ j = 1\ to\ k \tag{6}$$

For generalization, we can further add other contexts so that different constraints can be taken into consideration. Consequently, we append a parameter *C* to represent the additional information to be considered. Note that these extra constraints can be incrementally and selectively loosened or dropped according to their significance to a person of interest if no feasible solution can be obtained.

After the addition of these configurations, we have a complete LP problem which has at most 2(*k*+*h*) constraints to be optimized.

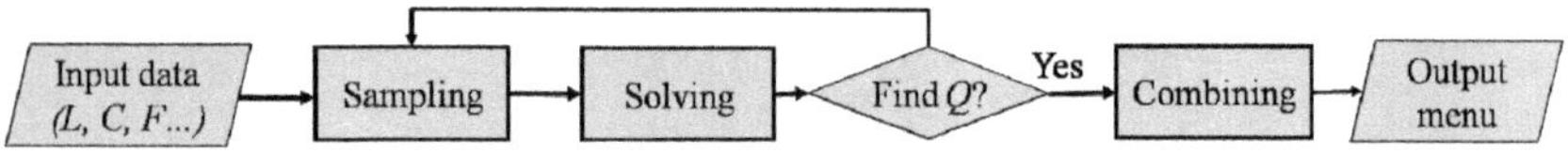

Fig. 2. The flow chart of the CPDSS

2.3 System Flowchart

As shown in Fig. 2, the diet suggestion of the CPDSS can be primarily divided into sampling, solving, and combing phases.

A. Sampling Phase

This phase is responsible for selecting an *F'* (a subset of foods) by sampling a food-searching space to increase food variability. We first have an empty *F'* and then sample foods in stock into *F'*. That is, we randomly select foods to *F'* so that there are at least some predefined portion of foods in each food type. That is, if there are 200 foods in the food type "starch" and the portion is 0.25, there will be 50 foods selected in *F'*, including those foods in stock. The random selection can be a non-uniform distribution. The sampling can also consider other information including user preference, cost to get the foods, and personal diet-inhibition.

B. Solving Phase

When the previous phase outputs the selected *F'*, the remaining work will be solving the LP problem with various context-related constrains. Firstly, the activity level (*L*), which is inferred by adding up the active degree of all activities performed by the user in a specific interval, and other contexts of interest (*C*) are integrated to determine some upper/lower bounds of the LP constraints. Secondly, we select utility functions for the optimization of the LP. Even though the selection of utility functions is flexible, currently we primarily focus on the following three kinds for implication, they are:

- Advisory utility: this utility is based on the evaluation of foods based on advice from nutrition specialists, and is often the most relevant to one's health. Intuitively, those foods that may cause harmful health effect will get negative utility values, and positive values if beneficial ones are chosen.
- Cost utility: this utility includes the price of foods, the scarcity of foods, and, most importantly, is whether the food is in stock. This utility returns a negative value since it is usually undesirable to get foods at higher cost, so that its sign has to be reversed before calculation. A food in stock will get positive cost utility (after sign reversion) because it is desirable to consume refrigerator stocking, while other foods get negative utility values under the same criterion.
- Preference utility: this utility is user-dependent and may be contradictory to the advisory utility. Patients who suffer obesity often prefer high-calorie and high-fat foods, but a dietician may suggest the patients stay away from those harmful foods. By default, the weight of the preference utility will always be lower than that of the advisory utility in the CPDSS.

For normalization, the above utility values will not exceed a predefined range. For example, we can scale all of our utility values within the interval [-10, 10] after normalization.

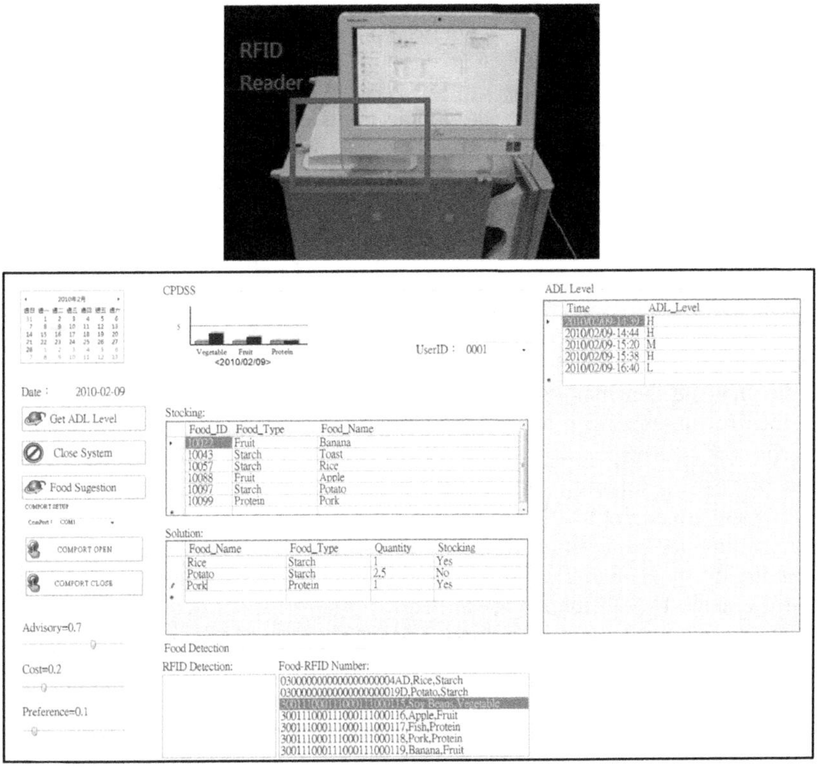

Fig. 3. Detailed CPDSS Fridge Interface (can be more simplified for an elder)

If a user does not like the suggestion or if the CPDSS cannot find a (primal) solution *Q* from *F'*, the system can always re-initiate the sampling phase and regenerate another *F'*. Since there is randomization involved in the sampling phase, it may eventually generate a feasible *F'* so that we can finally find a solution *Q*. If it is still not easy task to find a *Q*, we can try generating a larger *F'* while in the sampling phase so that there can be more candidate foods to choose from.

C. Combining Phase

This phase is an on-going yet significant task for improving system practicality. In the previous two phases, we already have our solution: a food list *F'* and its corresponding quantity list *Q*, but a user may feel confused if it comes to combining the resultant ingredients into useful and meaningful recipes. More important, a recipe itself also plays a role in improving one's health since seasoning and culinary methods are also among critical issue of diet suggestion, which will be discussed in section 4 of the paper.

3 System Implementation

We have implemented a prototype of the CPDSS which integrated a smart fridge as its user interface. The system incorporates the contexts regarding a user's activities from our ADL Inference Engine implemented by Bayesian Networks [11]. Based on the contexts, the system can in turn estimate the activity level of a user, which represents the vigorousness of the user in an interval of interest. Currently, the CPDSS skips the combining phase since its module is under development. In this prototype, we have equipped the fridge with an RFID reader to monitor the stocking status of the fridge as shown in Fig. 3. With the touch panel of the smart fridge, we can display summarized histogram charts for users to visualize their related history information.

On the right block of the interface lists the inferred activities along with the activity level (namely, the outputs from the ADL Inference Engine) in a time interval. A calendar and some operation buttons are laid on the left of the interface. The middle block lists all food in the fridge. All the user has to do is to press down a button on the left screen and the diet suggestion will be displayed in the bottom block where four columns indicate their names, food types, and corresponding quantities, and the current stocking status as a reference for later food replenishment. For simplicity, all items that their corresponding quantities are below 0.25 units will be ignored for optimization. After pilot simulations, these items generally have corresponding q equal 10^{-9} units and are negligible. In addition, the food quantity is approximated to multiple of 0.5 for simplicity to users. Currently, the system allows a user to set the weights of three utility functions. Initial setting of the weight for the advisory utility is 0.7, 0.2 for the cost utility, and 0.1 for the preference utility.

In the current implementation, foods consist of 24 nutrients including calorie, protein, vitamin, and mineral, etc. In addition, there are six food types, which are starch, protein (e.g. seafood, eggs, beans, and meats), dairy, oil (e.g. nuts and oil), vegetable, and fruit. In this implementation, the personal data includes user name, suggested amount of each nutrient from professionals' suggestion, and the lower/upper bound of nutrient limitations.

Table 1. CPDSS Output Food Suggestion List with different Activity Levels

Activity Level	LOW	HIGH
Food Suggestion	Wheat flakes, 2.5 units Sweet potatoes, 0.5 units Egg noodle, 1 unit Cereal flake, 1.5 units Bacon, 1 unit **Chicken liver, 2.5 units** **Gallbladder liver, 2.5 units** Low-fat milk powder, 2 units Sunflower oil, 0.5 units Low-calorie butter, 2.5 units Agar, 2.5 units Lavar, 2.5 units Preserved longan, 2.5 units Preserved starfruit, 2.5 units	Wheat flakes, 1.5 units Rice, 2.5 units Sago Rice, 2.5 units Buns, 0.5 units Salmon floss, 2.5 units Plumule bean noodle, 2 units **Salted eggs, 2.5 units** Full-fat milk powder, 2 units Salad oil, 0.5 units Low-calorie butter, 2.5 units Pumpkin, 2.5 units Bamboo shoots, 2.5 units **Orange, 2.5 units** Preserved pineapple, 2.5 units

Table 1. lists the simulated results suggested by the CPDSS based on a user's LOW and HIGH activity levels for the last 24 hours. Apparently, the major difference is the total quantities of each food type. In addition to this difference, the suggestion in fruit type is also different. The fruit with more water is weighted more when one's activity level changes from LOW to HIGH (in this case the orange is suggested). The suggestion in the list of HIGH activity level also suggests more intake in sodium quantity (in this case 2.5 units of the salted eggs are suggested).

Some may notice that the system chooses some scarce foods like liver or preserved foods. It may result from the wrong settings of unit-weight transformation since we are still working on the unit-weight transformation for the entire food database. As a result, those foods with small weight but high nutrition contents will be more likely to be selected.

4 Conclusion

In this paper we propose a context-aware personal diet suggestion system to help one improve quality of life through diet suggestion. With the consideration of various contexts (especially one's activity level), our goal is to provide healthier and satisfactory diet suggestions. In additional, the CPDSS has been integrated with an integration platform so that the system has the potential for future enhancement to cooperate with other appliances for better effect of a computer-aided diet regime. Al- though it is still a long way from providing diet suggestions to actual health improvement, the CPDSS is our first attempt toward more promising balanced diet. The functionality of the system can be further extended in the future if more information can be gathered or shared from outside of a smart home via a cloud-computing based services.

Acknowledgement

This work is sponsored by the Industrial Technology Research Institute of Taiwan, under project 99-EC-17-A-05-01-0626.

References

[1] Colavita, C., D'orsi, R.: Linear programming and pediatric dietetics. British Journal of Nutrition 64(2), 307–317 (2007)

[2] Fletcher, L., Soden, P., Zinober, A.: Linear programming techniques for the construction of palatable human diets. The Journal of the Operational Research Society 45(5), 489–496 (1994)

[3] Soden, P., Fletcher, L.: Modifying diets to satisfy nutritional requirements using linear programming. British Journal of Nutrition 68(3), 565–572 (2007)

[4] Henson, S.: Linear programming analysis of constraints upon human diets. Journal of Agricultural Economics 42, 380–393 (1991)

[5] Chamberlin, J.: A linear programming analysis of human diets based upon major staple crops: sensitivity of low cost formulations to caloric, protein and bulk constraints. Massachusetts Institute of Technology, Dept. of Mechanical Engineering (1971)

[6] Khan, A., Hoffmann, A.: Building a case-based diet recommendation system without a knowledge engineer. Artificial Intelligence in Medicine 27(2), 155–179 (2003)

[7] Ryu, B., Ryu, H.: Biological Measurement in Healthcare Refrigerator. City (2009)

[8] Suhuai Luo, S., Jesse, S., Jin, J., Li Jiaming, J.: A Smart Fridge with an Ability to Enhance Health and Enable Better Nutrition. International Journal of Multimedia and Ubiquitous Engineering (IJMUE) 4(2), 69–79 (2009)

[9] Gu, H., Wang, D.: A Content-aware Fridge Based on RFID in Smart Home for Home-Healthcare. City (2009)

[10] Liao, C.-F., Jong, Y.-W., Fu, L.-C.: Toward a Message-Oriented Application Model and its Middleware Support in Ubiquitous Environments. In: Proceedings of the 2008 International Conference on Multimedia and Ubiquitous Engineering, Korea, pp. 298–303 (2008)

[11] Lu, C.-H., Fu, L.-C.: Robust Location-Aware Activity Recognition Using Wireless Sensor Network in an Attentive Home. IEEE Transactions on Automation Science and Engineering 6(4), 598–609 (2009)

[12] United-States-Recommended-Daily-Allowances, `http://1stholistic.com/nutrition/hol_nutrition-RDA.htm`

Multimodal Situational Awareness for Eldercare

Weimin Huang[1], Aung Aung Phyo Wai[1], Siang Fook Foo[1], Jit Biswas[1], Chi-Chun Hsia[2], and Koujuch Liou[2]

[1] Institute for Infocomm Research, Singapore 138632
{wmhuang,apwaung,sffoo,biswas}@i2r.a-star.edu.sg
[2] Industrial Technology Research Institute, Tainan City 709, Taiwan
{shiacj,lioukj}@itri.org.tw

Abstract. Long term eldercare is often labor intensive. This paper addresses a multimodal sensing approach to situation awareness for elderly care using video and force sensitive resistor (FSR) sensor map. For elderly people, especially those with limited mobility, it is useful to keep care givers or family members known of their situations that may lead to abnormal patterns such as repeated action (get up and sit down) or hazardous result such as a falling from bed. By using multimodal sensing with video camera and FSR sensor, the situation awareness algorithm is proposed to detect and track human activities. Experiments have shown the effectiveness of the detection of primary situations for elderly care.

Keywords: Eldercare, Multimodal feature extraction, Multimodal situation awareness, Object tracking, Activity understanding.

1 Introduction

For the elderly who are living alone in their homes, or are unsupervised in nursing homes, it is quite frequently the case that simple and ordinary conditions may lead to life threatening situations. Mobility restricted elderly need constant supervision in the most simple of ambulant tasks [2]. Going from the bed to the toilet when the light is dim or the pathway impeded by an obstacle is one such situation which may lead to a potential fall. Even on the bed, hazardous situations abound. Geriatric practitioners are unanimous, in that the bed is a particularly dangerous area. Sitting up on the bed from a lying position has sometimes created situations of dizziness and fall [1,2]. In this paper we present a novel approach to the situation awareness for elderly in the daily living around a bed, where the hazardous events may occur due to the motion transit from different locations.

The force sensitive resistor (FSR) sensor and video camera are used for awareness of the situation of a person. Although we have installed Passive Infrared (PIR) sensor for motion detection which is good for position detection in a big range, but not good for activity recognition. The pressure sensing bed consists of FSR sensor matrix where pressure intensity readings are collected by an embedded sensing platform. To complement the pressure sensor in a manner that will provide capability that is not possible with pressure sensor alone and to facilitate care givers' observation of the situation, a video camera is also mounted so that the view of the scene is close to

Y. Lee et al. (Eds.): ICOST 2010, LNCS 6159, pp. 85–93, 2010.

the view point from a human observer and yet does not obstruct the daily activity of people living in the environment.

In this study, we focus on the situations that may lead to elderly falls to the ground. The ontology of the pre-fall motion has been designed by analysis of the free text description for falls that have been recorded in an establishment over the period of a year. Based on the analysis, situations of interests are identified as following:

S1. Person on bed, near edge of the bed
S2. Person sitting up (from lying position)
S3. Person getting up and leaving bed
S4. Walking around
S5. Care giver around

An automatic spatiotemporal registration of video camera and FSR sensor array is designed for data fusion and easy deployment. Both low level and high level data fusion are presented in the paper for feature extraction and situation awareness.

1.1 Related Works

Situation or context awareness is about what is going on around you, especially to the operators who concern about specific goals and tasks [6,7]. In eldercare, safety and well being of elderly are two of the main concerns to care givers and family members. To keep alerted about the situation of our beloved, there are research works started in Situation Awareness for healthcare with different methodologies and approaches.

Kanai et al developed systems using wearable sensors such as ultrasonic, active RFID sensors and accelerometer for dangerous situation awareness [3,5] followed by visual and sound notification. Krose et al adopted naïve Bayesian and HMM to recognize human activity [4]. In [8], Zhou et al designed a video based human activity analysis and visualization for home users, by silhouette extraction and motion tracking for single-person-living eldercare. In terms of representation of semantics, Mastrogiovanni et al presented a methodology that deals with the problem of representation of high level activities in context aware environments [9]. Chen et al presented a logical framework for behavior, reasoning and assistance in a smart home [10]. Both these approaches deal with the representation of common artifacts and common activities in the homes of elderly. Salmeri et al described a framework using body sensor networks for 'fall-illness' alarm, using waist and leg mounted motion sensors (accelerometers) to detect falls [11]. Peng et al used simple low cost multimodal sensors for human sleep/awake monitoring, with data fusion from video, PIR, accelerometer and heart rate sensors [12]. Zouba et al also presented a system to monitor elderly activity of daily living using video for human location and activity and other environment sensors, mainly using the sensors as binary sensor for location and usage of objects [13].

In many of the researches in the area, wearable sensors are used to measure human activities [11] which however may not be convenient to the users. The video based method on the other hand does provide rich information but it can not work well for some cases due to the constraints of the view, computation limits etc. Although the privacy concern for video is not the topic of this paper, there are ways addressing it been discussed in [8,12] and [14] by using extracted feature such as motion only feature, segmented silhouette or edge only feature. In this paper we focus on the combination of environment sensor, i.e. the FSR sensor and video camera and propose a new approach to bed around situation awareness for eldercare.

2 Data Capturing and Fusion Framework

A FSR sensor array is weaved together to fit to a single bed. The layout of the sensor array is shown in Fig.1.a, and the camera view with the sensor array mapping to the bed is shown in Fig.1.b. The sensor array is formed by 7x7 circular sensors and 7 long sensors in the center part and 4 long sensors at the side of the bed.

The framework of the data fusion is shown in Figure 2, with the spatiotemporal registration for data synchronization between different modalities. A Network Time Protocol server is used to provide time stamp for video and FSR data.

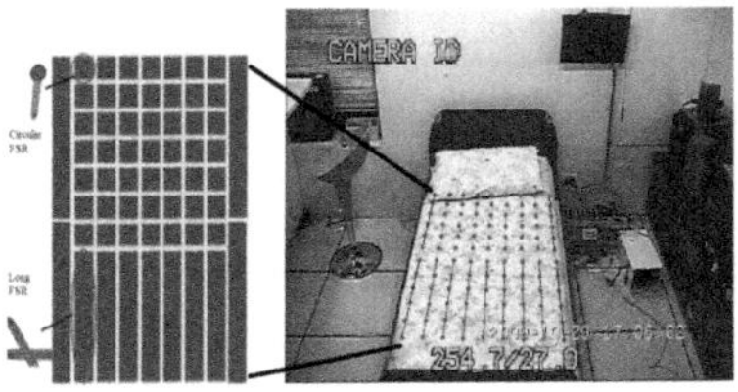

a. FSR layout b. Camera view of the room

Fig. 1. View of the bed and the FSR array fit on the bed

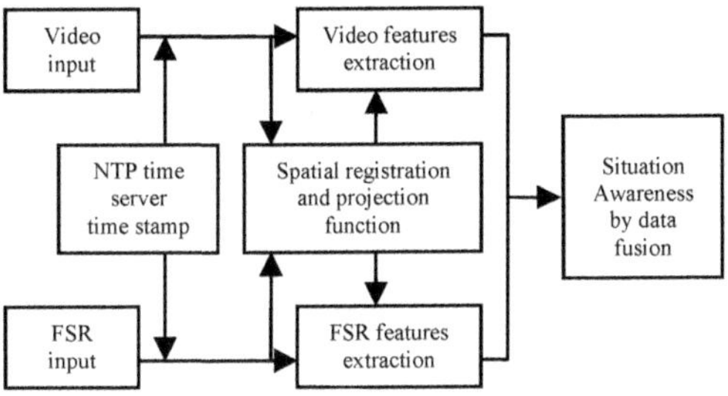

Fig. 2. Data fusion framework

The spatial registration is needed because the bed may be moved during the usage, usually when the user is sitting down on the bed or standing up. A landmark registration is adopted to register the bed position and a homography transform is used to map the physical sensor layout to the image view. The sensor matrix is shown in Fig.1.b by 'dots' and 'lines' on the bed after the registration.

3 Feature Extraction and Situation Awareness

Features from single modality may not be reliable or capable to represent the situation we are interested in due to the sensor's characteristics. Below we will describe the feature extraction as micro-context for video and FSR sensors first following the situation awareness using the multi-modal features.

3.1 Sensor Based Feature Extraction

The micro-context from FSR matrix can be characterized as: {*Bed occupancy*}, {*Near edge*}, {*Weight/Gravity center*} and {*Distribution range*}. The dynamic change of weight distribution will be represented by time sequences of the features at each time instance.

The FSR matrix in Fig.1.a can be represented as an image $p(j,i)$, $j=1,\ldots 12$, $i=1,\ldots 9$. Let the summed weight be $W = \sum p(j,i)$. The distribution P of the summed weight

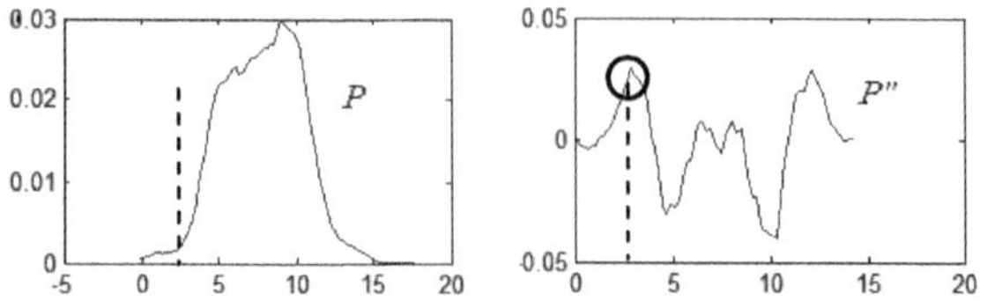

a. Weight distribution P b. Second derivative P'' of a.

Fig. 3. FSR weight force measurement

on the FSR matrix over different persons lying on bed is shown in Fig.3.a. Taken the second derivative P'', the *occupancy* is denoted as

$$O = \begin{cases} 1 & W \geq T_w \\ 0 & W < T_w \end{cases} , \quad P''(T_w) = \max_W P'' . \tag{1}$$

The {*Near edge*} can be measured accurately by computing the weight distribution in FSR image. First the FSR image is projected on to *i*-axis so we have a profile

$$p(i) = K \sum_j p(j,i), i = 1,\ldots,9 , \tag{2}$$

K is for normalization, $K=1/\sum_{j,i} p(j,i)$ .The $p(i)$ is then divided into three regions r_{left} = $\{p(i), i=1,2,3\}$, r_{center} = $\{p(i), i=4,5,6\}$, and r_{right} = $\{p(i), i=7,8,9\}$. Here a weighted sum of $p(i)$ is designed to better characterize the force distribution. Let the Gaussian kernel with σ=1.5 be $g_e(i)$ and $g_c(i)$ for the weighting,

$$g_e(i) = e^{-(|i-5|-4)^2/\sigma^2}, i = 1,2,3,7,8,9 , \tag{3}$$

$$g_c(i) = e^{-(i-5)^2/\sigma^2}, i = 4,5,6 . \tag{4}$$

The probability of the person near to the two edges or the bed center is defined as $p_{left} = \sum_{i=1,2,3} p(i) g_e(i)$, $p_{right} = \sum_{i=7,8,9} p(i) g_e(i)$, $p_{center} = \sum_{i=4,5,6} p(i) g_c(i)$ and

$$p_e = max\{p_{left}, p_{right}\} . \tag{5}$$

The micro context {*Near edge*} is defined as

$$N = \begin{cases} 0, & if \quad p_{center} \geq p_e \\ p_e, & if \quad p_{center} < p_e \end{cases} . \tag{6}$$

The {*Gravity center*} is simply the mean of the FSR image, {*Gravity center*} = {*x*, *y*}, where $x = \sum_{j,i} i \cdot p(j,i)/W$ and $y = \sum_{j,i} j \cdot p(j,i)/W$.

The distribution range is a feature to measure the force spread on the FSR matrix. Here we use the binarized FSR image b to measure the spread of the force,

$$b(j,i) = \begin{cases} 1 & p(j,i) \geq T \\ 0 & p(j,i) < T \end{cases} , \tag{7}$$

T is selected to remove the noise generated by the FSR sensor. The {*Distribution range*} D is defined as the standard deviation of image b.

The sensor based feature at time t is formed as

$$F_s(t) = \{W_t, O_t, N_t, x_t, y_t, D_t\} . \quad (8)$$

3.2 Video Feature Extraction

There are many methods for foreground objects segmentation, where Mixture of Gaussian (MoG) [15] is one of them. In our work we introduce the short term motion feature to compensate the foreground object segmentation. Fig.4 shows the result of the segmentation. (Details omitted here due to the space limitation.) By the introduction of the short term motion, we are able to reduce the fragments of objects.

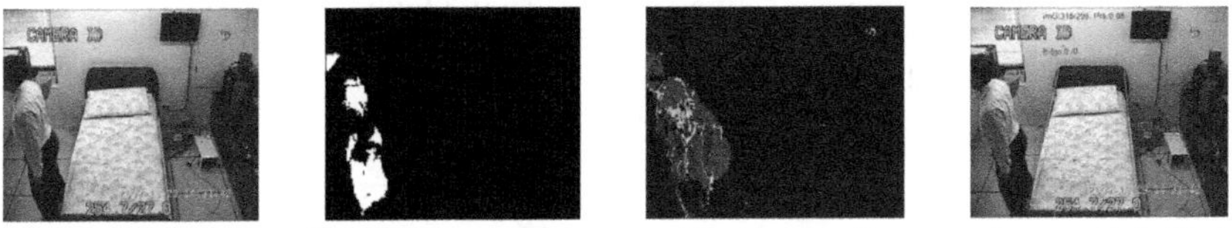

a. Original image b. MOG segmentation c. *Short term motion* *d. segmented object*

Fig. 4. Foreground segmentation using MoG and short term motion

Following the foreground object segmentation, the object tracking is started by combination of the group tracking [17] and mean shift tracking [16]. In our system, due to the constraints of networking and computing resource, the video frame rate is only at 8 fps and the FSR is 7 to 8 fps. With such frame rates the object tracking with mean shift is not reliable. In this work, we associate the FSR image with the motion cues to enhance the video object tracking, which is done in a sequential manner.

Assuming only one person on the bed each time and each video object is surrounded by a polygon (Fig.4.d). By counting the sensor $b(j,i)=1$ in the polygon, we can establish an association between the video object and the FSR map. Let the number of $b(j,i)=1$ associated to a video object $Q_m(t)$ at time t be $C_{FSR}(Q_m(t))$. We can use the changes of FSR images for object association. Given FSR image p_t at time t, we have

$$\alpha = |W_t - W_{t-1}| / max(W_t, W_{t-1}) , \quad (9)$$

$$N_{FSR}(Q_m(t)) = C_{FSR}(Q_m(t))/min(C_{FSR}, \sum C_{FSR}(Q_m(t))) . \quad (10)$$

The (9) is the relative weight change from time $t-1$ to time t and $N_{FSR}(Q_m(t))$ is normalized sensor number associated to each video object Q_m. The C_{FSR} is total number of sensors having $b(j,i)=1$. Let $V_{FSR}^m(t)$ be the association of video object Q_m with FSR map at time t. The update of $V_{FSR}^m(t)$ is

$$V_{FSR}^m(t) = \begin{cases} V_{FSR}^m(t-1), & \alpha < 0.5 \\ 1, & N_{FSR}(Q_m(t)) > 0.5 \\ 0, & N_{FSR}(Q_m(t)) < 0.5 \\ 0.5, & otherwise \end{cases} . \quad (11)$$

The $V_{FSR}^m(t) = 1$ means the object is associated with the FSR matrix, 0 means no association and 0.5 means uncertain of the association. It inherits the association from the same video object if the weight change α<0.5. If the inherent value is 0.5, the value of $N_{FSR}(Q_m(t))$ is further examined to decide the value of $V_{FSR}^{m}(t)$. The pseudo code is shown in Table 1, which combines the FSR object location and mean shift tracking.

In video tracking, we adopt the sequential object tracking [18] to tracking objects from most similar to least similar. With the video object tracking, many location related features can be extracted related to the situations of interests. Here we define an extra video features {*Inside bed*} I_{bed}.

The normalized intersection of the bed region and the object polygon is computed as the feature of {*Inside bed*},

$$I_{bed} = \frac{\{\,The\ object\ polygon\,\} \cap \{\,The\ bed\,\}}{\{\,The\ object\ polygon\,\}}\,. \tag{12}$$

The video feature for object Q_m is $F_m(t) = \{\, V_{FSR}^{m}(t), I_{bed}^{m}(t)\,\}$.

Table 1. Object tracking with video and FSR matrix

Object tracking algorithm
1. Object Initialization by object segmentation
2. For each object Q_m, assign $V_{FSR}^{m}(t)$ by association of FSR
3. For the object Q_m with $V_{FSR}^{m}(t) = 1$, assign the object ID as the one with $V_{FSR}^{m'}(t-1) = 1$, and adjust the position by *dx(t)=x(t)-x(t-1), dy(t)=y(t)-y(t-1).*
4. For each object Q_m, with $V_{FSR}^{m}(t) \neq 1$, tracking by assigning the object with an ID: a. New object ID if there is no spatial overlapping with any object at time t-1. b. Same ID of an object at t-1, if it is the only one spatially overlapped with Q_m. c. Mean-shift tracking using color histogram similarity if there are two or more objects merged into a group.
5. Go to step 2.

3.3 Situation Awareness with Video and FSR Sensor

In this section we describe the approach to situation awareness by fusion of FSR and video features. Some of the FSR and video features can be used directly for situation awareness, such as the {*Near edge*} feature in (6), while others will be derived by combination of the dynamics of the features.

{*Near edge*} is one of the situations caregivers would like to know since it often leads to fall of elderly from bed. The feature *N* in (6) is quite robust, so we can apply a threshold to *N* to infer the situation. The situation S1{*Near edge*} is triggered if $N>0.2$. We write it as

$$S1=1,\ \ if\ \ N>0.2. \tag{13}$$

S5 {*Care giver around*} is detected by counting how many persons in the scene including the one occupying the bed. If there are two or more persons, we will say there is a caregiver around. Similarly S4 {*Walking around*} is detected as moving object $\{Q_m, V^m_{FSR}(t)=0\}$.

Other situations rely on the transition of object within spatiotemporal windows. For simplicity, a naïve Bayesian is used to learn the dynamics of the FSR and video object location changes. For example, considering situations S3{*Getting up from bed*}, it is the cases many falls could occur especially for elderly with weak legs. Let the time window for the {*Getting up from bed*} be T_w, the changes of the posture of a human will result in the changes of the video object position in the image related to the bed position characterized by {*Inside Bed*} I_{bed}, the FSR weight *W*, and the {*Near edge*} measurement *N*. Within T_w, *W* and I_{bed} will reduce to zero, and *N* will increase to one. With the knowledge, we can reduce the data dimension by computing the mean value of the features over half of the time window. Given FSR measure $W(t)$, $t=1,\ldots,T_w$, the new feature set is defined as

$$W^1 = 2\sum_{t=1,\ldots,T_W/2} W(t)/T_w \ , \tag{14}$$

$$W^2 = 2\sum_{t=T_W/2,\ldots,T_W} W(t)/T_w \ . \tag{15}$$

In the same way we obtain a feature set $f=\{W^1, W^2, N^1, N^2, I_{bed}^{\ 1}, I_{bed}^{\ 2}\}$. For the time being, the time scale is not changed although it may vary for different persons. We can detect a situation with different time scale of T_w and report the situation whenever it is detected. By the Bayesian $p(S|f) = p(f|S)p(S)/p(f)$. For S3 (and S2), we have

$$S3=1, \ \text{if } p(S3|f)>p(\sim S3|f) \ . \tag{16}$$

The condition (16) can be written further as $p(f|S3)p(S3)>p(f|\sim S3)p(\sim S3)$.

4 Experiment and Discussion

We have tested 24 sets of collected sequences. Each sequence contains different situations. The dataset also includes 10 cases of {*Care giver around*}. Fig.5 shows some of the situations. From left to right the images show *walking*, *near edge*, *sitting up*, *getting up from bed*, and *care giver around*. The real caregiver ID may be detected by other modality such as RFID sensor, which is not addressed in this paper. The Table 2 summarizes the result of the detection accuracy.

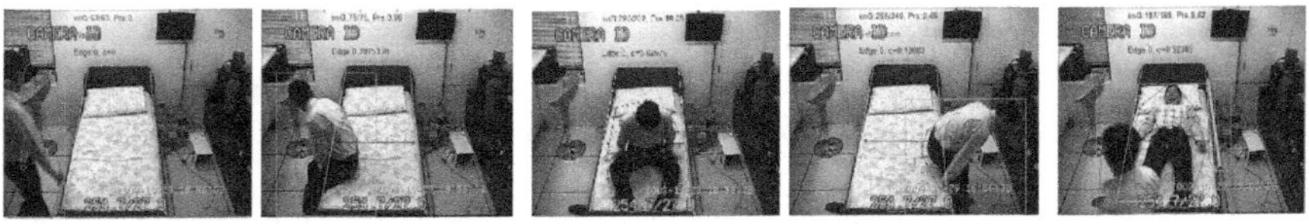

Fig. 5. Images of different situations

One of the problems in the experiments is how to precisely define a situation. E.g., in the situation of {*getting up from bed*}, it is difficult to identify an exact time to say it happens. We define it as a successful detection if the triggered alarm is falling within certain time window. For sitting up and getting up, the time window is 5 frames.

The result of {*Walking*} and {*Near edge*} are based on the detection per frame. The rest recognition result is based on detection per situation. The errors in {*Walking*} are mainly caused by person moving near bed, just before sitting. In {*Sitting up*} result, the false alarms are mainly caused by big motion of the person when he is still lying on the bed. The false alarm for caregiver around is relatively high. It was caused by the mean shift tracking which trapped the care giver ID with the lying person's ID due to the high degree of similarity between the appearances of the two objects using simple color histogram. It can be solved by incorporating of spatial information of color representation. The system also generates a few short term false alarms of *{Near edge}*. It may be removed by check the time sequence of the object.

Table 2. Experiment results

Situation	Walking	Sitting up	Near edge	Getting up	Caregiver
Detection(%)	98.5	93.75	99.86	100	100
False alarm(%)	22.78	14.29	7.21	5.88	20

5 Conclusions

This paper described a multi-modal feature extraction and situation detection approach to dangerous situation awareness for eldercare. The approach combines the FSR sensor and video camera for feature extraction and activity modeling, by associating the FSR and video with spatiotemporal synchronization for data fusion. The analysis of the experiment results of the situation awareness shows the robustness of the features and the efficiency of the multimodal approach. In this work the high level situations studied are limited to the bed and its surrounding areas. We believe the feature sets extracted can be useful for other situations, e.g. the sitting on and standing from a chair or sofa, the sleep quality measure with the motion. The future work is to conduct further experiments in this direction and expand the coverage to other scenarios such as lying on the floor.

References

1. Aung, A., et al.: Sleeping Patterns Observations for Bedsores and Bed-side Falls Prevention. In: EMBC 2009, Minnesota (2009)
2. Hsia, C.-C., et al.: An Approach for Incorporating End User Knowledge into Applications of Information Extraction Classification and Fusion in Institutional Eldercare. In: I-SPAN 2009 (2009)
3. Kanai, H., Tsuruma, G., Nakada, T., Kunifuji, S.: Notification of Dangerous Situation for Elderly People using Visual Cues. In: ACM-IUI 2008 (2008)

4. Kröse, B., van Kasteren, T., Gibson, C., van den Dool, T.: CARE: Context Awareness in Residences for Elderly. In: The 6th Int. Conf. of the Int. Society for Gerontechnology, pp. 101–105 (2008)
5. Kanai, H., Nakada, T., Hanbat, Y., Kunifuji, S.: A support system for context awareness in a group home using sound cues. In: Pervasive Health 2008, pp. 264–267 (2008)
6. Endsley, M.R.: Theoretical understandings of situation awareness: a critical review. In: Endsley, M.R., Garland, D.J. (eds.) Situation Awareness Analysis and Measurement. Lawrence Erlbaum Associates, Mahwah (2000)
7. Zaslavsky, A.: Smartness of Pervasive Computing Systems Through Context-Awareness. Keynotes Talk. In: ruSMART (2008)
8. Zhou, Z., Chen, X., Chung, Y.-C., He, Z., Han, T.X., Keller, J.M.: Activity Analysis, Summarization, and Visualization for Indoor Human Activity Monitoring. IEEE Trans. on CSVT 18(11), 1489–1498 (2008)
9. Mastrogiovanni, F., et al.: On the Problem of Describing Activities in Context-Aware Environments. Int. Journal of Assistive Robotics and Mechatronics 9(4) (2008)
10. Chen, L., et al.: A Logical Framework for Behaviour Reasoning and Assistance in a Smart Home. International Journal of Assistive Robotics and Mechatronics 9(4) (2008)
11. Salmeri, A., et al.: An Architecture to Combine Context Awareness and Body Sensor Networks for Health Care Applications. In: Mokhtari, M., Khalil, I., Bauchet, J., Zhang, D., Nugent, C. (eds.) ICOST 2009. LNCS, vol. 5597, pp. 90–97. Springer, Heidelberg (2009)
12. Peng, Y.-T., Lin, C.-Y., Sun, M.-T.: Multimodality Sensors for Sleep Quality Monitoring and Logging. In: Int Conf. on Data Engineering Workshops (2006)
13. Zouba, N., Bremond, F., Thonnat, M.: Multisensor Fusion for Monitoring Elderly Activities at Home. In: Proc. of AVSS 2009 (2009)
14. Chen, D., Chang, Y., Yan, R., Yang, J.: Tools for Protecting The Priavcy of Specific Individuals in Video. EURASIP Journal on Applied Signal Processing, 107–113 (2007)
15. Stauffer, C., Grimson, W.E.L.: Adaptive Background Mixture Models for Real-Time Tracking. In: CVPR 1999, vol. 2, p. 2246 (1999)
16. Comaniciu, D., Ramesh, V., Meer, P.: Kernel-based object tracking. IEEE Trans. on PAMI 25(5), 564–577 (2003)
17. Yang, T., Pan, Q., Li, J., Li, S.Z.: Real-time multiple objects tracking with occlusion handling in dynamic scenes. In: CVPR 2005, pp. 970–975 (2005)
18. Li, L., Huang, W., Gu, I.Y.-H., Luo, R., Tian, Q.: An Efficient Sequential Approach to Tracking Multiple Objects Through Crowds for Real-Time Intelligent CCTV Systems. IEEE Trans. on SMC-B 38(5), 1254–1269 (2008)

Mobile Personal Health Care System for Patients with Diabetes

Fuchao Zhou, Hen-I Yang, José M. Reyes Álamo, Johnny S. Wong, and Carl K. Chang

Department of Computer Science, Iowa State University, USA
{alanzhou,hiyang,jmreye,wong,chang}@cs.iastate.edu

Abstract. In this paper, we propose a personal diabetes monitoring system which integrates wearable sensors, 3G mobile phone, smart home technologies and Google Health to facilitate the management of chronic disease - diabetes. Our system utilizes wearable sensors and 3G cellular phone to automatically collect physical signs, such as blood glucose level and blood pressure. It allows users, especially seniors with diabetes, to conveniently record daily test results and track long term health condition changes regardless of their locations. It does so without having to ask users to manually input them into the system. Our system also utilizes Google Health to manage Personal Health Records (PHRs), which not only bridges the gaps between patients and different health care providers but enabling accesses to patients' PHRs anywhere and anytime by taking advantage of the universal accessibility of Google Health.

Keywords: diabetes monitoring, health care, behavioral modification, personal health record, Google Health, smart home.

1 Introduction

Diabetes is one of the most widely spread chronic diseases. In the United States, nearly 13 percent of adults aged 20 and older have diabetes. Diabetes is especially common in the elderly: nearly one-third of those aged 65 and older have the disease. It is suggested in a publication of the Department of Health and Human Services that in order to keep glucose at a healthy level, people with diabetes need to keep a balance between three important aspects: diet, exercise and diabetes medicine in daily routine [1, 2, 3]. Therefore, continuous self-monitoring of the blood glucose (blood sugar), daily diet, physical activity and medicine intake are crucial for the management of diabetes.

In recent years, small and wearable sensors have become widely available, which allows convenient and non-intrusive monitoring of patients' blood glucose, medicine intake and life styles, e.g., daily diet and exercise. In addition, contemporary 3G smart phones incorporate unforeseen computational powers which include internal database, voice recognition, GPS position and continuous access to local wireless networks and the Internet. The latest International Telecommunication Union (ITU) statistics reveals that there were about 4.6 billion mobile-phone users by the end of the year 2009

Y. Lee et al. (Eds.): ICOST 2010, LNCS 6159, pp. 94–101, 2010.

as compared to the total number of the Internet users was just above 1.5 billion [4]. This makes newer cellular phones a very promising mobile platform for advanced applications. To complete the picture, we observe that the growing popularity in the third-party online PHR management platform with security and privacy features, such as Google Health, Microsoft HealthVault and open-source project Dassia. The advantages of these PHR management platforms include: (1) facilitate information sharing between patients and multiple health care providers; (2) avoid unnecessary expenditures (i.e., duplicate lab test costs); (3) prevent adverse drug conflicts;(4) maintain comprehensive PHRs and provide easy access to the patient's own PHRs from any locations at any time [5].

There are many wearable and pervasive health monitoring systems in the market, and we summarizes some of their representative features. The mobile health monitoring systems for heart disease, using wearable ECG sensors and smart phone were developed in [6, 7]. Using mobiles with a multi-access service for the management of diabetic patients was proposed in [8],which was designed to collect data, either manually or automatically from the blood glucose meter; to monitor blood glucose levels; to suggest insulin dose adjustment when needed ;to deliver monitoring data to a health care center.

In our smart home lab at Iowa State University, several subsystems have already been developed to facilitate the people's daily activities, especially with respect to seniors' healthcare. For example, Smart Microwave and Smart Fridge can identify food and nutrition facts by scanning Universal Product Code (UPC) barcode with the help of U.S. Department of Agriculture (USDA) National Nutrition Database (USDA-NND) downloaded from USDA website, record the person's dietary history, and check conflicts with medicines taken. Watchdog is built not only for house safety but for reminder, like reminding the diabetic patient to carry the medicines and snack when leaving the house. The Medicine Information Support System (MISS) is designed for checking medicine conflictions and facilitating the person to take medicine in compliance to completeness and timeliness, with the support of a Global Medication Conflict Database (MCD) [9, 10].

The major contribution of this work is the design of personalized, integrated, and collaborative care system for self-monitoring and managing diabetes. Our mobile health care system has two major improvements compared to the system proposed in [8]. First, it not only monitors the blood glucose levels, but collects information about the daily diets, medicines taken and exercise done and makes it possible for patients to monitor their own health conditions, to receive warning and guidance to adjust their behaviors during their daily routines, and to be able to navigate intricate interactions among diet, exercise and medications. Second, it does not directly deliver data to a specific health care center. Instead it integrates mobile-based and smart home-based health monitoring systems with Google Health, breaking down the wall between the patient, patient's family members and different health care providers such that they can now provide collaborative care for the patient.

This paper is organized as follows. In Section 2, we describe the integrated architecture design including the software, hardware and communication interfaces between different components of the system. Section 3 gives the software architecture design in mobile phones and explains the implementation of web services in smart home. In Section 4, we describe behavioral modifications flowchart. Finally, summaries conclusions and future work are presented in section 5.

2 System Design

In this section, we introduce the sensors used, communication technologies between different components and functionalities of each component. Fig. 1 shows the overall picture of the system architecture of our proposed mobile personal health care system for patients with diabetes. We introduce this system in the following three levels:

(1) Wearable sensors which allows convenient, continuous and non-intrusive monitoring of people with diabetes for their test results, medicines, daily diet and exercise. In our prototype, Zephyr BT HxM with fabric sensors is used as an exercise tracker measuring the heart rate, speed and distance. Also, we are studying the UA-767PBT A&D Bluetooth Blood Pressure to trace the person's blood pressure and the Bluetooth-enabled blood glucose meter, MyGlucoHealth® Meter, to trace patients' blood glucose level. In our prototype, we simulated the blood glucose data.

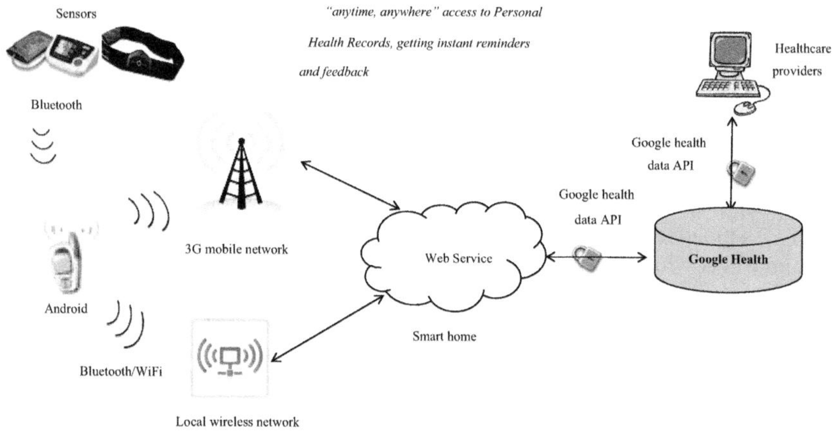

Fig. 1. System architecture of mobile personal health care system for people with diabetes

(2) 3G smart phone will gather, store and display statistical data from wearable sensors, update daily test results, diets and medicines taken, and get feedbacks and notifications from caregivers. There are two ways for smart phone to interact with Google Health. In LAN area, smart phone detect existing wireless Access Point (AP) and accesses Internet. Otherwise it resorts to 3G mobile network.

(3) Web services in smart home enable the interaction among the 3G smart phone, smart home subsystems and Google Health. Web service in smart home wraps Google Health data APIs and interacts with smart home subsystems like Smart Microwave and Smart Fridge for diet tracking. The smart phone utilizes KSOAP2 to interact with SOAP web service in smart home. Google Health is used to manage PHRs and facilitates information sharing between patients and multiple providers.

3 Software Framework

Multi-module software architecture is developed in Android mobile platform and integrates software components with web service technologies. Every module in the architecture is loosely coupled and is implemented by using Activities and Intents in the Android development simulator. Software Architecture of mobile personal health care system for diabetes is illustrated in Fig. 2, which includes GUI (Graphical User Interface) Module, Interface Module, Inference Module, Notification Module, common database operation interface with internal database Sqlite and KSOAP2 interface with SOAP web service in the home server.

GUI Module. The patient can retrieve or input data by interacting with GUI. The specific applications include: 1) Heath Care Team which contains the contact information of the person's health care team. 2) Health Care Goals includes the blood glucose, blood pressure, exercise and weight targets which are strictly set by the health care team. For example, the blood glucose target is 100mg/dL before a meal and is 140mg/dL after a meal. 3) Test Result Tracker displays daily, weekly or a custom time interval blood glucose test results in a graph that indicates whether the blood glucose is high, healthy or low. 4) Medicine Tracker, Exercise Tracker and Diets Tracker will track the information about medicine taken, exercise and diets. 5) Notification is for patient to check feedbacks from his or her health care team or family members and to read the reminders and suggestions from the scheduler in the smart phone.

Interface Module. Interface Module is responsible for gathering raw sensing data and transferring it into internal message format, which is implemented by using an experimental unofficial Bluetooth API for Android.

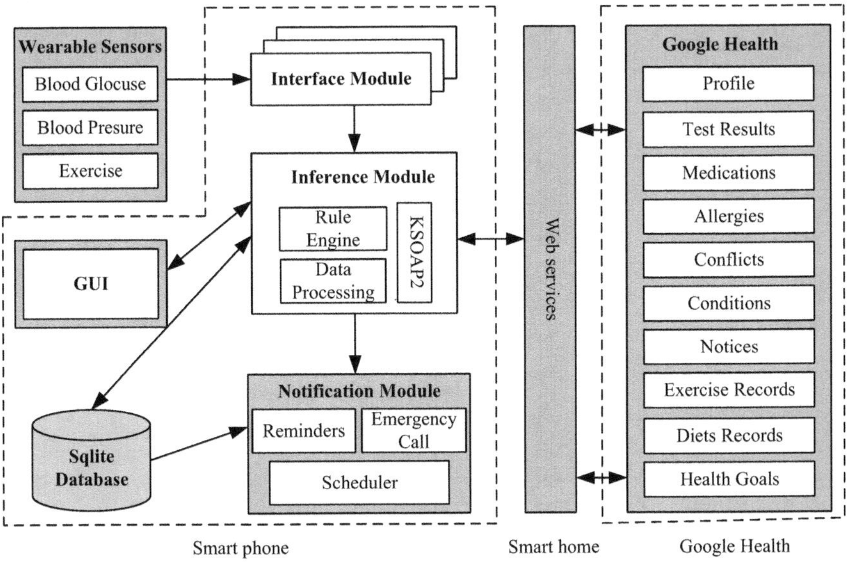

Fig. 2. Software Architecture of mobile personal health care system for people with diabetes

Inference Module. Inference Module is responsible for processing raw data from sensors via interface module and notices from Google Health through web service interface and interacting with GUI. After receiving the sensor data from the interface module, the inference module will store it into a database by calling the common database operation interface. It will also perform inference tasks based on pre-defined rules which are described in Section 4. The outcomes of the inference procedure are transformed into corresponding notification messages and then sent to the notification module. Inference module will periodically query if there are any notices updated from Google Health based on pull-based data consistency model. If there are notifications, it will trigger the corresponding action commands or notification messages. For example, when medications are updated in the Google Health by personal health team, inference module will get a notice whose message type is *MSG_ MEDICATONS_UPDATED*, and then it will release a command called *CMD_ DOWNLOAD_MEDICATIONS* to KSOAP2 interface. After getting the updated medications, it will notify the scheduler in the notification module to update the medicine taking schedule. Inference module also periodically updates the test results, diets and exercise records from wearable sensors or manual inputs into Google Health.

Notification Module. Based on the outputs from inference module, Notification Module will post reminders to the person or notices to health team. In emergency situations like when blood glucose is very high or the user has not taken medicine or blood glucose test for several days, notification module will make an emergency call to the person's health team. The scheduler in the notification module will post a text or voice reminder to remind the user to take medicine or anything pre- scheduled.

Web service. A Web service deployed in the smart home enables communications between 3G smart phone and Google Health. This Web service wraps Google Health data APIs to interact with Google Health. It also cooperates with other subsystems in home system, for example, to interact with MISS in smart home for medicine

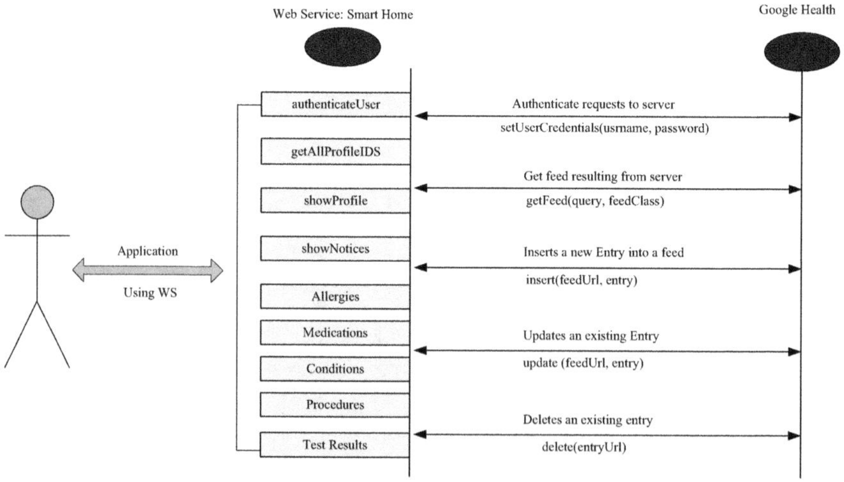

Fig. 3. Use case for interacting with Google Health

conflicts checking and interact with Smart Microwave and Smart Fridge Subsystems for diets management. Fig.3 shows a use case for interacting with Google Health.

Google Health. Google Health is a free online service for patients to maintain their personal electronic health records while allows appropriate access as needed with the permission of the patient to different health care providers.

4 Behavioral Modifications Flowchart

Through web service, we integrate smart phone, smart home and external systems like Google Health, MCD and Weather web service. With the help of these subsystems and wearable sensors, the mobile health care system traces the person's activities in exercise, diets and medications taken, and gives warnings and suggestions for preventing accidents and improving the person's behaviors during his or her daily routine. The behavioral modifications flowchart is illustrated in Fig.4. In our design, we use Google Health as PHR management system which breaks down the wall between the patient, patient's family members and different health care providers such that they can work together to continuously refine targets for blood glucose levels control, exercise and nutrition intake and give a prescription to the patient. The behavioral modifications steps are the following:

(1) When the person takes a blood glucose test, the system will automatically make an emergency call to prevent potential accidents if the blood glucose level is dangerously high or low. If it is relatively low or high, the person is suggested to eat food or take medicine under the guidance of the system.

(2) The system will remind the person to take medicines based on the prescription or whenever needed. With the helps from MISS and Google Health, the system will check whether there are conflicts or allergies among medications the person is taking. If there are any medicine conflicts or allergies, the system will suggest the person to consult with his or her doctors. The system can also indicate whether the person needs to take medicine with food and whether he or she is complying with completeness (right dose) and timeliness (right time) [10].

(3) Diet is an extremely important factor affecting a patient's diabetes. Based on the personal health situations, food allergies and other dietary restrictions, the health care providers make a list of prohibited foods. With the support of Smart Microwave and Smart Fridge Subsystems at smart home and barcode reader embedded in cell phone, the health care system can check whether the food is in the prohibited food list. If it is not in the list, then the system further identifies nutrition facts of the food, checks the person's daily consumption history and then takes different actions based on the percentages of carbohydrates and fats accounting for the person's daily caloric intake respectively. Also, by checking the person's medicine intake history, it can check whether there are conflicts with medicines taken.

(4) The system can suggest the person to exercise either indoor or outside based on weather information from the weather web service. When the person goes outside, he or she will lock the door by scanning a RFID tag identification. The Watchdog then will learn the fact that the owner will go outside and thus remind him or her to scan the RFID tag attached to the medicine bottle and the barcode on the snack packets to make sure the person brings the right medicine and snack. During exercise, the

exercise tracker sensor will monitor the person's heart rate. If the heart rate is more than 85% target heart rate, the system will give an alert and may suggest the person to slow down or even stop exercising.

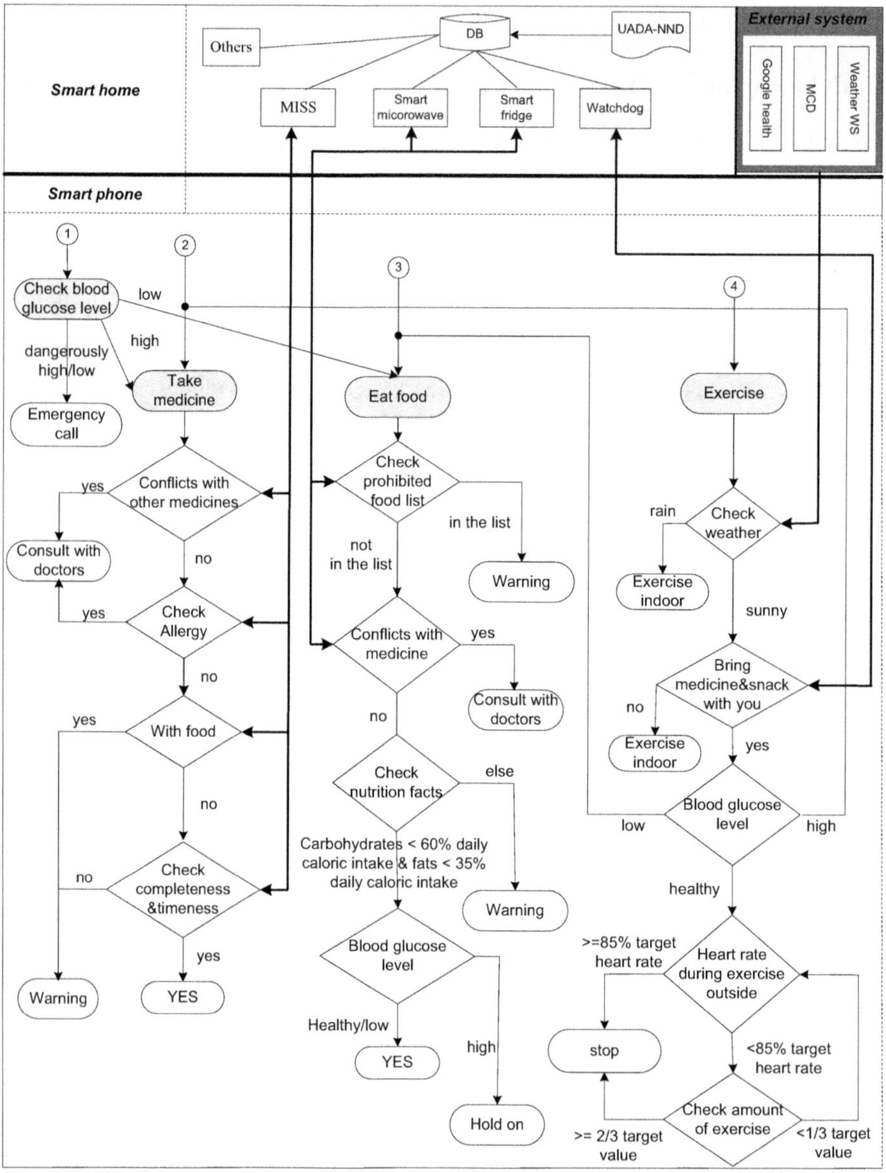

Fig. 4. Behavioral modifications flowchart

5 Conclusions and Future Work

This paper presents a personal diabetes monitoring system which integrates wearable sensors, 3G mobile phones, smart home technologies and Google Health to facilitate the management of diabetes conditions. This diabetes monitoring system not only assist with the tasks of diabetes management, but also improves the medicine and food safety by taking full advantage of features in existing subsystems in smart home and Google Health. Since there exists imprecision when collecting the exact data of diets and exercise (for instance, when a patient dines out or go to a gym), our prototype system supports both automatic and manual inputs of diets, medicine and exercise information.

We are currently working on 1) to improve the accuracy of automatically collected dietary and exercise information; 2) to enhance the accuracy and completeness of reasoning. One of our ongoing efforts is to explore the use of data mining tools, such as Intelligent Miner, DataMiner, Clementine, and 4Thought, to find the implicit relations between blood glucose, medicine, diets and exercise; 3) to establish a dynamic model of exercise, diets, medicine and weigh effects on the blood glucose level. Our goal is to establish a more comprehensive model than the current one on the effects of exercise on plasma glucose and insulin levels described in [11].

References

1. New Survey Results Show Huge Burden of Diabetes, U.S. Department of Health and Human Services NIHNews National Institutes of Health (2009) (accessed January 26)
2. Centers for Disease Control and Prevention, `http://www.cdc.gov/diabetes/pubs/pdf/tctd.pdf` (accessed January 20, 2009)
3. National Institutes of Health National Diabetes Education Program, `http://ndep.nih.gov/` (accessed January 20, 2009)
4. `http://www.itu.int/newsroom/press_releases/2009/39.html` (accessed January 26, 2009)
5. eHealth Strategies with Microsoft and Google in the Game, LLC, 9/30/2008 (2008)
6. Leijdekkers, P., Gay, V., Barin, E.: Trial Results of a Novel Cardiac Rhythm Management System Using Smart Phones and Wireless ECG Sensors. In: Mokhtari, M., Khalil, I., Bauchet, J., Zhang, D., Nugent, C. (eds.) ICOST 2009. LNCS, vol. 5597, pp. 32–39. Springer, Heidelberg (2009)
7. Chung, W., et al.: A Cell Phone Based Health Monitoring System with Self Analysis Processor using Wireless Sensor Network Technology. In: 29th EMBC, pp. 3705–3708 (2007)
8. Lanzola, G., Capozzi, D., D'Annunzio, G., Ferrari, P., Bellazzi, R., Larizza, C.: Going Mobile with a Multiaccess Service for the Management of Diabetic Patients. Journal of Diabetes Science and Technology 1(5) (September 2007)
9. Álamo, J.M.R., Wong, J., Babbitt, R., Chang, C.: MISS: Medicine Information Support System in Smart Home Environments. In: Helal, S., Mitra, S., Wong, J., Chang, C.K., Mokhtari, M. (eds.) ICOST 2008. LNCS, vol. 5120, pp. 185–199. Springer, Heidelberg (2008)
10. Álamo, J.M.R., Yang, H.-I., Babbitt, R., Wong, J., Chang, C.: Support for Medication Safety and Compliance in Smart Home Environments. International Journal of Advanced Pervasive and Ubiquitous Computing (2009)
11. Roy, A., Parker, R.S.: Dynamic Modeling of Exercise Effects on Plasma Glucose and Insulin Levels. Journal of Diabetes Science and Technology, YMPOSIUM 1(3) (May 2007)

Estimation of Instantaneous Bandwidth and Reconstruction of Noisy ECG Signal Measured by a 24-Hour Continuous Healthcare System for the Elderly and People with Disabilities

Heyoung Lee[1] and Z. Zenn Bien[2],

[1] Department of Control & Instrumentation Engineering, Seoul National University of Technology, Seoul 139-743, Korea
[2] School of Electrical & Computer Engineering, Ulsan National Institute of Science and Technology, Ulsan Metropolitan City 689-798, Korea

Abstract. In this manuscript, a case study is conducted on bio-signals of time-varying spectral content with the purpose of developing a quality of life engineering product. The study deals with noise reduction of electrocardiogram (ECG) for detecting abnormality of the heart system during daily life. Instantaneous bandwidth (IB) of ECG is estimated and is used adaptively as IB of variable bandwidth filter (VBF) for suppressing noise whose Fourier spectrum overlaps with that of ECG and estimating more accurately parameters such as onsets, ends, rates, intervals and durations on the six principal waves of ECG measured during daily life. The proposed method based on the VBF improves the SNR on the P, Q and T waves without damaging the QRS complex, different from, the methods based on the Fourier spectral analysis.

Keywords: ECG, variable bandwidth filter, instantaneous bandwidth, instantaneous frequency, motion artifacts, continuous healthcare system.

1 Introduction

Signals with time-varying spectral content can be found in many biomedical applications [1][2][3]. We consider, as an example, a 24-hour continuous health care system in which various bio-signals such as electrocardiogram (ECG), electroencephalogram, electromyogram, blood pressure and voice are measured and processed. In the system, changes on physical and mental states, if any, are observed and analyzed to diagnose and predict abnormality of the human body. Note that a bio-signal measured from a human's body is a set of components that can be considered as some transmuted versions of primitive signals through some complex biomechanical and electrochemical processes. For example, a measured ECG signal is a modulated version of a true one by muscular movements of organs in the chest. Each cardiac beat of ECG is associated with a sequence of the six principal waves named as P, Q, R, S, T and U. Some characteristic parameters on the six principal waves, such as rate, interval, duration, amplitude and waveform of segment and

Y. Lee et al. (Eds.): ICOST 2010, LNCS 6159, pp. 102–112, 2010.

combinations, are known to be relevant to the states of the heart system and are used for clinical purposes [8][9]. The QT interval which refers the time interval between the QRS complex onset and the T wave end is currently considered as an index of the ventricular repolarization time [8][9]. Abnormal QT values are associated with ventricular pro-arrhythmicity [8][9]. Also, it is known that ischemic heart disease can be assessed based on abnormality of the ST segments [9].

ECG is a typical example of signals with time-varying instantaneous bandwidth (IB). ECG of a healthy individual exhibits a quasi-periodic variation in beat-to-beat intervals [9]. According to the analysis of the rhythmic phenomena known as the respiratory sinus arrhythmia, the instantaneous heart rate (IHR) fluctuates along with the respiration phases, namely, cardio-acceleration phase during inspiration and cardio-deceleration phase during expiration [9][10][11][12]. It is known that the sympathetic and parasympathetic nerve systems modulate the cardiac activity. Not only the spontaneous rhythmic activity but also body motions and mental loads during daily life cause some fluctuations to the IHR. For example, it is known that postural changes and mental loads of complex decision-makings cause significant variations in the IHR [9]. In fact, several studies have suggested a link between negative emotions (such as anxiety and hostility) and reduced IHR [9]. The heart rate variability (HRV), which refers a measure on a variation of the IHR [9], is used as a predictor of risk after acute myocardial infraction and as an early warning sign of diabetic neuropathy [9]. Thus, in clinical assessment of the heart system during daily life, it is important to measure some relevant quantities such as IHR, HRV, PR interval, QT interval and ST segment in a very reliable way, which is possible by removing noise whose Fourier spectrum overlaps that of ECG [12][13][14].

A measured ECG during daily living activities has some corruption of various noises caused by muscular activities, incomplete contact of electrodes, base line drift and electrical interference of the power line, etc [13]. In particular, motion artifacts disturb assessing functions on the heart system in high physical exercise phase since motion artifacts appear in the measured ECG as a superimposed and/or modulated form [9][14]. Motion artifacts are usually believed to be the most difficult form of noises to be eliminated from ambulatory ECG since Fourier spectra of motion artifacts and ECG overlap almost completely, and the morphology of motion artifacts often resembles that of the six principal waves [8][9][14]. Thus, rejection of motion artifacts is highly desirable to extract reliable features that are clues for assessing abnormal states of the heart system [8][9][14].

In this study, a noisy ECG signal is cleaned through off-line processing and on-line processing by a 24-hour healthcare system for the elderly and disabled. In off-line processing, one beat of IB corresponding to RR segment of ECG is estimated. In on-line processing, firstly, IHR and R-peak instants are estimated. Secondly, the estimate of one beat of IB is linearly scaled, shifted and synchronized with the estimates of R-peak instants to form IB of variable bandwidth filter (VBF) that is capable of coping with a quasi-periodic variation of ECG. Finally, a clean ECG signal is obtained from the output of VBF whose IB is adaptive to spectral variation of ECG, due to the spontaneous rhythmic activity and the physical load on the heart system. It is remarked that the linear scaling can be modified, depending on the relationship between the loads of the heart system and the corresponding time-scaling to each of the six principal waves.

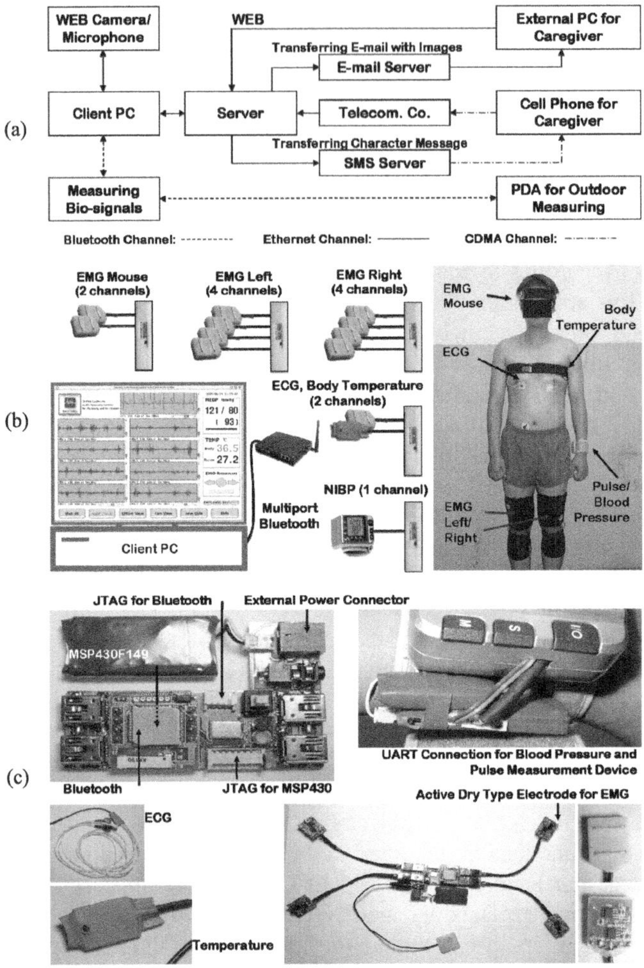

Fig. 1. A 24-hour continuous healthcare system. (a) Overall connection diagram. (b) Experimental setup and graphic user interface. (c) Wearable measurement devices.

2 A 24-Hour Continuous Healthcare System

As background information of our case studies, we describe briefly a 24-hour continuous health care system that we have been developing as a quality of life engineering product for the elderly and people with disabilities [4]. The system shown in Fig. 1 measures and processes five kinds of bio-signals (ECG, electromyogram, body temperature, blood pressure and voice) continuously for extracting information on health status of a subject [4]. The system is composed of three parts: (i) a wearable subsystem with functions of amplification, A/D conversion and communication, (ii) an interaction subsystem for providing alarms on health status to a pre-arranged caregiver, and (iii) client and server computers for processing and maintaining data.

Data, alarm and control command are transferred through Ethernet, CDMA, and Bluetooth channels. The measured bio-signals during movements are transferred to client PC through Bluetooth channel. A pre-arranged caregiver observes and checks on experimental conditions through CDMA and Ethernet channels when the caregiver receives a character message or an e-mail with still images. The wearable subsystem consists of two parts: (i) an active electrode part that performs amplification and filtering of analog bio-signals, and (ii) a common hub part that performs A/D conversion and transmission of data through Bluetooth channel. The wearable subsystem measures Lead I ECG of the bipolar limb leads configuration, which is sampled at rate 1 [kHz] and quantized at 12-bit resolution after being amplified 500 times [4].

3 Variable Bandwidth Filter (VBF) with Variable Gain

Physically, the variable bandwidth filter (VBF) can be implemented by combining time-varying resistors, time-varying capacitors and operational amplifiers. A time-varying capacitor can be manufactured by varactor diode, switched capacitor and MEMS capacitor [5][6]. MEMS capacitor of a metalized membrane (top electrode) suspended above a heavily doped silicon bulk (bottom electrode) has variable capacitance when it is pumped by a large signal voltage [5][6].

To be specific, we consider an example circuit composed of a time-varying capacitor $c(t)$ and a resistor $r(t)$ shown in Fig. 2(a). The $i-v$ relation of the circuit is described as follows:

$$\begin{aligned} i(t) &= i_r(t) + i_c(t) \\ &= c(t)Dv(t) + (1/r(t) + Dc(t))v(t) \\ &= g_1(t)Dv(t) + g_0(t)v(t), \qquad D = d/dt. \end{aligned} \tag{1}$$

That is, $i(t) = Gv(t)$, where $G = g_1(t)D + g_0(t)$, $g_1(t) = c(t)$ and $g_0(t) = 1/r(t) + Dc(t)$. In the circuit, we assume that $g_1(t)$ and $g_0(t)$ are changed independently by controlling $c(t)$ and $r(t)$. For notational simplicity, we denote $m_0(t)$ and $m_1(t)$ as

$$m_0(t) = \int_0^t g_0(\tau)/g_1(\tau)d\tau, \quad m_1(t) = \int_0^t 1/g_1(\tau)d\tau .$$

For frequency analysis of VBF, we define an extended Fourier transform (EFT) and an inverse EFT (IEFT) as follows:

$$\begin{aligned} \widetilde{F}[x(t), g_1(t), g_0(t)] &\equiv \int_{-\infty}^{\infty} [x(t)/g_1(t)]e^{-i\omega_{g1}m_1(t)+m_0(t)}dt \\ &= X(\omega_{g1}), \end{aligned} \tag{2}$$

$$\begin{aligned} \widetilde{F}^{-1}[X(\omega_{g1}), g_1(t), g_0(t)] &\equiv (1/(2\pi))e^{-m_0(t)}\int_{-\infty}^{\infty} X(\omega_{g1})e^{i\omega_{g1}m_1(t)}d\omega_{g1} \\ &= x(t). \end{aligned} \tag{3}$$

To conform that (3) is the inverse of the EFT of (2) symbolically, we consider a function $X(\omega_{g1}) = 1$. Then, let $X_n(\omega_{g1})$ be a sequence function such that

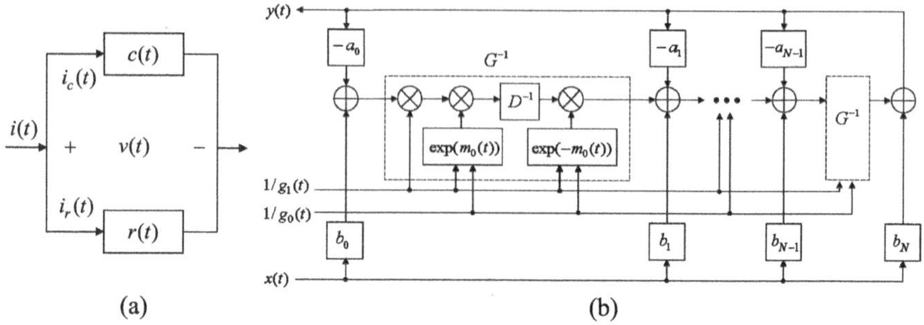

Fig. 2. Block diagrams of VBF circuits. (a) An example of elementary circuit G. (b) A canonical block diagram of VBF with variable gain.

$$X_n(\omega_{g1}) = X(\omega_{g1})\chi_{[-n,n]},$$

where $\chi_{[-n,n]}$ is the characteristic function of the interval $[-n,n]$. From (3), we obtain that

$$\begin{aligned} x_n(t) &= \widetilde{F}^{-1}[X_n(\omega_{g1}), g_1(t), g_0(t)] \\ &= \delta_n(m_1(t))\exp(-m_0(t)), \end{aligned}$$

where $\delta_n(m_1(t)) = \sin(m_1(t)n)/(m_1(t)\pi)$. The function $\delta_n(m_1(t))$ converges to the Dirac delta function $\delta(m_1(t))$ as n goes to ∞ if $m_1(t)$ is asymptotically proportional to t [7]. From (2), $\widetilde{F}[x_n(t), g_1(t), g_0(t)]$ converges to unity as n goes to ∞, that is,

$$\begin{aligned} \lim_{n\to\infty} \widetilde{F}[x_n(t), g_1(t), g_0(t)] &= \lim_{n\to\infty} \widetilde{F}[\widetilde{F}^{-1}[X_n(\omega_{g1}), g_1(t), g_0(t)], g_1(t), g_0(t)] \\ &= X(\omega_{g1}). \end{aligned}$$

This means that (3) is the inverse of EFT in (2) since $X_n(\omega_{g1})$ converges to $X(\omega_{g1}) = 1$ as n goes to ∞. A simple computation gives the following relation:

$$\widetilde{F}[G^k x(t), g_1(t), g_0(t)] = (i\omega_{g1})^k \widetilde{F}[x(t), g_1(t), g_0(t)],$$

where $G^k = G(G^{k-1})$ and $G^0 = G$. In (2), the function $\exp(m_0(t))$ is inside of the integral, whereas the function $\exp(-m_0(t))$ in (3) is outside of the integral. This means that VBF constructed by G has the variable gain $\exp(-m_0(t))$. The gain is controlled by $g_0(t)$ and the IB is controlled by $1/g_1(t)$. The notion on the operator $G = g_1(t)D + g_0(t)$ makes it possible to implement an amplifier with time-varying IB and time-varying gain that can lead to various applications in biomedical engineering.

Next, we derive a canonical block diagram of VBF as:

$$\sum_{k=0}^{N} a_k G^k y(t) = \sum_{k=0}^{N} b_k G^k x(t), \quad a_N = 1,$$

where $x(t)$ is the input and $y(t)$ is the output. For notational simplicity, let G^{-1} denote the abbreviation of $G^{-1}_{(-\infty,t]}$,

$$G^{-1}_{(-\infty,t]} x(t) = e^{-m_0(t)} \int_{-\infty}^{t} [x(\tau)/g_1(\tau)] e^{m_0(\tau)} d\tau.$$

Then, $G^{-1}Gx(t) = x(t)$ if $x(t)\exp(m_0(t))$ converges to zero as t goes to $-\infty$. A canonical block diagram of VBF with variable gain is shown in Fig. 2(b).

4 Estimation of Instantaneous Bandwidth of ECG Signal

For a band-limited signal $x(t)$ in the sense of EFT, the $1/g(t)$ is the IB of $x(t)$, if, and only if, $e(t) = x(t) - y(t)$ is equal to zero and $1/g(t)$ is minimal, where $y(t) = x(t) \otimes h(t)$ and $h(t)$ is the impulse response of VBF with $1/g(t)$. The symbol $\otimes$ represents the extended convolution operation [15] and $Y(\omega_g) = X(\omega_g)H(\omega_g)$. Since ECG signals are of nearly band-limited, we adopt this idea to derive an iterative routine for estimating IB of ECG. We consider a noisy ECG signal $x(t)$, which is measured during daily activities,

$$x(t) = s(t) + noise\,. \tag{4}$$

Processing the $x(t)$ directly for estimating IB, the noise may cause some large distortion to the estimate. To obtain a better estimate of IB, we use a less noisy T-periodic signal $r(t)$ (dashed curve) shown in Fig. 3(a), with zero mean and $T = 750$ [msec]. The peak of amplitude is equal to 100. The $r(t)$ is obtained by the off-line processing: (i) dividing a noisy ECG signal into RR segments, (ii) scaling width of each RR segment to mean width T, (iii) averaging the scaled RR segments over time, (iv) linking the average RR segment, and (v) denoising at level 5 based on Daubechy D1 wavelet.

Let $V = \{-MT,\cdots,0,T,\cdots,MT\}$ be R-peak instants of $r(t)$. In the iterative routine for estimating IB of $r(t)$, the $1/g_k(t)$ at the kth iteration is updated with the constraint (5),

$$(1/(2MT))\int_{-MT}^{MT} 1/g_k(t)dt = c_0\,, \quad k = 1,2,\cdots,K\,, \tag{5}$$

to the direction of decreasing the quantity P_k defined by

$$P_k = \max_t |e(t)|\,, \quad -MT \le t < MT\,, \tag{6}$$

where

$$e(t) = r(t) - y_k(t)\,. \tag{7}$$

With $1/g_k(t)$, the $y_k(t)$ is computed from VBF. The parameter c_0 is the mean value of the estimated IB. In the kth iteration, the $1/g_k(t)$ is revised with a step $\Delta_k(t)$ of (12) computed from $e(t)$ as follows:

$$1/g_k(t) = (c_0/c_k)(1/g_{k-1}(t) + \Delta_k(t))\,, \tag{8}$$

where

$$c_k = (1/(2MT))\int_{-MT}^{MT} [1/g_{k-1}(t) + \Delta_k(t)]dt\,, \quad c_0 = 1/g_0(t)\,.$$

Since $e(t)$ includes a part of ECG signal as well as noise and spectral band of $e(t)$ is fairly wide, the routine may fail to converge and which results in large estimation error. To avoid divergence of the routine, the step $\Delta_k(t)$ in (8) is computed through

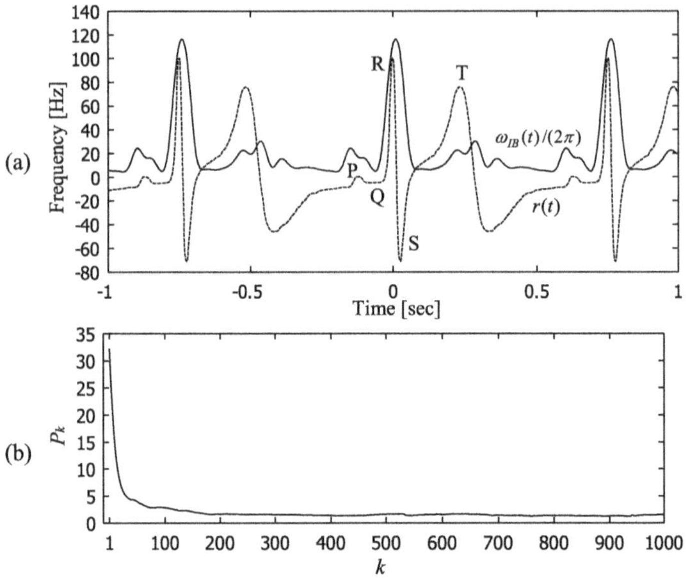

Fig. 3. Estimation of IB. (a) Estimated IB (solid curve) corresponding to P, Q, R, S and T waves of ECG (dashed curve). c_0=42π and σ_0=2π. (b) Peak error P_k vs. iteration number.

the off-line processing: (i) saturation, (ii) soft-threshold, (iii) normalization, and (iv) smoothing.

Let t_n denote the nth zero crossing of $e(t)$ and $\chi_{[t_n,t_{n+1})}$ denote the characteristic function of the interval $[t_n,t_{n+1})$. Then, we divide $e(t)$ into segments as follows:

$$e(t)=\sum_n e_n(t)\,,\qquad e_n(t)=e(t)\chi_{[t_n,t_{n+1})}\,.$$

Next, we compute the function

$$\bar{e}(t)=\sum_n \bar{e}_n(t)\,,\qquad \bar{e}_n(t)=\max_t(|\,e_n(t)\,|)\chi_{[t_n,t_{n+1})}\,. \tag{9}$$

That is, the amplitude of each segment $|\,e_n(t)\,|$ is saturated to its peak value to avoid introducing error due to high frequency noise to the estimate of IB. With the mean μ of $\bar{e}(t)$, we apply a soft-threshold operation to (9) and compute the function

$$\tilde{e}(t)=\sum_n \tilde{e}_n(t)\,, \tag{10}$$

where

$$\tilde{e}_n(t)=\begin{cases}\bar{e}_n(t)-\mu, & \text{if } \bar{e}_n(t)\geq\mu,\\ 0, & \text{otherwise,}\end{cases} \tag{11}$$

and $\mu=(1/(2MT))\int_{-MT}^{MT}\bar{e}(t)dt$. Let κ_n denote length of time support of the nth $\tilde{e}_n(t)$. Then, we normalize $\tilde{e}_n(t)$ with κ_n and compute the function

$$\hat{e}(t)=\sum_n \tilde{e}_n(t)/\kappa_n\,.$$

In the k th iteration, the step $\Delta_k(t)$ for updating $1/g_{k-1}(t)$ as (8) is computed as follows:

$$\Delta_k(t) = \sigma_0 \overline{\Delta}_k(t) / \max_t(\overline{\Delta}_k(t)), \qquad -MT \le t < MT , \tag{12}$$

where the parameter $\sigma_0 > 0$ is a step magnitude and $\overline{\Delta}_k(t)$ is a smoothed version of $\hat{e}(t)$ by a moving average filter using the Blackman window of width 100 [sec]. The operations on soft-threshold, normalization and smoothing avoid increasing $1/g_k(t)$ rapidly on the intervals with large noise. Finally, an estimate ${}^s\omega_{IB}(t)$ of one beat of IB corresponding to RR interval of $r(t)$ is obtained as follows:

$${}^s\omega_{IB}(t) = \omega_{IB}(t)\chi_{[0,T)} \,. \tag{13}$$

Figure 3 shows an estimated $\omega_{IB}(t)$ corresponding to $r(t)$ and Fig. 3(b) shows the variation of P_k. From Fig. 3, we find that the estimated IB for P, Q and T waves is below 30 [Hz]. This means that P, Q and T waves can be reconstructed without influence of power line interference and damage of QRS complex when VBF is used. Waveform on not only ECG but also IB is a personalized feature of the heart system. In the case of the subject, the end of T wave is vague and U wave is not observed. The onsets of P, Q, R and T waves and the ends of P, Q, S and T waves can be estimated reliably since the IB is very low near the onsets and the ends, if the estimated IB is used for cleaning noisy ECG signals.

5 Estimation of R-Peak Instants, Scaling and Synchronizing

Fluctuations of IHR disturb to obtain accurate estimate of R-peak instants. To reduce the estimation error, firstly, IHR is estimated through a running correlation operation between $x(t)$ of (4) and its segment that is updated continuously at every time instant. Secondly, a template including two RR segments is obtained from $r(t)$ shown in Fig. 3 and which is scaled with the estimate of IHR. Finally, R-peak instants are estimated through a cross-correlation operation between $x(t)$ and the scaled version of the template.

At every time instant t, the running correlation function $\Psi(t,\eta)$ is computed as follows:

$$\Psi(t,\eta) = \int_{-\infty}^{\infty} x(\tau)\, {}^s x_t(\tau-\eta) d\tau \,, \qquad -d \le \eta \le d \,, \tag{14}$$

where ${}^s x_t(\tau)$ is a segment of $x(\tau)$ and its time support is equal to $[t - W/2, t + W/2]$ centered at t. The constant W is taken as 2 seconds here, which includes two or three cardiac beats, typically. The segment ${}^s x_t(\tau)$ is updated continuously to cope with variation of the heart rate. For a fixed t, the $\Psi(t,\eta)$ has several peaks spaced almost equally along the η axis since ECG signal is quasi-periodic. Let $\eta_k(t)$ denote the trajectory of the k th peak of the $\Psi(t,\eta)$ on the $t-\eta$ plane. The function $1/\eta_1(t)$ is the forward IHR and the function $1/\eta_{-1}(t)$ is negative of the backward IHR.

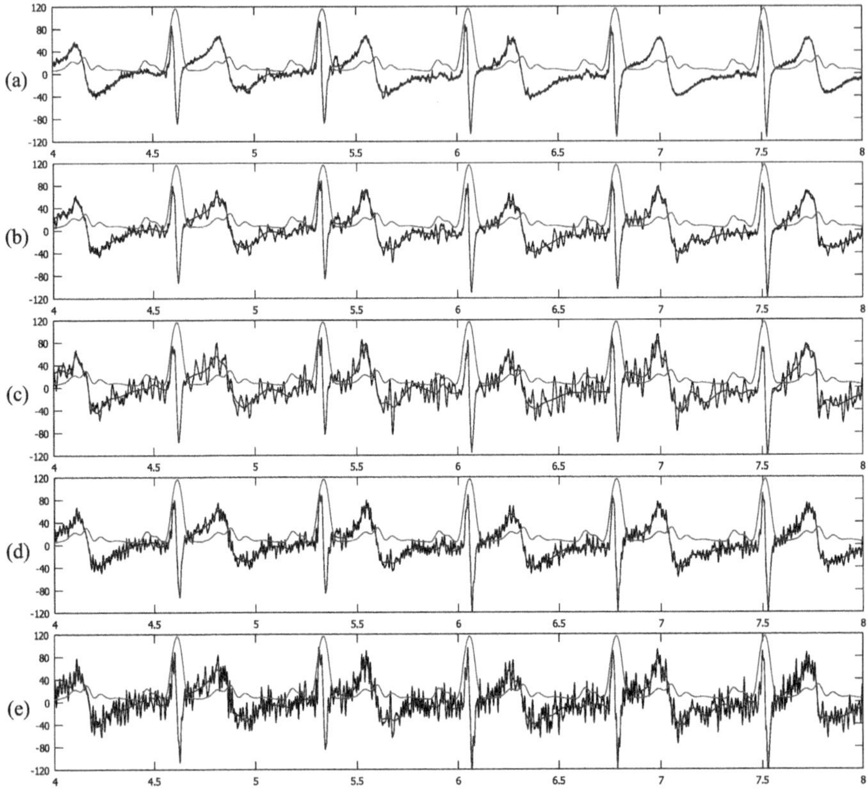

Fig. 4. Reconstructions of ECG signal. The unit of the horizontal axes is [sec]. (a) Reconstruction of ECG without adding noise. (b) With a white Gaussian noise limited to 50 [Hz], SNR=12 dB. (c) With a white Gaussian noise limited to 50 [Hz], SNR=6 dB. (d) With a white Gaussian noise limited to 100 [Hz], SNR=12 dB. (e) With a white Gaussian noise limited to 100 [Hz], SNR=6 dB.

For the cross-correlation operation in (16), we compute a template ${}^{s}r_0(t)$ centered at $t=0$ from $r(t)$, which includes two RR segments, as follows:

$$ {}^{s}r_0(t)={}^{s}r_{back}(t)+{}^{s}r_{forw}(t)\,, \qquad -T \le t < T\,, $$

where T is the RR interval. The ${}^{s}r_{back}(t)$ is the RR segment of $r(t)$ on interval $[-T,0)$ and the ${}^{s}r_{forw}(t)$ is the RR segment of $r(t)$ on interval $[0,T)$. To cope with fluctuations of IHR, the ${}^{s}r_0(t)$ is scaled with $\eta_1(t)$ and $\eta_{-1}(t)$ as follows:

$$ {}^{s}\bar{r}_t(\tau)={}^{s}r_{back}((\tau-t)(T/|\eta_{-1}(t)|))+{}^{s}r_{forw}((\tau-t)(T/\eta_1(t)))\,. \tag{15} $$

That is, every time instant t, the template ${}^{s}r_0(t)$ is shifted and scaled to fit it into instantaneous period of $x(t)$ in both directions of backward and forward. Then, R-peak instants $\bar{t}_n$ of $x(t)$ are computed from the peak of the cross-correlation function (16),

$$\Xi_X(t) = \int_{-\infty}^{\infty} x(\tau)^s \bar{r}_t(\tau) d\tau . \tag{16}$$

Finally, the $1/g(t)$ whose peaks are synchronized with R-peaks of $x(t)$ is constructed by shifting and scaling ${}^s\omega_{IB}(t)$ in (13)

$$1/g(t) = \sum_n {}^s\omega_{IB}(v_n t + \rho_n), \qquad 0 \le t < \infty , \tag{17}$$

where $v_n = T/(\bar{t}_{n+1} - \bar{t}_n)$ and $\rho_n = -v_n \bar{t}_n$.

Figure 4 shows five reconstructions of ECG computed by VBF with the $1/g(t)$ of (17). Figure 4(a) shows comparison of a reconstruction and a noisy ECG measured by the 24-hour continuous health monitoring system [4]. In Fig. 4(a), we find that VBF removes effectively noises without introducing severe distortions to the reconstructed signal.

Ordinarily, the spectral range of motion artifacts is in between 0 and 100 [Hz] [14]. For examining performance of the proposed method, we conduct four experiments under contaminating the measured ECG signal with white Gaussian noises, as shown in Fig. 4. Traditional methods based on LTI filter framework may fail to suppress noises in between 0 and 100 [Hz] without damaging QRS complex. The proposed method suppresses noises effectively included in P, Q and T waves without damaging QRS complex severely since IB ranges between 5 [Hz] and 30 [Hz] for P, Q and T waves.

6 Conclusions and Further Studies

In this manuscript, a study is conducted on reconstruction of a noisy ECG signal corrupted by motion artifacts whose spectra overlap with the spectrum of ECG. The proposed method based on the VBF improves the SNR of the P, Q, T and waves without damaging the QRS complex, different from, the method based on the LTI filter. The reduction of motion artifacts will enable us to estimate more accurately parameters such as onsets, ends, rates, intervals and durations on the six principal waves of ECG, which are used for diagnosing possible heart diseases.

The case study of application conducted in this manuscript demonstrates excellent feature extraction methods that can be used for a 24-hour continuous health monitoring system. One of the major goals of the investigations presented in this manuscript is to develop a method to diagnose and predict abnormal health states of the human body in real time during daily life. As demonstrated by our experiments based on the numerical model of VBF, the real time processing is promising if we use a hardware-defined VBF.

References

1. Otto, C., Milenkovic, A., Sanders, C., Jovanov, E.: System architecture of a wireless body area sensor network for ubiquitous health monitoring. J. Mobile Multimedia 1, 307–326 (2006)
2. Milenkovic, A., Otto, C., Jovanov, E.: Wireless sensor networks for personal health monitoring: issues and an implementation. Computer Communications 29, 2521–2533 (2006)

3. Stridh, M., Sornmo, L., Meurling, C.J., Olsson, S.B.: Characterization of atrial fibrillation using the surface ECG: time-dependent spectral properties. IEEE Tr. on Biomedical Engineering 48, 19–27 (2001)
4. Lee, H., Kim, Y., Jung, J.-W., Park, K.-H., Kim, D.-J., Bang, B., Bien, Z.: A 24-hour health monitoring system in a smart house. Gerontechnology 7, 22–35 (2008)
5. Raskin, J.-P., Brown, A.R., Khuri-Yakub, B.T., Rebeiz, G.M.: A novel parametric-effect MEMS amplifier. J. Microelectromechanical Systems 9, 528–537 (2000)
6. Girbau, D., Otegi, N., Pradell, L., Lazaro, A.: Study of intermodulation in RF MEMS variable capacitors. IEEE Tr. on Microwave Theory and Techniques 54, 1120–1130 (2006)
7. Arfken, G.B., Weber, H.J.: Mathematical Methods for Physicists. Academic Press, London (1995)
8. Almeida, R., Gouveia, S., Rocha, A.P., Pueyo, E., Martinez, J.P., Laguna, P.: QT variability and HRV interactions in ECG: quantification and reliability. IEEE Tr. on Biomedical Engineering 53, 1317–1329 (2006)
9. Task Force of The European Society of Cardiology and The North American Society of Pacing and Electrophysiology, "Heart rate variability,". European Heart Journal 17, 354–381 (1996)
10. Link, A., Endt, P., Steinhoff, U., Goedde, P., Trahms, L.: Analysis of QRS shape variability and short-term heart rate variability of CAD patients. Computers in Cardiology 25, 385–388 (1998)
11. Barros, A.K., Ohnishi, N.: Heart instantaneous frequency (HIF): an alternative approach to extract heart rate variability. IEEE Tr. on Biomedical Engineering 48, 850–855 (2001)
12. Kotani, K., Hidaka, I., Yamamoto, Y., Ozono, S.: Analysis of respiratory sinus arrhythmia with respect to respiratory phase. Methods of Information in Medicine 39, 153–156 (2000)
13. Ziarani, A.K., Konrad, A.: A nonlinear adaptive method of elimination of power line interference in ECG signals. IEEE Tr. on Biomedical Engineering 49, 540–547 (2002)
14. Hamilton, P.S., Curley, M.G., Aimi, R.M., Sae-Hau, C.: Comparison of methods for adaptive removal of motion artifact. Computers in Cardiology 27, 383–386 (2000)
15. Lee, H., Bien, Z.: On the eigenstructure of linear quasi-time-invariant systems. International Journal of Systems Science 29, 873–887 (1998)

Changing ICT for Client/Patient Management and Clinical Information in Residential and Community Aged Care Services in Regional Australia: Structured Interviews with Service Managers

Jeffrey Soar[1,*] and Rob Eley[2]

[1] Collaboration for Ageing & Aged-care Informatics Research, School of Information Systems, Faculty of Business, University of Southern Queensland, Australia
[2] Centre for Rural and Remote Area Health, University of Southern Queensland, Australia

Abstract

Aims: To determine the degree of change in investment in ICT (Information and Communication Technologies) in residential and community aged care services in regional Queensland.

Methodology: a convenience sample using structured telephone interviews of senior executives or managers of service providers

Findings: Aged care providers were found to have made significant recent investment in ICT. A major driver was to improve patient care. There were investments in clinical systems and systems for administration.

Summary: Aged care is not generally seen to be a sector that has taken advantage of ICT; that appears to be changing and there is now significant investment in clinical systems and other systems to assist staff in providing care.

Keywords: information technology, computing, aged care, seniors, workforce.

1 Introduction

The interest internationally in the adoption of ICT to assist in the delivery of care for the frail elderly [1] is shared in Australia. The aged and community care sector in Australia is facing many challenges including those related to rising consumer demand, workforce availability and skill levels, and providing services across the vast geographical spread of the aged care population and location of services. These challenges promote the need to investigate and implement new models of care delivery through ICT.

In 2009 a telephone survey was undertaken of residential and community aged care service managers across regional Queensland, a geographically large state with

* Corresponding author.

Y. Lee et al. (Eds.): ICOST 2010, LNCS 6159, pp. 113–120, 2010.

particular challenges of distance for serving remote communities. The aim of the research was to explore the level of use of ICT and recent changes that may have occurred in greater availability and adoption. A baseline for the survey was a national survey of nurses and ICT that was previously undertaken by the same authors [2] [3]. There was interest in refreshing this previous work to get an understanding of changes that may be occurring in ICT in aged care.

2 Ageing

Australia shares the concerns of most countries regarding the impact of an ageing population. Increasing pressures on health and aged care services are associated with the interest in new solutions for care planning and delivery.

Technology is anticipated to offer significant potential for equipping societies to respond to these pressures [4], [5]. Applications include assisting aged people in extending active and independent lives, maintaining consumer productivity, better managing and supporting the care workforce and in delivering and increasing the quality of care in home, community and residential care settings. Globally there is an increasing level of activities, strategy development, research projects, and adoptions of telecare, telehealth, smart homes and assistive technologies by consumers and care provider organisations [6]. Technologies offer an array of benefits including a reduction in hospital admissions and length of stay. [7], [8].

3 Technology

There is interest in better supporting aged care services to meet increasing challenges. There are particular issues of workforce availability and skilling. Few carers are supported by ICT tools for sharing of client information, communications with other members of the care team and for enhancing workforce productivity.

There is recognition of the potential for technology to enhance the safety and independence of frail older people, enable access to care services and to extend their ability to remain in lower levels of care such as their own home or other independent living arrangements. Intelligent monitors can keep a continuous watch on vital signs, activity patterns, their safety and security. The technology can monitor indicators of their state of health, provide alerts to events such as falls, and give early warnings of potential problems. The technology can notice changes in activities and alert a carer. Monitoring devices can be more accurate guides to the health risks such as a heart attack than are the patient's symptoms, providing advance warnings and reducing unnecessary emergency callouts [9]. Automation is expected to enhance security, safety and independence [10]. This could help maintain quality of life and decrease the demand for carer support hours.

There is much research or demonstration models with the aim of promoting the adoption of ICT for care [11], [12]. In a state of Australia a system of referrals away from hospital admission to community aged care is in use [13]. There are similar initiatives around most Australian health jurisdictions for managing Emergency

Department demand. Aged and Community Care service providers are actively investigating the use of assistive technologies to ensure effective service delivery.

Research into adoption issues, return on investment, realisation of benefits, integration and interoperability is required to ensure a sustainable system. Current evidence indicates that the level of adoption of technology in aged care services remains low. There appears to be many factors influencing this and these are seen to include awareness, attitudes to technology, design issues, telecommunications capacity, technical support, overall cost and uncertainty that benefits will be realised.

An indication of the extent of new technologies available to ageing services and related research is available from the web-site of the Center for Aging Services Technologies [14]. A new centre in Ireland, Technology Research for Independent Living (TRIL) is using ethnographic approaches to better understand seniors' attitudes to technology [15].

4 Residential and Community Aged Care Services

In Australia the frail aged can be supported in their own homes or in institutional settings. The latter include retirement villages which may provide minimal support such as security, social activities and some other services. RACFs (Residential Aged Care Facilities) or nursing homes offer two levels of care – low care for residents capable of some independence and high care for people needing help with many of the basic activities of daily living. The latter includes dementia wards. People needing support may also receive services in their own homes. RACFs and some aged care services in people's homes funded mostly by the federal Department of Health and Ageing subject to assessment of the individual. RACFs can be one of several owned by a large organization or can be independent. They can be for profit or not-for-profit. Major for profit operators include BUPA and Tricare; NFP includes Blue Care, RSL Care, Baptist Care, Lutheran Care and Spiritus.

5 Methodology

A purposive sample design was employed and a convenience sample of 50 aged care facilities were invited to participate with the aim of achieving a 50% or better response. Starting with facilities in and around the Queensland regional city of Toowoomba (which has a population of 100,000 people) the area was broadened to encompass most of rural and regional southern Queensland to achieve this desired number.

The project officer telephoned facility managers who were invited to participate in a 10 minute semi-structured telephone interview. Managers who agreed to participate were then sent the consent form by email or fax for signature and return. Of the 50 facilities that were contacted three declined. Of the 47 who agreed 30 were interviewed at their convenience. Data collection was stopped at 30 when data saturation had been reached.

6 Findings

Participants were asked about the use of IT applications for patient/client management. Responses to this question are given in Table 1. All but two facilities use their computers to generate care plans for patient management. Four of these had made no changes; the two facilities that did not use computers for patient management offered no further comment.

Table 1. Changes in patient/client management

	Type of Care Facility				Independent		Financial Status	
Change	High	Low	Both	Total	Yes	No	Profit	NFP
Yes	4*	2	18	24	6	17*	4	19*
No	0	1	5	6	2	4	0	6
Total	4	3	23	30	8	22	4	26

* Indicates the location of public facility response.

One facility noted their recent utilisation of "internet-based programs". Two that indicated partial use of the client management software commented "*to a certain extent*" and "*don't use resident care site; only [the] finance [part]*". One facility indicated that care plans were prepared on the computer but kept in hard copy. The one public facility contributing to the study also indicated partial use of their computerised patient management systems.

6.1 Use of IT Applications for Clinical Use

Only four facilities did not use this type of software and one of those had purchased the software but had not implemented it yet. Changes in IT applications for clinical use are given in Table 2. Of the 26 facilities that used the software 23 had implemented change. This also includes the one public facility interviewed. One respondent indicated that "*all carers have access*" to this system.

Table 2. Changes in clinical use

	Type of Care Facility				Independent		Financial Status	
Change	High	Low	Both	Total	Yes	No	Profit	NFP
Yes	3	3	17	23	10	13	4	19
No	1*	0	6	7	3	4*	0	7*
Total	4	3	23	30	13	17	4	26

* Indicates the location of public facility responses.

Five further comments were recorded from those using the software. One facility indicated they utilise incontinence software only and another indicated the use of eMIMS (a commonly-used medicines-reference database). Improvement in the use of clinical software was noted with three comments can be summed up by one respondent who noted "*Computers are now a big part of our clinical care*".

6.2 Requirement of Nursing Staff to Use Computers

Of the 30 facilities 17 stated that their staff were required to use computers (Table 3). One offered the comments that "*everybody has to use a computer as nothing is handwritten*". Two facilities noted that the requirement of nursing staff to use computers is dependent on the staff position. Both indicated that while registered staff (registered and enrolled nurses) were required to use computers this was not expected of the unregistered staff at assistant in nursing or personal carer level.

Table 3. Facilities requiring nursing staff to use computers

	Type of Care Facility				Independent		Financial Status	
Change	High	Low	Both	Total	Yes	No	Profit	NFP
Yes	1	2	14	17	7	10	2	15
No	3	1	7	11	5	6*	2	9*
Unsure	0	0	2	2	1	1	0	2
Total	4	3	23	30	13	17	4	26

* Indicates the location of public facility responses.

6.3 What Is the Driving Force (If Any) for Increased Adoption of IT?

Respondents were asked what is the driving force (if any) for increased adoption of IT. Four options were provided to this question with the opportunity also to add others. Comments were also solicited. Responses are tabulated in Table 4. In many cases more than one driving force for the increased adoption of IT was offered resulting in 68 responses from the 30 respondents. The public facility manager indicated all options.

Table 4. Driving force for the increased adoption of IT

	Type of Care Facility				Independent		Financial Status	
Change	High	Low	Both	Total	Yes	No	Profit	NFP
Patient	3	2	11	16	7	9	2	14
Patient administration	2	0	10	12	2	7	0	12
General administration	2	0	9	11	5	9	0	11
Parent Organization	1	1	11	13	0	13	0	13
Other	3	2	11	16	7	9	2	14

Patient care

Eight comments supported the 16 responses to this area and included improvement of systems whilst reducing paperwork which therefore enabled more hands on care to be administered. One respondent proposed that whilst patient care is the current driving force, originally IT was adopted in their facility to look more professional.

The adoption of IT has enabled all patient records to be kept together and it was also suggested that could also be increased if computers were available on trolleys to instantly record information as it is measured. One facility indicated that demands to better support patient care came from the medical professionals.

Patient administration

Of the twelve respondents who indicated they believed this was the driving force for IT, only one offered an additional comment. This comment reported that the introduction of IT has facilitated the ability to easily access patient notes and reports as well as referring to reports prepared by the patient's doctor. In addition adoption of IT enables the facility to get online and retrieve other important patient information.

General administration

Eleven respondents believed that general administration was a factor in the driving force for the increased adoption of IT. Two very different comments highlighted two areas of improvement that the adoption of IT has offered their facilities. One facility indicated it has reduced the amount of paperwork being produced which in turn has reduced the amount of storage space required to store this paperwork. The other facility proposed to use IT in their facility to monitor data for accreditation purposes.

Directives from parent organisations

Of the 17 facilities interviewed that were representative of a larger organisation, 13 believed that the increased adoption of IT was the initiative of their governing body. One of these facilities however indicated that the directive from the parent organisation was not solely responsible for their improvement in IT. They noted that staff time management had been improved as there is no longer the need for manual reporting. One interviewee felt that if parent organisations did not promote advances in IT then facilities would not effect changes.

Other

A total of 16 other responses were recorded and presented in Table 15. In addition to presenting a professional appearance, one respondent also believed that in future the level of IT adopted in the workplace may be a determining factor in where staff decides to seek employment. In addition this respondent also indicated that IT may provide an 'edge' for facilities to promote themselves. One individual proposed that

Table 5. Other comments described as the driving force for the adoption of IT

Comment description	Number
Efficiency or time management associated with better provision of professional care services.	6
Provides the ability to link with other organisations or health care professionals.	2
Facilitates communication between accrediting bodies regarding current compliance and regulatory directives.	2
Keeping informed of constant advances in technology in aged care and other related industries.	2
Present a professional appearance.	2

IT will be used to keep up-to-date with current advancements in aged care. It was also indicated by one respondent that having staff that are confident as well as proactive in the use of IT is integral to its implementation within a facility. One facility described their initial integration of IT into their facility was a direct result of government funding, and that despite this the adoption of IT is now centred on clinical care.

7 Conclusion

Most people have become familiar with and have adapted to technologies that are now pervasive across industries. This research set out to refresh previous research and to determine the degree of change in investment in ICT in residential and community aged care services in regional Queensland. A convenience sample using structured telephone interviews of senior executives or managers of service providers was undertaken.

The research found that aged care providers have made significant recent investment in ICT. A major driver was to improve patient care. There were investments in clinical systems and systems for administration. Aged care is not generally seen to be a sector that has taken advantage of ICT; that appears to be changing and there is now significant investment in clinical systems and other systems to assist staff in providing care.

References

[1] Essen, A., Conrick, M.: Visions and realities: developing 'smart' homes for seniors in Sweden. eJHI - electronic Journal of Health Informatics 2(1), e2

[2] Eley, R., Fallon, A.B., Soar, J., Buikstra, E., Hegney, D.: Nurses' confidence and experience in using information technology. Australian Journal of Advanced Nursing 25(3), 23–35 (2008)

[3] Eley, R., Fallon, A.B., Soar, J., Buikstra, E., Hegney, D.: Barriers to use of information and computer technology by Australia's nurses: a national survey. Journal of Clinical Nursing 18, 1151–1158 (2008)

[4] Bowes, A., McColgan, G.: West Lothian Interim Report, West Lothian Council and the Department of Applied Social Science, University of Stirling (2005)

[5] Soar, J.: Information Management in Modern Healthcare Organisations. In: Proceedings IBIMA, Marrakesh, Morocco, January 4-6 (2008)

[6] CSCI 2006, Time to Care? An overview of home care services for older people in England, report published by Commission for Social Care Inspection, London (October 2006), http://www.csci.org.uk

[7] Soar, J., Livingstone, A., Wang, S.-Y.: A Case Study of an Ambient Living and Wellness Management Health Care Model in Australia. In: Mokhtari, M., Khalil, I., Bauchet, J., Zhang, D., Nugent, C. (eds.) ICOST 2009. LNCS, vol. 5597, pp. 48–56. Springer, Heidelberg (2009)

[8] Darkins, A., Ryan, P., Kobb, R., Foster, L., Edmonson, E., Wakefield, B., Lancaster, A.E.: Care Coordination/Home Telehealth: The Systematic Implementation of Health Informatics, Home Telehealth, and Disease Management to Support the Care of Veteran Patients with Chronic Conditions. In: Telemedicine and e-Health, December 2008, pp. 1118–1126 (2008)

[9] Soar, J., Seo, Y.: Health and Aged Care Enabled by Information Technology. Annals of the New York Academy of Sciences 1114, 154–161 (2007)
[10] Philipson, G., Roberts, J.: Caring for the future: The impact of technology on aged and assisted living (Invited Paper). eJHI - electronic Journal of Health Informatics 2(1), e3 (2007)
[11] Bowes, A., McColgan, G.: Smart technology at home: users' and carers' perspectives, Interim report, by Department of Applied Social Science. University of Stirling (February 2005)
[12] SOPRANO - Service-oriented Programmable Smart Environments for Older Europeans, `http://www.soprano-ip.org/` (accessed December 5, 2008)
[13] Soar, J., Yuginovich, T., Whittaker, F.: Reducing avoidable hospital admissions of the frail elderly using intelligent referrals. eJHI - electronic Journal of Health Informatics 2(1), e3 (2007)
[14] CAST, Center for Ageing Services Technologies, `http://www.agingtech.org` (accessed January 28, 2009)
[15] TRIL, Technology Research for Independent Living, `http://www.trilcentre.org/` (accessed January 28, 2009)

An Action-Based Behavior Model for Persuasive Telehealth

Duckki Lee[1], Sumi Helal[1], and Brian David Johnson[2]

[1] Mobile & Pervasive Computing Laboratory, Computer & Information Science & Engineering Department, University of Florida, Gainesville, FL 32611, USA
{dlee,helal}@cise.ufl.edu
[2] Digital Home Group, INTEL, 20270 NW AmberGlen Ct., AG1-112
Beaverton, OR 97006
brian.david.johnson@intel.com

Abstract. Technological advances in telehealth systems are primarily focused on sensing, monitoring and analysis. Intervention, behavior alternation and in general affecting change could use additional research and technology development. Many people, especially the elderly, are resistant to change. Such resistance diminishes the impact factor of telehealth systems. Persuasion technology and mechanisms are urgently needed to counter this resistance to change and promote healthy lifestyle. In this paper, we propose an action- based behavior model to enable persuasion. We also review existing technologies we believe are most suitable for enabling persuasive telehealth. We present our ongoing work in the domain of behavior alteration for obese and diabetic individuals.

Keywords: Remote monitoring and intervention, behavior alteration, persuasive computing, persuasive technology, persuasive telehealth, behavior change theory, behavior change model.

1 Introduction

Advances in healthcare have led to longer life expectancy so that the elderly population is increasing rapidly. By 2030, the number of US adults aged 65 years or older will more than double to about 71 million. Moreover, about 80% of the elderly age with at least one chronic condition and 50% age with at least two. Chronic diseases disproportionately affect older adults and are associated with disability, diminished quality of life, and increased costs for health care and long-term care [3]. Many elderly people prefer independent living without caretakers. Industry and academia put forth considerable effort to support independent living as well as to provide cost-effective solutions for successful healthy aging [1,2,4,5,6,8,9].

Telehealth systems are a cost-effective approach that could support independent living. However, many of these systems are asymmetric - they mostly provide capabilities to monitor and collect medical data but offer very limited means to affect change or alter the user behavior. Research for sensing, monitoring and tele-care has been conducted for over a decade and has recently matured. What remains to be

Y. Lee et al. (Eds.): ICOST 2010, LNCS 6159, pp. 121–129, 2010.

urgently needed is research and supportive technology to enable effective intervention. Simple and naïve approaches for intervention and behavior alteration do not seem to work (e.g. just telling what people need to do). What we really need is persuasive power to make this intervention and behavior alteration more effective.

In order to help break initial research barriers, we propose an action-based behavior model that promotes persuasion and the use of persuasive technologies. We present existing telehealth systems and discuss their limitations before we introduce our model. We then review promising technologies for persuasive telehealth and briefly discuss our ongoing work in persuasive telehealth in the domain of obesity and diabetes.

2 Present Telehealth Systems and Limitations

Personal medical devices are highly available and affordable and their accuracy of measurement is improving. Thanks to emerging standards such as the Continua Health Alliance [4], building highly interoperable telehealth systems using personal medical devices is becoming a pleasant reality. This will hopefully lead to improved quality of care. Also, there have been joint efforts between industry and academia on middleware enablers for telehealth systems. For instance, STEPSTONE [2] is a joint project between IBM and the University of Florida to create technology that would enable the scalable, "friction-free" integration of device-based healthcare solutions into enterprise systems using a Service Oriented Device Architecture (SODA) [7].

The Center for Connected Health [8], a division of Partners HealthCare in Boston, develops innovative and effective solutions for delivering quality patient care outside of the traditional medical setting. Two representative efforts for health record interoperation are Microsoft Healthvault [5] and Google Health [6]. Through these two web portals (services), patients can easily manage their health records and share them with medical professionals. In Europe, the EU funds programs such as the Ambient Assistive Living (AAL) [9] to enhance the quality of life for older people and strengthen the industrial base in Europe through the use of Information and Communication Technologies (ICT).

However, many present telehealth systems are limited in that they only emphasize sensing and monitoring. Some system even utilized social networks as a collective sensor [1]. While sensing and monitoring are crucial and important, we believe that intervention and behavior alteration for affecting changes are equally important and need to be further developed and researched. One possible reason behavior alteration is not adequately addressed is because we don't have powerful tools for persuasion and affecting change. Another reason could simply be that it is difficult for computer scientists to understand the necessary behavioral and social theory. Obviously, social and behavioral scientists are domain experts who understand the theory, the clinical practice and how to perform outcome assessments. However, these two communities need to collaborate more closely to create more effective telehealth systems.

3 A Framework for Persuasive Telehealth

Most telehealth systems follow the framework shown in Figure 1, with the exception that intervention is assumed to be simply informing and advising the user. In this framework we explicitly define the necessary steps and processes of this framework. We emphasize the intervention step in preparation for presenting our action-based model in the next section. The framework consists of 6 steps or stages as shown in Figure 1. We next described each stage in some details.

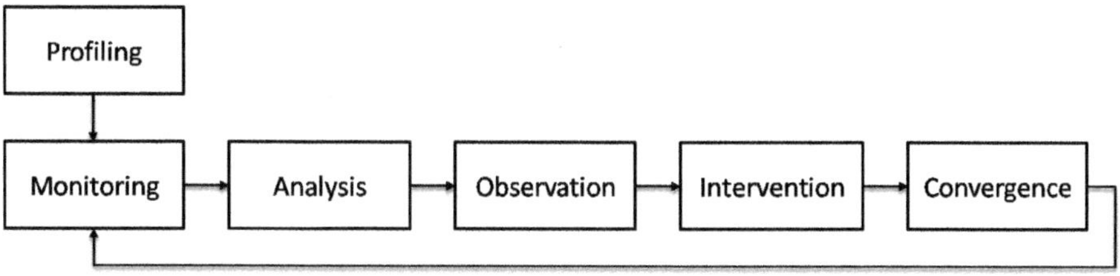

Fig. 1. A Framework for Persuasive Telehealth

Profiling. In this stage, user information and domain-specific knowledge are collected. User information is any predefined or existing information related to the user such as age, gender, medical history, disabilities, chronic conditions, preference/interest, among other parameters. Domain-specific knowledge gives guidelines for analysis. Without this stage, the system would struggle to infer this information dynamically using error-prone machine learning techniques.

Monitoring. Data most pertinent to a specific domain is monitored through a sensory sub-system. This data could range from physical statuses (e.g., vital signs, level and type of activities, food consumption, etc.) to mental statuses (e.g., mood, feeling, etc.) Monitoring of the environment and other non-user conditions could also be pertinent to the goal of the telehealth system.

Analysis. Domain-specific analysis is performed based on the gathered data from the monitoring stage qualified by the personalized/customized information of the end user. For example, daily caloric expenditure could be calculated from analysis of activities over the day based on a patient's height and weight. In order to analyze raw sensed data, some level of domain knowledge of that data is required.

Observation. Domain experts (e.g., medical professionals) diagnose current user health status, behavior and areas of concerns by drawing conclusions out of the analyzed data. Such observations should drive the specifics of what needs to be changed.

Intervention. Many behavior theories and models emphasize the importance of motivation and ability [15,16,17,18,19,20,21,22,23,24,25]. Fogg states that three factors (motivation, ability and trigger) are necessary for behavior change in his behavior model [11,26]. In our action based behavior model in section 4, we utilize Fogg's work in the intervention process along with other popular persuasion approaches such as goal setting and rewarding.

Convergence. Here, outcome assessment is performed and a determination is made if any behavior change has actually materialized. Convergence to the desired goals of the telehealth system will be measured by the change of the user behavior and status over time. Based on assessment outcomes, adaptation rules are applied in an attempt to stimulate convergence.

4 Action-Based Behavior Model

Existing behavior change theories and models [15,16,17,18,19,20,21,22,23,24,25] explain how people change their behaviors. Each theory and model focuses on different factors such as self-efficacy, intention, social, environmental and personal factors. However, these models are not easily utilizable as is by health Telematics researchers especially engineering and computer scientists. In this paper we contribute a behavior change model that we believe is more palatable and utilizable by the health Telematics researcher community. The model is based on collective knowledge we gained by studying the various social and behavioral science theory. Specifically, we propose an Action-based Behavior Model (ABM) that focuses on the intervention and convergence processes in the framework presented in section 3.

In this model, we first increase the users' awareness about their conditions by informing them about their current health status. This should increase their motivation by giving them the reasons for change. Next, we set goals. In this stage, we can utilize several types of goal setting: self-setting, assigned, participatory [13], as well as guided and group setting [14]. This process makes the user understand the details of the goals and the benefits of achieving them. Then, we educate the patients about how to achieve the goals. The next stage is reminding the user to act toward the goal. Even if the user is highly motivated and is capable to act and achieve the goal, he/she might simply forget. There are two manifestations to the reminding process. The first reminds the user to get him/her started acting towards the goal. The second is released gradually while achieving the goal, to let the users know their progress toward the goals so they know where they stand. The final step is rewarding based on the achievement progress. Rewarding can be intrinsic (e.g., praise), extrinsic (e.g., gifts, credit, gift cards) or virtual reward (e.g. virtual credit as well practiced in game).

In our proposed ABM model shown in Figure 2, each step (represented as a rectangle) is an action and a state, which can be easily understood and applied to the technological intervention channel. The model partitions the telehealth system into a cyber system and a set of user actions. The cyber part is further divided into cyber sensing and a cyber influence parts to sense and influence exactly the set of actions prescribed by our model. The possible influence "acts" that our model can prescribe are currently being finalized and include: *inform, exemplify, simulate (e.g., play of what if scenarios) [27], tailor, educate, remind, monitor, morally support, analyze and observe*. These acts are shown above the influence/sense arrows in Figure 2. Some acts may support different actions. For instance, simulation increases self and goal awareness and provides effective education through virtual experience.

In our model, cyber sense learns about the user's actions (or inactions) and in general senses any relevant vitals and status information. It also learns once (initially) about the user profile and preferences. Cyber influence, on the other hand, is where technological channels are used to manufacture controlled persuasion, of course within ethical guidelines [12]. Actions in the model consist of human actions (solid rectangles) and cyber actions (dotted rectangles). The intuition behind our model is that we designed it so that we guarantee progress of persuasion factors as the user (guided by the cyber system) steps through it. In fact, each human (and one cyber) action increases persuasion through one or more of its elements [11] (motivation, ability and trigger). Figure 2 shows which element is contributed to by which action (see Figure legend).

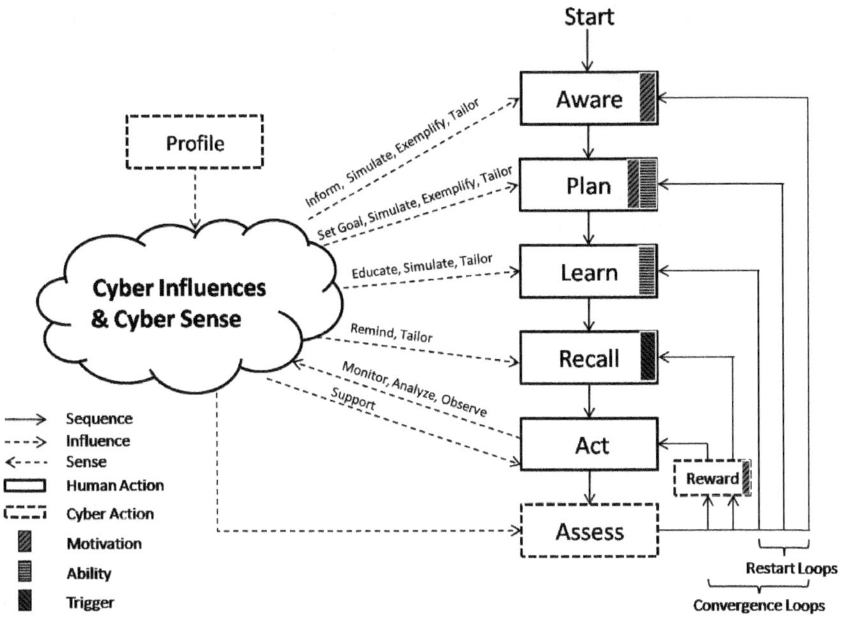

Fig. 2. Action-based Behavior Model

From "Start", a user goes through each step's action from Aware to Act. Cyber influence will affect and help the user to make each action. While the user acts toward the goals, cyber sense will monitor, analyze and observe the user's action. After some rounds of acting, the Assess cyber action will evaluate the achievements of the goals and will guide the user to either continue, or rolls the user back to the appropriate action based on the achievement and deficit of each action. For positive achievements, the Reward cyber action may give intrinsic, extrinsic or virtual rewards to reinforce the motivation.

5 Promising Technologies for Persuasive Telehealth

Successful implementation of our proposed Action-based Behavior Model relies on an effective technology to implement the cyber influence and to achieve persuasion. We review existing technologies and discuss their suitability for persuasion.

House calls (old fashion care) and AVR (Automated Voice response) are not adequate for persuasion and intervention. There are not enough health care professionals to make house calls, and if they do, there are no guarantees the user is available at the time of call or that the user will be persuaded. AVR had always been confusing and require much more patience than many users can afford.

Web portals are a pull technology that requires the user's attention and initiative to use. They can convey much more accurate and personalized data, but they pose challenges to usability especially for those who do not or cannot use computers (e.g., certain disabilities or older adults). Mobile messaging (e.g., SMS) could be used as a technology channel for persuasion but again, messages can get ignored especially as the user gets overwhelmed with the management of these messages (reading, deleting, etc).

Domestic robots (Figure 3) are a new technology that we have recently evaluated and which we consider to be a promising persuasive technology for persuasive telehealth. A recent survey of domestic robots can be found in [28]. Let us first describe domestic robots' unique features compared to other devices. One of the reasons some technologies are difficult to use in persuasion is because they require user to spend effort learning and getting familiarized with the technologies. Domestic robots are much easier to use through their natural human-like communication, which is not only easy but also fun (pleasure) to use them. Their friendliness create an emotional link and makes the user (e.g., elderly) more comfortable using them. Domestic robots are in fact effective informers, educators, reminders and even readers of the users' feelings and thoughts, which are hard to detect by other devices.

Social networks can be an effective tool to set the right goal and find solution for many problems or hindrances toward completing the goal. The problems or hindrances could be related to many different fields that require experts who have different knowledge and background. Social networks can be the cheapest way to bring experts like doctors, psychologists and nutritionists with friends and family of patients. If we utilize this social network effect well, then social networks could be a powerful persuasive tool. In this case, the domestic robot interacts with and abstracts the social network to the user.

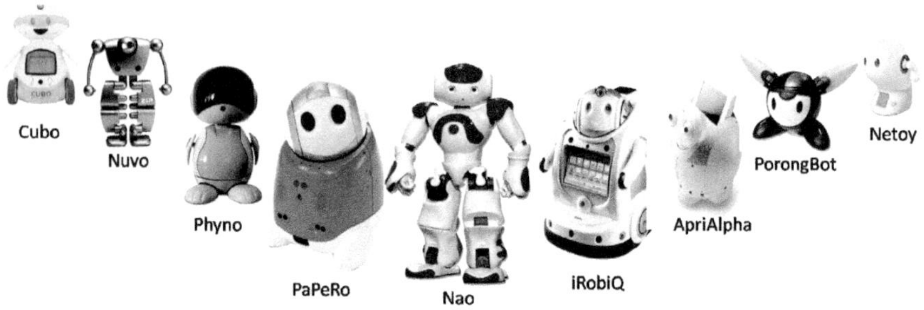

Fig. 3. Robotic Companions

6 Persuasive System for Obese and Diabetic Patients

We are currently working on a Persuasive Healthcare Framework for obesity and diabetes management, a project funded by the National Institutes of Health (NIH). The framework employs robots and social networks, which will be deployed in the Gator Tech Smart House (GTSH) [10], a real-world test-bed for persuasive telehealth field studies. Figure 4 shows the architecture of the Framework.

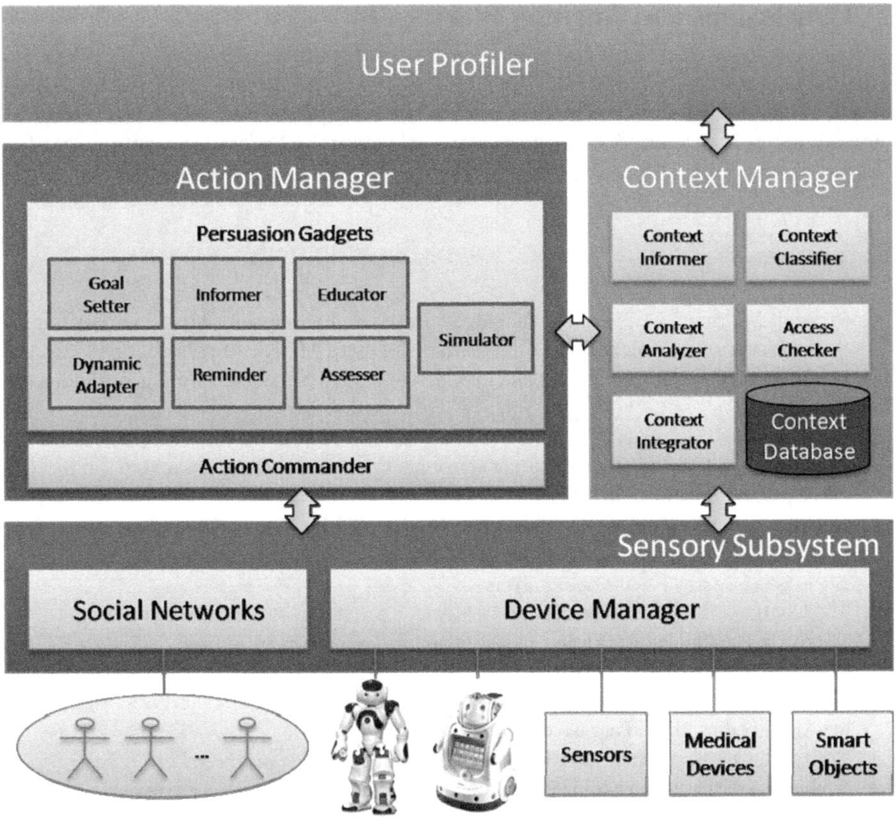

Fig. 4. Persuasive Healthcare Framework

From the bottom, the sensory subsystem consists of Social Networks and Device Manager. Social Networks are utilized for goal setting and dynamic adaptation. Caregivers such as physicians, nurses or psychologists as well as family, friends and/or neighbors who are close to the user can individually or collaboratively assist in setting the appropriate goals. Device Manager controls all different kinds of devices including medical devices, smart objects and domestic robots. They provide significant sensing capability to the cyber system. It also provides raw context information to the Context Manager in the higher layers.

Context Manager consists of components for integrating, analyzing, informing and classifying contexts and controlling access for security and privacy. Context Integrator gathers raw context information from the Device Manager and synthesizes it to make additional contexts. The Context Analyzer uses contexts from Context Integrator and derives or infers contexts through context reasoning.

The Action Manager consists of Persuasion Gadgets and Action Commander. The gadgets correspond to the influence acts used by the cyber influence system. The Action Commander puts acts in motion by coordinating the sensing and the act interactions with the user.

7 Conclusions and Ongoing Work

This paper presented a framework for Persuasive Telehealth and proposed an Action-based Behavior Model (ABM) to support behavior alteration. Also, we briefly reviewed technologies suitable for persuasive telehealth and provided a summary of an ongoing research in persuasive telehealth in the domain of obesity and diabetes.

References

1. Weitzel, M., Smith, A., Lee, D., Deugd, S., Helal, S.: Participatory Medicine: Leveraging Social Networks in Telehealth Solutions. In: Mokhtari, M., Khalil, I., Bauchet, J., Zhang, D., Nugent, C. (eds.) ICOST 2009. LNCS, vol. 5597, pp. 40–47. Springer, Heidelberg (2009)
2. Helal, A., Bose, R., Chen, C., Smith, A., de Deugd, S., Cook, D.: STEPSTONE: A SODA Case Study in Personal Tele-Health Management. Submitted to the Journal of Ambient Int elligence and Smart Environments
3. Healthy Aging: Improving and Extending Quality of Life Among Older Americans: At a Glance (2009), `http://www.cdc.gov/chronicdisease/resources/publications/AAG/aging.htm`
4. The Continua Health Alliance, `http://www.continuaalliance.org`
5. Microsoft Health Vault, `http://www.healthvault.com`
6. Google Health, `https://health.google.com/health`
7. de Deugd, S., Carroll, R., Kelly, K.E., Millett, B., Ricker, J.: SODA: Service-Oriented Dev ice Architecture. IEEE Pervasive Computing 5, 94–97 (2006)
8. The Center for Connected Health, `http://www.connected-health.org`
9. Ambient Assisted Living Joint Programme, `http://www.aal-europe.edu/`
10. Helal, S., Mann, W., Zabadani, H., King, J., Kaddoura, Y., Jensen, E.: The Gator Tech Sm art House: A Programmable Pervasive Space. IEEE Computer 38, 50–60 (2005)
11. Fogg, B.J.: A behavior model for persuasive design. In: PERSUASIVE (2009)
12. Berdichevsky, D., Neunschwander, E.: Towards an Ethics of Persuasive Technology. Com munications of the ACM 42(5), 51–58 (1999)
13. Locke, E.A., Latham, G.P.: Building a Practically Useful Theory of Goal Setting and Task Motivation: A 35-Year Odyssey. American Psychologist 57(9), 705–717 (2002)
14. Shilts, M.K., Horowitz, M., Townsend, M.S.: Goal Setting as a Strategy for Dietary and Ph ysical Activity Behavior Change: A Review of the Literature. American Journal of Health Promotion 19(2), 81–93 (2004)
15. Glanz, K., Rimer, B.K., Lewis, F.M.: Health Behavior and Health Education. In: Theory, Research and Practice. Wiley & Sons, San Fransisco (2002)
16. Becker, M.H. (ed.): The health belief model and personal health behavior. Health Educ. M onogr. 2, 324–508 (1974)
17. Rosenstock, I.: Historical Origins of the Health Belief Model. Health Education Monograp hs 2(4) (1974)
18. Prochaska, J.O., Velicer, W.F., Rossi, J.S., Goldstein, M.G., Marcus, B.H., et al.: Stages of change and decisional balance for 12 problem behaviors. Health Psychol. 13(1), 39–46 (1994)
19. Prochaska, J.O., DiClemente, C.C., Norcross, J.C.: Search of how people change applicati ons to addictive behaviors. American Psychologist 47(9), 1102–1114 (1992)

20. Sbeppard, B.H., Hartwick, J., Warshaw, P.R.: The theory of reasoned action: A meta- anal ysis of past research with recommendations for modifications and future research. Journal of Consumer Research 15, 325–343 (1988)
21. Fishbein, M.: A Theory of Reasoned Action: Some Applications and Implications. In: Ho we, H., Page, M. (eds.) Nebraska Symposium on Motivation, pp. 65–116. University of Ne braska Press, Lincoln (1980)
22. Ajzen, I.: The Theory of Planned Behavior. Organizational Behavior and Human Decision Processes. Special Issue: Theories of Cognitive Self-Regulation 50(2), 179–211 (1991)
23. Mearns, J.: Social learning theory. In: Reis, H., Sprecher, S. (eds.) Encyclopedia of human relationships, vol. 3, pp. 1537–1540. Sage, Thousand Oaks (2009)
24. Bandura, A.: Social cognitive theory: An agentive perspective. Annual Review of Psychol ogy 52, 1–26 (2001)
25. Rotter, J.B.: The development and applications of social learning theory. Prentice Hall, En glewood Cliffs (1982) (selected papers)
26. Fogg, B.J.: Persuasive Technology: Using Computers to Change What We Think and Do. Morgan Kaufmann Publishers, CA (2003)
27. King, P., Tester, J.: The Landscape of Persuasive Technologies. Communications of the A CM 42(5), 51–58 (1999)
28. Lee, D., Yamazaki, T., Helal, S.: Robotic Companions for Smart Space Interactions. IEEE Pervasive Computing 8(2), 78–84 (2009)

Real-Time Monitoring of Potential Effects of Neuroprotection by Acupuncture in Global Ischemic Model of Hyperglycemic Rats

Samjin Choi[1], Gi-Ja Lee[1], Su-Jin Chae[1], Sung Wook Kang[1], Seok Keun Choi[2], Seung-Hoon Lee[3], Jeong-Hoon Park[1], Kyung-Sook Kim[1], Ilsung Cho[1], and Hun-Kuk Park[1,4,*]

[1] Department of Biomedical Enginerring, College of Medicine, Kyung Hee University, 1 Hoegi-dong, Dongdaemun-gu, Seoul 130-701, South Korea
[2] Department of Neurosurgery, Kyung Hee University Medical Center, Seoul, South Korea
[3] Department of Acupuncture and Moxibustion, College of Oriental Medicine, Kyung Hee University Medical Center, Seoul, South Korea
[4] Program of Medical Enginerring, Kyung Hee University, Seoul, South Korea
sigmoidus@khu.ac.kr

Abstract. Acupuncture is known to be effective in ischemia treatment, and glutamate excitotoxicity is an important factor in neuronal cell death. We observed the effect of acupuncture on cerebral blood flow and Δglutamate in the ischemic stroke rat model of hyperglycemia. A global ischemia was induced using the eleven vessel occlusion method in ten Sprague-Dawley rats: the control group and the acupuncture-treatment group. Extracellular Δglutamate was assessed using an intra-cerebral biosensor system measuring 256-Hz sampling frequency, simultaneously with cerebral blood flow and electroencephalogram. Acupuncture stimulation was applied to acupuncture points, Yang Tomb Spring (GB34) and Suspended Bell (GB39) during the ischemic period. 23 diagnostic parameters were proposed first for a detailed analysis of changes in cerebral blood flow and glutamate release during ischemia and reperfusion. Acupuncture rats showed a significant decrease in ischemic ($p < 0.05$) and reperfusion cerebral blood flows ($p < 0.0001$) than control rats, and a significantly larger decrease in ischemic Δglutamate ($p < 0.05$) and peak level of reperfusion Δglutamate ($p < 0.005$) than control rats. From these results, we suggest that acupuncture stimulation is responsible for the potential protection of neurons through suppression of %cerebral blood flow response in the increased plasma osmolality and extracellular Δglutamate in diabetic rats under ischemic conditions.

Keywords: Acupuncture; Eleven vessel occlusion animal model; Ischemic condition; Hyperglycemia; Glutamate; Cerebral blood flow.

1 Introduction

Acupuncture, an ancient art derived from East Asian medical tradition, has been one of the primary modalities applied to stroke patients in Korea. Reports on acupuncture

* Corresponding author.

Y. Lee et al. (Eds.): ICOST 2010, LNCS 6159, pp. 130–137, 2010.

in the medical literature have been anecdotal [1]. Based on its widespread use, promising results, relatively fewer severe adverse effects, relatively low cost, and the insufficient quality of past research, a recent review recommended further research on acupuncture for stroke rehabilitation [2].

Hyperglycemia was reported to lead to an increase in morphologic brain damage and severity of neurologic deficits in animal models of global ischemia [3]. In addition, pre-ischemic hyperglycemia aggravates brain damage caused by transient global or forebrain ischemia [4]. Several studies have concluded that hyperglycemia can be an independent risk factor for cerebrovascular events in diabetes. However, because the role of glucose concentration and neurological damage during brain ischemia in diabetes is not completely understood, the effects of hyperglycemia on ischemia are controversial [5].

In this study, we observed the potential effects of manual acupuncture on cerebral blood flow (CBF) and extracellular glutamate concentration throughout induction of ischemic and reperfusion conditions in hyperglycemic rats, using a ten-minute eleven vessel occlusion (11VO) rat model. Changes in glutamate release were monitored with electroencephalography (EEG) and two channels CBF.

2 Materials and Methods

2.1 Animal Preparation

Male Sprague-Dawley rats (225 ± 25 g) were used in the experiment, and were housed in a 22-24°C and 12hr light/dark cycle controlled environment. The animals were fed commercial rat chow and water ad libitum. Adequate injection and anesthesia were planned as a measure to minimize pain or discomfort. All animal use procedures were approved by the Ethical Committee of the Kyung Hee University College of Medicine and were in strict accordance with the National Institutes of Health Guide for the Care and Use of Laboratory Animals.

Hyperglycemia was induced by a single intraperitoneal injection of streptozocin (Sigma Chemical, St Louis, Mo, USA), which was freshly dissolved in a 0.1 M citrate buffer at pH 4.5 and delivered at a dose of 60 mg/kg body weight. Blood glucose levels and body weights were determined 48 hr after streptozocin injection. Animals with a blood glucose concentration > 300 mg/dl were assigned to the hyperglycemic group. There were two experimental groups; five hyperglycemic rats without acupuncture treatment (control group) and five hyperglycemic rats with acupuncture treatment (acupuncture group).

2.2 Monitoring Setup

Animals were anesthetized with an intraperitoneal injection of 350 mg/kg chloral hydrate. Rectal temperature was maintained regularly at 37.1°C using a heating pad. An 11VO was used as the global ischemia model [6]. After dividing the omohyoid muscle, a pair of occipital arteries, the superior hypophyseal artery, ascending pharyngeal artery, and pterygopalatine artery were coagulated with bipolar electrocautry. The ventral clivus just caudal to the basioccipital suture was then drilled and exposed to a 3-mm diameter. Next, the basilar artery was permanently coagulated. Rats were placed in prone position using a stereotactic frame, and the skin was incised with a midline along the superior sagittal suture. Eight burr holes were made for real-time measurements of brain temperature, two channels EEG, glutamate release, and two channels CBF. In detail, two burr holes were made 4-mm apart from the midline and 1-mm in front of the coronal suture for insertion of probes for glutamate and brain temperature. At 2-mm intervals from these holes, three burr holes were made on each side for two EEG probes and one CBF probe. Specifications of EEG, CBF, glutamate used in this study are summarized in Tables 1 to 3.

In the acupuncture group, acupuncture stimulation was applied throughout the ischemic period. Four acupuncture needles with a length of 40 mm and a diameter of 0.25 mm were manually inserted about 5 mm deep into acupuncture points just anterior and inferior to the fibular head (Yang Tomb Spring) and distal 4/5 sites on the imaginary line connecting the lateral side of the knee and the lateral malleolus of the tibiofibula (Suspended Bell). The needles were slowly rotated at a couple of alternate rotations of 180 deg/sec, in such a fashion that one needle is rotated for 10 sec, and the next needle is then rotated, while other needles remain inserted.

Table 1. Specifications of 511 AC Amplifier for monitoring EEG signals

Input impedance (MΩ)	20
Common mode rejection ratio (dB)	90
Input noise (μV peak-to-peak)	4
Output impedance (Ω)	500
Band pass filter: Gain (dB)	12

Table 2. Specifications of BLF21D laser Doppler flow meter for monitoring CBF response

Laser: Optical power output (mW)	< 2
Laser: Wavelength (nm)	780
Field of measurement (mm^3/mm)	1
Doppler signal band (Hz)	24 - 24 k
Output range (ml/min/100g)	0 - 100

Table 3. Specifications of micro-dialysis electrode for monitoring glutamate release

Dialysis type	20-10-4-4
Standard glutamate solution (μM)	50-450
Sensitivity (nA/μM)	0.23
linear regression (R^2)	0.999

2.3 Analysis and Statistics

Waveforms obtained from laser Doppler flowmetry, EEG, and potentiostat for Δglutamate were displayed using the DASYLab data acquisition system (National

Instruments, USA) and were analyzed with both Matlab 6.5 and DADiSP 2002 Evaluation Version B18 (DSP development Co., USA). According to reports found in the literature, we proposed 23 diagnostic parameters for a detailed analysis of changes in %CBF and glutamate release during conditions of ischemia and reperfusion. Of these 23 diagnostic parameters, 11 were defined for analysis of changes in %CBF levels, and 13 were defined for analysis of changes in glutamate release. The definitions of these parameters are given as follows:

Parameter	Description
For CBF	
$\%CBF_{zero}$ (%)	Zero level of %CBF
$\%CBF_{pri\text{-}base}$ (%)	Base level of pre-ischemic %CBF
$\%CBF_{i}$ (%)	Ischemic %CBF level
$\%CBF_{rep\text{-}max}$ (%)	Maximum level of reperfusion %CBF
T_{pri} (sec)	Time of pre-ischemia induction
$T_{i\text{-}fall}$ (sec)	Time elapsed to real ischemia induction after manipulation
T_{i} (sec)	Time of ischemia induction
$T_{rep\text{-}rise}$ (sec)	Time elapsed to reach $\%CBF_{rep\text{-}max}$ after the onset of reperfusion period
$T_{rep\text{-}fall+base}$ (sec)	Reperfusion time - $T_{rep\text{-}rise}$
$S_{Ci\text{-}dec}$ (%/sec)	Decrement slope in ischemic period
$S_{Crep\text{-}inc}$ (%/sec)	Increment slope in reperfusion period
For glutamate (GLU)	
ΔGLU_{zero} (μM)	Zero level of GLU release
$\Delta GLU_{pri\text{-}base}$ (μM)	Base level of pre-ischemic GLU release
$\Delta GLU_{i\text{-}max}$ (μM)	Maximum level of ischemic GLU release
$\Delta GLU_{rep\text{-}max}$ (μM)	Maximum level of reperfusion GLU release
T_{pri} (sec)	Time of pre-ischemia induction
$T_{i\text{-}release}$ (sec)	Time delay of the beginning of GLU release after the onset of ischemia
$T_{i\text{-}rise}$ (sec)	Time elapsed to reach $\Delta GLU_{i\text{-}max}$ after the beginning of GLU release
$T_{rep\text{-}delay}$ (sec)	Time elapsed to reach $\Delta GLU_{rep\text{-}max}$ after the onset of reperfusion period
$T_{rep\text{-}fall}$ (sec)	Time elapsed to return to $\Delta GLU_{rep\text{-}base}$ in reperfusion period
$T_{rep\text{-}base}$ (sec)	Time of $\Delta GLU_{rep\text{-}base}$ in reperfusion period
$S_{Gi\text{-}inc}$ (μM/sec)	Increment slope in ischemic period
$S_{Grep\text{-}inc}$ (μM/sec)	Increment slope in reperfusion period
$S_{Grep\text{-}dec}$ (μM/sec)	Decrement slope in reperfusion period

Statistical analysis was performed to compare the mean changes in %CBF and glutamate release between control and acupuncture groups using the two-tailed Student's t-test. P-values < 0.05 were regarded as statistically significant.

3 Results and Discussions

Figures 1 and 2 show representative waveforms with respect to changes in %CBF and extracellular glutamate release during an 11VO model ischemia/reperfusion.

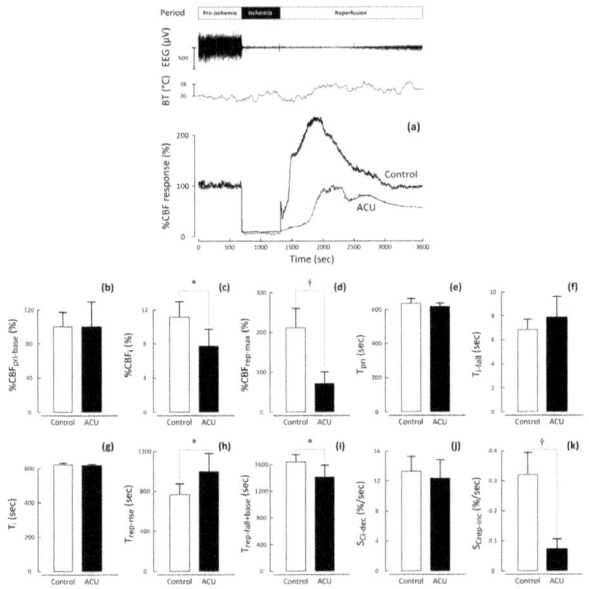

Fig. 1. Representative real-time changes in ischemia-evoked EEG, brain temperature (BT) and %CBF (a) during use of an 11VO model in the control and acupuncture (ACU) groups, measured using a laser Doppler flow meter. Quantitative results (b to k) for the diagnostic parameters proposed for analysis of changes in %CBF throughout the experimental protocol: 10-min pre-ischemic (control) period, 10-min ischemic period, and 40-min reperfusion period. Each result is expressed as mean ± standard deviation of five control rats and five acupuncture rats. *$p < 0.05$; †$p < 0.0001$.

3.1 Changes in CBF Response

As shown in Fig. 1, the change pattern of ischemia-evoked %CBF responses in the 11VO model of hyperglycemic rats with acupuncture treatment was similar to that without acupuncture treatment. Mean time intervals ($S_{Ci\text{-}dec}$) between induction of ischemia and the beginning of the %CBF plateau in the control group (13.26 ± 3.12 s) were similar to those than in the acupuncture group (12.35 ± 2.97 s). After onset of ischemia, %CBF decreased rapidly to near 10% of original levels, and the EEG response became flat. These changes were maintained throughout the 10 min ischemic period. Decreases in ischemic %CBF (%CBF_i) were 11.10 ± 2.91% and 7.71 ± 2.55% for the control and acupuncture groups, respectively. After reperfusion in the controls, %CBF increased considerably, and then returned to the level of the baseline, along with an accompanying EEG recovery. Acupuncture-treated rats showed patterns similar to those without acupuncture treatment. However, the maximum reperfusion %CBF response (%$CBF_{rep\text{-}max}$) in the control was approximately three times that of the acupuncture group ($p < 0.0001$). Also, the time elapsed to reach the maximum %CBF level ($T_{rep\text{-}rise}$) showed a significant increase ($p < 0.05$) in hyperglycemic rats with acupuncture treatment, 763.46 ± 173.28 s, compared to hyperglycemic rats without acupuncture treatment, 994.96 ± 237.39 s. Thus, the increment slope during the reperfusion period ($SC_{rep\text{-}inc}$) associated with $\%CBF_{rep\text{-}max}$ and $T_{rep\text{-}rise}$ also showed a significant decrease in the acupuncture group compared to the control group ($p < 0.0001$).

Commonly, %CBF increases after onset of ischemia, and considerable reactive oxygen is produced during the reperfusion period as a result of increased oxygen supply and metabolism, or reperfusion injury. Some studies [7] have shown that diabetic stroke might be associated with a decrease in reperfusion %CBF. Although there may be negative reports showing no significant neuroprotective effects, acupuncture stimulation in diabetic stroke might be responsible for cellular protective effects and improvement in CBF. Therefore, reduced reperfusion %CBF, taken together with the present results, suggest the likelihood that acupuncture stimulation during the ischemic period suppresses hyperemia in the increased plasma osmolality [8], and/or decreased levels of adenosine [3] under diabetic conditions, and that suppression leads to effects of a potential neuroprotection by acupuncture stimulation.

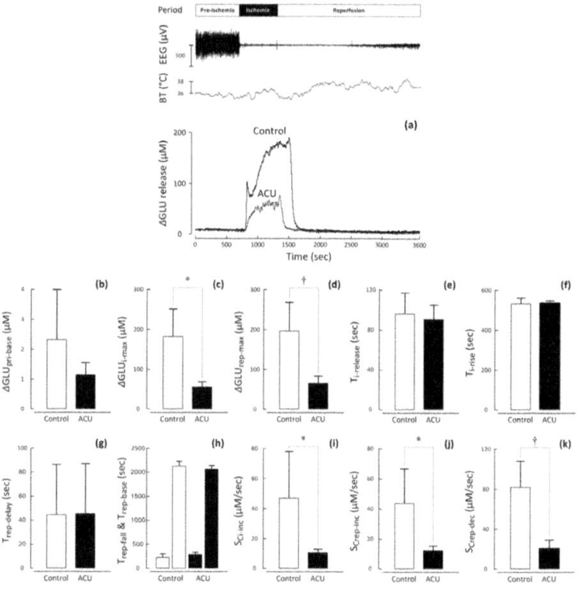

Fig. 2. Representative real-time changes in ischemia-evoked EEG, BT and extracellular Δglutamate (a) during use of an eleven-vessel occlusion model in the control and ACU groups, measured using a micro-dialysis electrode. Quantitative results (b to k) of the diagnostic parameters proposed for analysis of changes in glutamate release throughout the experimental protocol: 10-min pre-ischemic (control) period, 10-min ischemic period, and 40-min reperfusion period. Each result is expressed as mean ± standard deviation of five control rats and five acupuncture rats. *$p < 0.05$; †$p < 0.005$.

3.2 Changes in Glutamate Release

As shown in Fig. 2, the change pattern of ischemia-evoked Δglutamate in an 11VO model of hyperglycemic rats with acupuncture treatment was also similar to that without acupuncture treatment. The mean time delay at the beginning of Δglutamate after onset of ischemia ($T_{i\text{-release}}$) in the control group (96.14 ± 22.56 s) was similar to that in the acupuncture group (90.40 ± 15.95 s). In both groups, rapid elevation of Δglutamate began at $T_{i\text{-release}}$ after onset of ischemia, and continued to rise throughout the 10 min ischemic period. Following reperfusion, Δglutamate showed a considerable decrease, and was then restored to the level of the pre-ischemic period at $T_{rep\text{-delay}}$ + $T_{rep\text{-fall}}$ after reperfusion, along with accompanying EEG recovery. The time elapsed to reach $\Delta GLU_{rep\text{-max}}$ after onset of the reperfusion period ($T_{rep\text{-delay}}$) and the time elapsed to return to $\Delta GLU_{rep\text{-base}}$ during the reperfusion period ($T_{rep\text{-fall}}$) were not significant in either group. However, elevation of glutamate release was suppressed in the acupuncture group, resulting in a decrease of approximately 70%. Maximum changes in extracellular Δglutamate during the ischemic period ($\Delta GLU_{i\text{-max}}$) were 182.24 ± 73.91 μM in the control group and 56.23 ± 13.93 μM in the acupuncture group ($p < 0.05$), while those of extracellular glutamate release during the reperfusion period ($\Delta GLU_{rep\text{-max}}$) were 196.70 ± 77.58 μM in the control group and 65.92 ± 19.40 μM in the acupuncture group ($p < 0.005$). Three slopes showed a significant decrease ($p < 0.05$) in the acupuncture group: a 77.60% decrease in $S_{Gi\text{-inc}}$ ($p < 0.05$), a 72.18% decrease in $S_{Grep\text{-inc}}$ ($p = 0.0164$), and a 74.68% decrease in $S_{Grep\text{-dec}}$ ($p = 0.001$), compared to the control group.

Our previous study also showed that the two groups, normal rats with and without acupuncture stimulation, showed a significant difference in extracellular Δglutamate, while the reduction of %CBF and reperfusion hyperemia were not significantly different between the two groups. Results were consistent with those reported previously in that stroke might be associated with a decrease in ischemic/reperfusion Δglutamate by acupuncture stimulation [9]. Suppression of Δglutamate could be an important mechanism explaining the effect of acupuncture on ischemic stroke. Glutamate excitotoxicity is a major mechanism of neuronal cell death in diabetic rats under ischemic conditions, and is a probable target of therapeutic intervention. Therefore, these results suggest that ischemic acupuncture stimulation contributes to potentially the neuroprotective effect, saving neurons from acute and/or delayed neuronal cell death induced by ischemia in diabetic rats [9].

4 Conclusions

This study has demonstrated the neuroprotective effects of acupuncture stimulation under hyperglycemic conditions. A reproducible 11VO ischemia model was induced as a global ischemia. Patterns of change in %CBF and EEG during ischemia and reperfusion indicate that the surgical setup and 11VO model are suitable for monitoring the effect of acupuncture under conditions of diabetic ischemia. The real- time monitoring system used in our laboratory highlights new possibilities for a detailed analysis of the *in vivo* dynamics of changes in the neurotransmitter glutamate after ischemia. From the proposed 23 diagnostic parameters for a detailed analysis of changes in %CBF and glutamate release during ischemia and reperfusion, we found that a significant decrease ($p < 0.05$) in the maximum responses to ischemic and reperfusion %CBF was observed in acupuncture rats. Compared with control rats, a significantly larger increase ($p < 0.05$) in the time elapsed to reach maximum %CBF levels during reperfusion was observed in acupuncture-treated hyperglycemic rats. Furthermore, a significant decrease ($p < 0.05$) in maximum levels of ischemic and reperfusion Δglutamate was observed in acupuncture-treated hyperglycemic rats. Compared with control rats, a significant decrease ($p < 0.05$) in the increment slope during the ischemic period, and increment and decrement slopes during the reperfusion period was observed in acupuncture-treated hyperglycemic rats. We conclude that the decrease in %CBF and Δglutamate during diabetic ischemia is responsible for the potential neuroprotective effects of acupuncture stimulation in a rat model. Additionally, it is anticipated that the results obtained from this study will help the patients care management, particularly the effects of acupuncture on the diabetes.

Acknowledgments. This study was supported by a research fund from Seoul R&BD (grant #CR070054).

References

1. Erickson, R.J.: Acupuncture Therapy for Stroke: Approaches from the Acupuncture Literature. Acupunct. Med. 18, 48–53 (2000)
2. Yang, Z.J., Shen, D.H., Guo, X., Sun, F.Y.: Electroacupuncture Enhances Striatal Neurogenesis in Adult Rat Brains After a Transient Cerebral Middle Artery Occlusion. Acupunct. Electrother. Res. 30, 185–199 (2005)
3. Guyot, L.L., Diaz, F.G., O'Regan, M.H., Song, D., Phillis, J.W.: The Effect of Streptozotocin-Induced Diabetes on the Release of Excitotoxic and Other Amino Acids from the Ischemic Rat Cerebral Cortex. Neurosurgery 48, 385–390 (2001)
4. Muranyi, M., Ding, C., He, Q., Lin, Y., Li, P.A.: Streptozotocin-Induced Diabetes Causes Astrocyte Death After Ischemia and Reperfusion Injury. Diabetes 55, 349–355 (2006)
5. Zasslow, M.A., Pearl, R.G., Shuer, L.M., Steinberg, G.K., Lieberson, R.E., Larson Jr., C.P.: Hyperglycemia Decreases Acute Neuronal Ischemic Changes After Middle Cerebral Artery Occlusion in Cats. Stroke 20, 519–523 (1989)
6. Caragine, L.P., Park, H.K., Diaz, F.G., Phillis, J.W.: Real-Time Measurement of Ischemia-Evoked Glutamate Release in the Cerebral Cortex of Four and Eleven Vessel Rat Occlusion Models. Brain Res. 793, 255–264 (1998)
7. Kawai, N., Keep, R.F., Betz, A.L., Nagao, S.: Hyperglycemia Induces Progressive Changes in the Cerebral Microvasculature and Blood-Brain Transport during Focal Cerebral Ischemia. Acta. Neurochir. 71, 219–221 (1998)
8. Duckrow, R.B.: Decreased Cerebral Blood Flow during Acute Hyperglycemia. Brain Res. 703, 145–150 (1995)
9. Pang, J., Itano, T., Sumitani, K., Negi, T., Miyamoto, O.: Electroacupuncture Attenuates both Glutamate Release and Hyperemia After Transient Ischemia in Gerbils. Am. J. Chin. Med. 31, 295–303 (2003)

Interactive Web-Phone Technology to Support and Optimize Care Plans for Aging and People with Disabilities

Dick Schoech

University of Texas Arlington
School of Social Work, POB 19129, 211 S. Cooper, Arlington Texas, USA
Ph.: 817-272-3964
Schoech@uta.edu

Abstract. This paper presents and discusses the Teleherence system that uses web and phone technology to optimize care plans. It uses text-to-speech and speech recognition along with landline, cell, smart, SMS (text messaging), and VOIP phone technology. Teleherence delivers surveys that can inform, remind, suggest, persuade, encourage/motivate, teach, reward, query and branches, and query and alert. Specific uses and considerations for use of Teleherence with the elderly will be discussed. Preliminary findings will be discussed at ICOST 2010.

Keywords: Adherence to treatment plans, Web- phone technology, automated calling, SMS, branching surveys.

1 Problem

While most segments of society use technology to improve their operations, the human services lag behind in the use of technology. Technology is especially needed that supports care managers with large caseloads. Technology has the capacity to identify clients at high risk, support the client's change process, follow-up with booster information, personalize agency monitoring, predict success, and gather evaluation data that can improve treatment effectiveness.

2 System Being Developed

Researchers at The University of Texas Arlington Schools of Social Work and Computer Science and Engineering are developing a web-phone system to support care managers and optimize client outcomes. Called Teleherence, this system calls a client at agreed upon times, delivers reminders and messages, asks questions, graphs responses, sends desired alerts, and flags potential problems or opportunities using smart algorithms. It uses text-to-speech and speech recognition along with landline, cell, smart, SMS (text messaging), and VOIP phone technology. The system can also deliver pre-recorded audio files such as motivational messages from the care manager.

Y. Lee et al. (Eds.): ICOST 2010, LNCS 6159, pp. 138–143, 2010.

The Teleherence system is being developed in partnership with Mental Health Mental Retardation of Tarrant County with support from the National Institute of Health, National Library of Medicine.

3 Description of System Modules

The proposed system has five modules.

1. A client module where care managers specify client information, appointment schedules, when the client wants to be called, how often to call the client, who else to call in the care management process (e.g., a spouse), etc. This module sits on an agency server so that client information does not have to reside outside the agency. The remaining modules reside on an independent university based server that contains no client identifiable information. Separating the two parts of the system allows agencies to keep control over their client data.
2. A survey development module where care managers or their superiors design the survey items which are messages containing information, questions and possible answers, text messages, and prompts to capture client recordings that are sent to care managers and others. The module allows users to arrange survey items into a series of standard templates, such as a template for following up with a client after that client missed an appointment. The module also allows users to string together one or more templates in to a client-customized survey, assign repeat schedule, and set alerts that are triggered based on client responses.
3. A survey delivery module that delivers audio or text messages to inform, remind, suggest, persuade, encourage/motivate, teach, reward, query and branches, and query and alert. The messages can be triggered based on client readiness stage, phase of treatment, analyses of previous survey data, or predictions of treatment plan success or failure. Basic survey questions (in italics) for a care management plan objective involving medication adherence could be:
    i. (After a pin number is entered) This is the Teleherence System calling. *Did you take your 9:00 A.M. medication?* If yes, Teleherence could end or go to item ii and ask the next questions once a week. If no, Teleherence delivers a motivational message and schedules a call back at a specified time, e.g., 9:30.
    ii. *Do you feel your medication is working?* If no, Teleherence asks the client to record the problems associated with the medication and emails the recording to the care manager.
    iii. *Do you need an appointment with your care manager?* If yes, Teleherence gives the phone number of the appointment desk and alerts the care manager.
    iv. *Do you want to leave a message for your care manager?* If yes, Teleherence records and emails the recorded message. Note that clients can press a keypad key to repeat an item, skip an item, or go back to the previous item.

A basicsurvey for a care management plan objective to monitor an elderly homebound client could be the following. It could be delivered in the voice of a loved one if needed.

i. *This is the Teleherence System calling for your weekly checkup. How are you doing this week?* Press 1 or say fine. Press 2 or say average. Press 3 or say poor. If poor, Teleherence email an alert to the care manager.
ii. *Can you enter a number or say about how many people have visited you this week?* Teleherence records the number on a graph (see report module).
iii. *Do you have enough food available for your meals?* If the client indicated they were doing poor, had no visitors, and had no food, an alert could be sent to a local police station or to someone who could quickly check on the client. The client could be informed that someone is coming and given a number to cancel the visit.
iv. *Do you want to leave a message for your care manager?* If yes, Teleherence records and emails the recorded message to the care manager.

5. A report module that graphically displays survey results over time to those needing to see the results, e.g., the care manager, client, spouse, or others in a client's support group. Currently, a line graph is used.
6. A prediction module that uses techniques such as data mining to predict adherence and non-adherence to objectives and flag risks and opportunities. This module makes the system smarter with use, i.e., able to better predict and give rationales for the prediction as more data is collected during use. This module is not yet developed.

4 Current Uses of the System

The system is currently being implemented in four different programs. Preliminary results will be presented where they are available.

1. A rehabilitation alternatives program for parolees and probationers
2. An addictions recovery program for probationers
3. A program supporting veterans returning to college
4. A family Intervention program for women and families who are juggling the demands of parenting while trying to stay clean and sober at the same time.

The Teleherence system has applicability for anyone following a plan of care. It can be used to deliver "booster" messages on key intervention concepts, for delivering cognitive behavioral interventions, for explaining what to expect in treatment each week, for involving a client's support system in their treatment, or for client follow-up. Many other uses are anticipated.

5 Potential Uses of the System with the Elderly and for People with Disabilities

Teleherence system is most applicable for clients who are familiar with technology and do not have problems answering phone messages in a recorded or computer generated voice. It is most relevant for client whose care plans concern maximizing their independent living at home or in more structured environments.

One obvious use of the Teleherence system concerns medication management. Clients could be called as needed with instructions for taking medications. These calls could be followed 10 minutes later asking if the person took the pill. These followup calls could continue until a yes response was received. Since pills are usually to be taken as precise intervals, the Teleherence system could be set up once to deliver reminders repeatedly. Reminders can be delivered via a computer-generated voice, a recorded voice of a trusted person, or using a text message.

Another use of Teleherence would be to provide education on important topics for a client. Using medication management example above, if the client had a phone capable of handling video, video instructions for taking a pill could be delivered. If the care plan objective concerned safety, a video for checking on home safety could be provided. These videos could be replayed as often as needed and rescheduled to reinforce the education whenever necessary. The concepts of "Just in Time Training" could be used in the design of these educational surveys.

An additional use is to involve a client's support system in their care. For example, someone who visits the elderly person could be called periodically and asked for their input on how well the client is doing. If the discrepancy between what the client is reporting and what the support system person is reporting becomes too great, an alert could be triggered to the care manager or a more extensive check up survey could be triggered that tries to determine what is happening in this particular situation. Teleherence is able to chart responses over time and these charts could be available online to family or support group members. These charts can provide a visual record that graphically displays small differences over time that may not be noticeable by a busy caretaker or frequent visitor. These charts might be especially important if benchmarks exist in areas such as cognitive disabilities where certain benchmarks or tests are able to detect that additional services are needed by a client. Having a set of objectives related to each specific elderly problems would allow Teleherence to help carry out structured care according to established protocol.

Another use of Teleherence is for delivering measurement instruments for benchmarking and evaluation, and following up at periodic intervals such as 3 and 6 months. Since Teleherence is inexpensive to operate, follow- up could be scheduled for much shorter intervals, such as every 2 weeks, with notification sent whenever relapse seems likely. Once the prediction module is developed, the potential for relapse could be predicted from previous cases.

Use of the Teleherence system for staff of nursing homes or supported living environments is also feasible. For example, busy staff could be reminded with text messages tasks, paperwork, or reports are due. Clients could also receive reminders via text messages, etc., for important gatherings and even that meals are ready if they were forgetful. Periodic surveys of client satisfaction could be charted and if satisfaction fell below a certain level, alerts could be sent to key administrators.

A final use of systems like Teleherence is for the education of new employees and even the education of students in universities programs such as social work. Having students putting themselves into the Teleherence system with a specific treatment regime would allow the student to experience how the regime might be implemented from a client perspective. This experience could be similar to having students spend a day in a wheel chair to see what life is like for a person with a mobility disability.

The Teleherence system does not have to be used as a stand along system. Teleherence system would work well as the client interface for an environment with extensive health monitoring and measurement. Decision rules could be established that triggered treatment plan routines based on monitoring profiles. For example, if a motion sensor recorded significantly less movement over a defined period, Teleherence could trigger a call to the client that asked about the client's well being and encouraged the client to exercise more. The Teleherence system is a natural complement with the growing field of home health monitoring.

6 Special Considerations When Using Teleherence with the Elderly

The elderly pose special challenges if they are suffering from cognitive impairment or if they are easily confused by computer generated structured messages. Different tactics might need to be used to work around these special challenges. For example, messages might be best presented in a voice with which the cognitive impaired are familiar. A son or daughter's voice could be used in any daily pill reminder message. These messages can easily be recorded using the Teleherence to request recordings from loved ones using a landline telephone system. Similarly, an introductory message in the care manager's voice might be necessary to assure the elderly person that replying to messages and pressing numbers is safe. Teleherence can currently personalize surveys by pulling in the client's name, appointment date, time, and location, and other key pieces of information stored in the database. Another technique that might need to be used with clients with a cognitive impairment would be to provide limited audio instructions with each call and to make many small simple message calls rather than fewer messages that are more complex. Research is needed in these areas to determine how best to address the special issues that the elderly and people with disabilities present to automated phone interaction.

7 Contact Information

Dick Schoech, PhD., Professor, University of Texas Arlington School of Social Work, Schoech@uta.edu 817-272-3964 (ICOST presenter & author).

Gergely Zaruba, Ph.D, and Manfred Huber, Ph.D., Professors, University of Texas Arlington Computer Science & Engineering Department, zaruba@uta.edu; huber@exchange.uta.edu (Co-developers).

References

1. Bush, N., Donaldson, G., Moinpour, C., Haberman, M., Milliken, D., Markle, V., Lauson, J.: Development, Feasibility and Compliance of a Web-Based System for Very Frequent Qol and Symptom Home Self- Assessment After Hematopoietic Stem Cell Transplantation. Quality of Life Research 14(1), 77–93 (2005)
2. Cramer, J.A., Rosenheck, R.: Compliance with Medication Regimens for Mental and Physical Disorders. Psychiatric Services 49, 196–201 (1998)

3. Day, J.: How Reflections on Concordance in Mental Health Can Affect Research and Clinical Practice in Adherence. The Pharmaceutical Journal 27, 505–507 (2003)
4. Dolder, C.R., Lacro, J.P., Jeste, D.V.: Adherence to Antipsychotic and Nonpsychiatric Medications in Middle-Aged and Older Patients with Psychotic Disorders. Psychosomatic Medicine 65, 156–162 (2003)
5. Editors: Seniors with CHF Embrace Monitoring System Based on Automatic Voice Technology. Disease Management Advisor 7(3), 40–44 (2001)
6. Grunebaum, M., Luber, P., Callahan, M., Leon, A.C., Olfson, M., Portera, L.: Predictors of Missed Appointments for Psychiatric Consultations in A Primary Care Clinic. Psychiatric Services 47(8), 848–852 (1996)
7. Magura, S., Laudet, A.B., Mahmood, D., Rosenblum, A., Knight, E.: Adherence to Medication Regimens and Participation in Dual-Focus Self-Help Groups. Psychiatric Services 53(3), 310–316 (2002)
8. Mundt, J.C., Bohn, M.J., King, M., Hartley, M.T.: Automating Standard Alcohol Use Assessment Instruments Via Interactive Voice Response Technology. Alcoholism: Clinical & Experimental Research 26(2), 207–211 (2002)
9. National Institute of Mental Health: Research on Adherence to Interventions for Mental Disorders (2003), `http://grants.nih.gov/grants/guide/pa-files/PA-03-111.html`
10. Nose, M., Barbui, C., Gray, R., Tansella, M.: Clinical Interventions for Treatment Non-Adherence in Psychosis: Meta-Analysis. The British Journal of Psychiatry 183, 197–206 (2003)
11. Owen, R.R., Fischer, E.P., Booth, B.M., Cuffel, B.J.: Medication Noncompliance and Substance Abuse among Patients with Schizophrenia. Psychiatric Services 47(8), 853–858 (1996)
12. Schneider, S.J., Schwartz, M.D., Fast, J.: Computerized, Telephone-Based Health Promotion:I and II Stress Management Program. Computers in Human Behavior 11/2, 205–214 (1995)
13. Záruba, G.V., Kamangar, F.A., Huber, M., Levine, D.: CONNECT – A Personal Remote Messaging and Monitoring System to Aid People with Disabilities. IEEE CommunicationsMagazine, 101–109 (September 2005)

Use Cases for Abnormal Behaviour Detection in Smart Homes

An C. Tran, Stephen Marsland, Jens Dietrich, Hans W. Guesgen, and Paul Lyons

School of Engineering and Advanced Technology, Massey University
Palmerston North, New Zealand
{a.c.tran,s.r.marsland,j.b.dietrich,h.w.guesgen,
p.lyons}@massey.ac.nz

Abstract. While people have many ideas about how a smart home should react to particular behaviours from their inhabitant, there seems to have been relatively little attempt to organise this systematically. In this paper, we attempt to rectify this in consideration of context awareness and novelty detection for a smart home that monitors its inhabitant for illness and unexpected behaviour. We do this through the concept of the Use Case, which is used in software engineering to specify the behaviour of a system. We describe a set of scenarios and the possible outputs that the smart home could give and introduce the SHMUC Repository of Smart Home Use Cases. Based on this, we can consider how probabilistic and logic-based reasoning systems would produce different capabilities.

Keywords: Abnormal behaviour detection, context awareness, use case, smart home.

1 Introduction

During the last twenty years, the 'smart' in 'smart home' has become more important [1, 2], with a focus on behaviour recognition and subsequent abnormal behaviour detection. There have been many proposed frameworks and algorithms for behaviour recognition [3], but little discussion of what precisely a smart home that monitors behaviour should do. Here we focus on smart homes for elderly care monitoring, discuss Use Cases that describe a situation, and then propose suitable outputs from the smart home.

Software Engineers specify systems by employing Use Cases to define their features in normal language without any preconception of how the system is implemented. Use Cases specify the participants in the task (the 'actors'), their (single) goal, preconditions, triggers and postconditions. We believe that applying this methodology to smart homes may help to identify what precisely we desire from a smart home. Informal enough to be understood by naive users and formal enough to be used as system specifications by developers, they are popular with standards bodies and developer communities such as W3C and the OMG consortium [4].

Y. Lee et al. (Eds.): ICOST 2010, LNCS 6159, pp. 144–151, 2010.

Independent sets of Use Cases have been used not only in computer science, but also in business to describe business cases to compare and evaluate heterogeneous approaches [5, 6].

Our Use Cases identify abnormal behaviours, and present the reasoning behind the smart home's choice of reaction. They have been selected to identify some of the context awareness and behaviour recognition needed by an intelligent smart home. We have identified some Use Cases and suggest that many in the smart home research community could identify others. We aim to stimulate discussion of the desired behaviours of a monitoring smart home. In this paper, it is impossible to present all the Use Cases we have developed; instead we refer the reader to the online, editable repository at `http://muse.massey.ac.nz/shmuc`, a canonical resource that other researchers can draw upon, add to, and modify.

Use Cases can assist smart home researchers to make principled choices between methodologies such as logic-based algorithms [7–9], and probabilistic machine learning algorithms [7, 10], and to benchmark different implementations: an informed evaluation can be made quickly and easily by testing implementations on the Use Cases.

The Use Cases discussed here focus on detecting abnormal behaviour by the inhabitant. The smart home monitors, identifies behaviours, and isolates those that are unusual. We use the classification of abnormal behaviour presented in [11, 12]: (1) statistical abnormality, (2) violation of socially-accepted standards, (3) based on theory of personal development, (4) subjective abnormality, and (5) biological injury. A behaviour's novelty often derives from its context: using the heater is unusual if the temperature is warm, sleeping is unusual behaviour in the kitchen, etc. Therefore, context awareness is important in the detection of abnormal behaviour, as in much smart home research [13].

2 The Use Cases

In our Use Cases, daughter Debbie has a mother Mary who lives alone, but has dementia. Debbie has decided to set up a smart home system to look after her mother so that she can continue in full-time work. This smart home system aims to detect any unusual actions by Mary and send appropriate alerts to Debbie and Carita, a carer who will check up on Mary if required. Fig. 1 show a taxonomy of six classes of smart home Use Case that we have identified to help Debbie to care for her mother by passively observing Mary and detecting abnormal and potentially dangerous behaviour without 'crying wolf' (i.e., producing false positives) too often. We consider only a small number of possible outputs by the system: (1) do nothing and wait for further data, (2) raise an alarm to alert Mary (3) record a message for Debbie to view later, and (4) send an urgent alert to Carita. For space reasons, we include one example only of each of four of the Use Cases in the repository at `http://muse.massey.ac.nz/shmuc`

2.1 Abnormality in Duration

SHMUC Use Case A1. *An over-long shower*

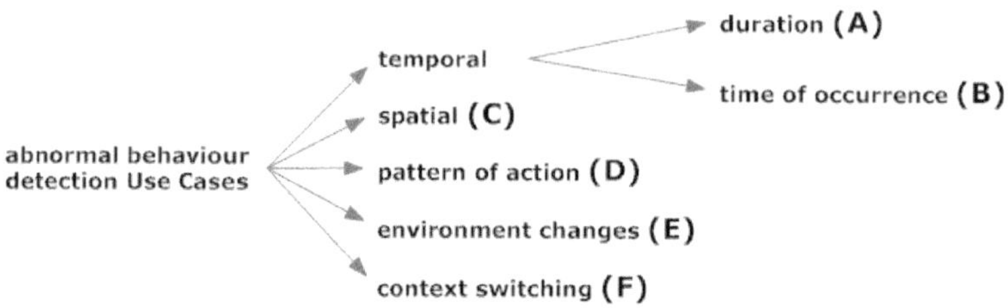

Fig. 1. Classification of the subsets of Use Cases presented in this paper

Goal: To detect an unusually extended activity. **Initial state:** Mary was at home alone. **Description:** Mary woke up at 0800. She began her morning shower at 0810, as usual, but at 0840 the motion sensor in the bathroom still indicated movement, and the shower tap was still on, so her shower had lasted for 30 minutes. **Norm:** Mary normally showers for 10 to 20 minutes. **Outcome:** An alert message was sent to Debbie, who called Carita. Carita discovered Mary confused and cold in the shower, having forgotten what she was doing. **System design implications:** An excessively long activity may put the smart home inhabitant at risk. This poses the following questions: When does a shower become longer than usual? 1 minute over the average? 5? 10? Or is the amount of overrun relative (1%? 5%? 10%)? Perhaps a more sophisticated statistic is appropriate (>1 standard deviation from the mean).

Note that Use Cases are an informal documentation tool; their structure can best be described as semi-standardised. The structure above is consistent with the spirit of Use Case design, but adapted to suit the particular requirements of Smart Homes. The most notable innovation is the inclusion of a section labelled Norm which presents the 'normal' behaviour that should occur in this case.

There are two other Use Cases in this category, **SHMUC Use Case A2:** A justifiably short shower, and **SHMUC Use Case A3:** A Long Nap. These cases are not presented here in full. A2 demonstrates that some abnormal behaviours must be detected before they are complete if a suitable response is to occur. A3 examines a behaviour where abnormal duration is more difficult to categorise, and demonstrates the high degree of world knowledge that a Smart Home may need if its responses are to be appropriate.

An activity's start time is meaningful: an inappropriate activity start time could imply illness or even dementia, but a forgetful person may only need a reminder to function normally.

2.2 Anomaly in Time of Occurrence

An activity's start time is meaningful: an inappropriate activity start time could imply illness or even dementia, but a forgetful person may only need a reminder to function normally. Use Cases in SHMUC category B concern anomalies in time of occurrence. As with category A, we present one Use Case as an example, and a very brief summary of the others contained in the repository.

SHMUC Use Case B1. *Variation in shower start time*

> **Goal:** To recognise acceptable variation in the start time of an activity.
> **Initial state:** Mary is home alone.
> **Description:** One cold winter morning, Mary awoke at 0800. She decided to wait until 0830 before taking her shower. The system noticed that Mary did not take a shower from 0800 to 0820 as had previously occurred, and generated a reminder for Mary and a warning message for her daughter, Debbie. Mary ignored the reminder, and waited until 0830 as she had intended. After work, Debbie checked the system and recognised that the system had made an incorrect inference that had occurred because it had not observed this activity in the winter. Debbie then provided feedback to the system to update this activity start time.
> **Norm:** Mary's shower starts in the time-range 0800 - 0820.
> **Outcome:** Mary's shower time was accepted at 0830.
> **System design implications:** In general, it is probably safe to assume that activity start times more than 1 standard deviation from the mean are interesting but not inherently problematic behaviours. Therefore it is acceptable to request external (human) input regarding the classification of the behaviour, and it may not be necessary for the Smart Home to rely on pre-loaded world knowledge.

There are currently two other Uses Cases in category B: **SHMUC Use Case B2:** Taking Medicine After Midnight, and **SHMUC Use Case B3:** Late for Church. B2 deals with explicitly scheduled events, and B3 presents a situation in which there is some data that the system cannot possibly know, and which will cause it to reason incorrectly.

As with the abnormal duration, the abnormal start times presented in the three Use Cases in Category B seem easy to detect. However, context and other issues may be important:

i) Some people have quite variable schedules. And even the most regular people, move behaviours from their normal times in response to unexpected events such as an upset stomach. It may be that behaviours will need to be categorised into regular and irregular ones.

ii) Identifying contextual factors may help to increase the detection accuracy. For example, after Debbie's feedback, the start time of Mary's shower would be from 0800 to 0830. However, the system would be more useful if it used the seasonal context to estimate start times: 0800 to 0820 in summer, 0830 to 0850 in winter, updatable as more situations were observed.

iii) As with duration, there are questions about how long the system should wait before issuing an alert and what constitutes a suitable alert. For example, if the system could interact with Mary rather than just raising an alarm, then it could ask her if she had forgotten to go to church, or issue other reminders.

2.3 Performing Activities in the Wrong Places

Performing an action in the wrong place (e.g., jumping on the bed or lying on the kitchen floor) may be dangerous or signify that something has gone wrong. Use Case category C concerns the relationship between an activity's location and abnormal behaviour.

SHMUC Use Case C1. *Lying down in the kitchen*

Goal: To react to some abnormal behaviours immediately, as they are potentially very significant.
Initial state: Mary was at home alone.
Description: At 0815, Mary went to the kitchen to prepare her breakfast. She got some bread and put it in the toaster. She walked around the kitchen while she was waiting, and then suddenly lay down on the floor. The behaviour was recognised, and then the spatial properties of the activity checked. As this behaviour should not be seen in the kitchen, an alert was created, and marked urgent as the behaviour was potentially serious.
Norm: Inhabitants do not lie down in the kitchen.
Outcome: An alert message was sent to both Debbie and Carita.
System design implications: There is a class of activities that fall outside the bounds of normal behaviour and can be prima facie assumed to be both interesting and problematic. This should reduce the computational effort involved in deciding how to react to an observed activity. However, complementing that is the difficulty of foreseeing all possible inappropriate behaviours. It's difficult enough to build a world model that allows for normal behaviours, but the size of the problem is potentially much larger if the system has to detect all possible dangerous abnormal behaviours.

Detecting abnormality of activity spatial property requires the spatial data to be stored by the system and attached to behaviour. In comparison to the previous Use Cases, this is more static; the information does not change frequently.

2.4 Abnormality in a Behaviour Pattern

The sensor patterns generated by 'standard' behaviours are variable. Evidence from various smart home datasets suggest that cooking dinner involves between 4 and 58 actions (e.g. MIT Activity Recognition Data, MavLab Sensor Data [14]), and other behaviours exhibit similar variation. In such situations it is difficult to decide what a smart home should be able to detect, and how to avoid false positives. We use tea-making to illustrate the complexity of identifying errors even in simple task.

SHMUC Use Case D1. *Making tea with sugar*

Goal: Mary wishes to make a cup of tea.

Initial state: Mary was at home alone.

Description: During the training phase, the system identified a tea making behaviour that consisted of the following actions (where $[\cdot]_{0,1}$ describes an activity that occurs 0 or 1 times):

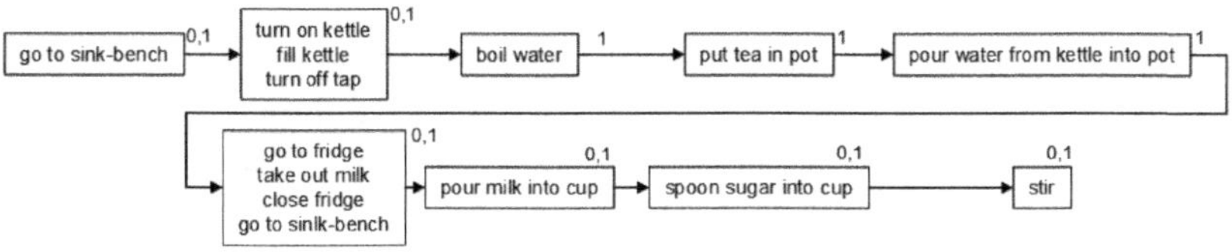

After training, this system was ready to monitor Mary's activity. One afternoon Mary made a cup of tea, using the following set of actions:

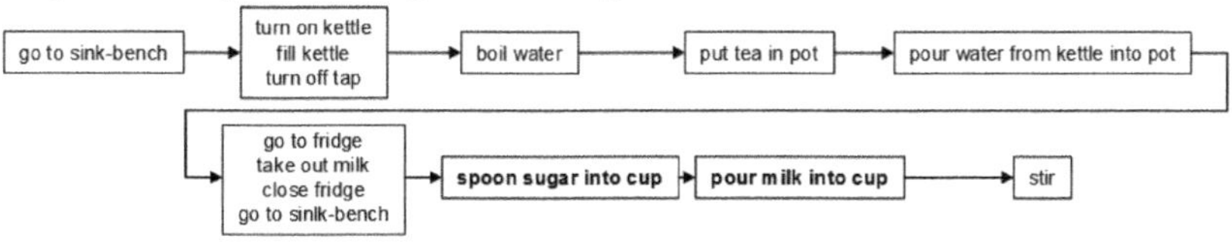

The system treated this sequence as a novelty, as the items in bold are reversed in order with respect to the syntax created during training. However, it did not cause an immediate alarm, as the system identified that the order of two actions, i.e. "get sugar" and "get hot water", does not affect on the final state of the activity. Therefore, the system did not create an alert, but modified its representation of tea-making instead.

Norm: The tea-making sequence conforms to the syntax specified by the Finite State Machine (FMS).

Outcome: The activity pattern was automatically updated, a notification was issued.

System design implications: Activities often comprise a partially ordered sequence, and there is no guarantee that observation of any number of instances will reveal all the orderings. The system should therefore be able to distinguish between abnormal event sequences and previously unseen, but valid event sequences. The system may be unable to infer this without external input from a competent source (which might rule out the inhabitant, if the inhabitant were dementing).

The Use Cases in category D demonstrate massive potential variation in behaviour presentation and the difference between a 'safe' one and one that demonstrates illness can be subtle. They also highlight differences between using logic-based methods and probabilistic-based methods. The valid but unusual order of tea-making activities in the first scenario, is reasonable, but it can be a challenge to recognise it depending on how behaviours are represented. A Markov-based approach may ignore the difference, while an FSM would have to learn this and store the updated syntax. In order for the learning to be as trivial as suggested by the description in the Use Case, some kind of knowledge-based reasoning system would need to identify the importance of order; clearly removing the cup from the cupboard after the water has been poured would not be valid. A hierarchical knowledge base that associated the essential tea-making goals (dissolving tea in hot water) with the actions required to achieve the individual goals might facilitate this. An alternative could be to use partial orders for the patterns.

3 Discussion and Conclusion

We seek to demonstrate that Use Cases can expose behavioural requirements of a smart home, not to document them all within an 8-page format. Our Use Cases address the following questions: (1) what types of abnormal behaviour may occur? (2) how does the system reason about its inhabitant's behaviour? (3) how should it react to abnormal behaviour? (4) what information should be involved in abnormality detection?

Use Cases are implementation-independent, but they can guide implementation choices between, say, probabilistic methods, and techniques based on symbolic logic and reasoning. They have clarified some of the common types of abnormality. Although we have not addressed some types of abnormality included in the psychological definition of novelty that we reported earlier, those related to biological injury are implicit in some of the use cases that we have presented.

The discussion has identified some ways that smart homes can reason about unusual behaviour. Temporal abnormalities can be detected using statistical analysis of prior observation (e.g. a training phase). Contextual data is also important, but it can conjure up the 'curse of dimensionality', as isolating important factors is a very difficult machine learning problem. We suggest that it may be appropriate to combine statistical machine learning methods and logic, e.g., inductive logic programming [15]. From examples, the system could learn some rules with context awareness: 'Mary usually goes out around 1500 to 1530 at the weekend if she is not sick and it is not raining'. Obviously, this would allow learnt rules to be used to detect abnormality more accurately than current approaches based solely on abnormal start time detection. However, problems of performance remain to be solved for this technique, which is still a research focus for us.

There are also many different approaches to detecting abnormality in behaviour patterns such as Markov models (Hara et al. [7]), and temporal logic (Jakkula and Cook [16]). The above scenarios on abnormal presentation of behavioural patterns show that abnormality in patterns depends on many factors other than the order of actions. We have followed the line of NAF ('negation as failure', i.e. unidentifiable patterns are abnormal), with feedback to teach the system about failed cases that are in fact normal. In addition, the wide variety of normal ways to accomplish a 'standard' task such as making a cup of tea makes isolating an abnormal pattern of observations difficult. The NAF approach is limited, as it relies on complete coverage in the training data. A system that can generalise from examples may compensate for limited training sets.

The Use Cases presented here would be improved by the inclusion of non-functional aspects such as scalability and Total Cost of Ownership; the latter would improve system evaluation and comparison. While it might be easier with a logic-based system to address many of the requirements discussed, such a system would require comprehensive and expensive initial setup work. On the other hand, logic-based systems might be easier to maintain as they offer users reflection and introspection facilities such as explanations (such as derivation logs) and configuration options (such as customising thresholds).

Acknowledgements. We acknowledge the support of the other members of the Massey University Smart Environments group (`http://muse.massey.ac.nz`).

References

1. Giroux, S., Pigot, H.: From Smart Homes to Smart Care: ICOST 2005 (Assistive Technology & Research). IOS Press, USA (2005)
2. Carlos, A., Paul, M.: Ambient Intelligence: Concepts and applications. Computer Science and Information Systems 4(1), 1–27 (2007)
3. Chua, S., Marsland, S., Guesgen, H.: Spatio-temporal and context reasoning in smart homes. In: Proceeding of COSIT Workshop on Spatial and Temporal Reasoning for Ambient Intelligence System, pp. 9–20 (2009)
4. Jacobson, I.: Object-Oriented Software Engineering, A Use Case Driven Approach. Addison-Wesley, Reading (1992)
5. Intel: Intel vPro technology Microsoft Windows 7 Microsoft SCCM better together use cases, `http://communities.intel.com/servlet/JiveServlet/download/3232-3-2124/Windows7vProUsecases.pdf` (last visited: 22/10/2009)
6. The Business Rules Group: Defining business rules - what are they really?, `http://www.businessrulesgroup.org/first-paper/br01ad.htm` (last visited: 22/10/2009)
7. Hara, K., Omori, T., Ueno, R.: Detection of unusual human behavior in intelligent house. In: Proceedings of the 12th IEEE Workshop on Neural Networks for Signal Processing, vol. 4 (2002)
8. Augusto, J., Nugent, C.: The use of temporal reasoning and management of complex events in smart homes. In: Proceedings of the 16th European Conference on AI, pp. 778–782 (2004)
9. Chen, L., Nugent, C., Mulvenna, M., Finlay, D., Hong, X., Poland, M.: Using event calculus for behaviour reasoning and assistance in a smart home. In: Helal, S., Mitra, S., Wong, J., Chang, C.K., Mokhtari, M. (eds.) ICOST 2008. LNCS, vol. 5120, pp. 81–89. Springer, Heidelberg (2008)
10. Rivera-Illingworth, F., Callaghan, V., Hagras, H.: Detection of normal and novel behaviours in ubiquitous domestic environments. The Computer Journal (2007)
11. Dewey, R.A.: Psychology: An introduction, `http://www.intropsych.com/` (last visited: 22/10/2009)
12. Kardas, E.P.: What is abnormal behavior? `http://www.purgatory.net/merits/abnormal.htm` (last visited: 22/10/2009)
13. Meyer, S., Rakotonirainy, A.: A survey of research on context-aware homes. In: Proceeding of the Australasian Information Security Workshop Conference on ACSW Frontiers 2003, pp. 159–168 (2003)
14. University, W.S.: Smart home datasets, `http://ailab.wsu.edu/casas/datasets.html` (last visited: 22/10/2009)
15. Lavrac, N., Dzeroski, S.: Inductive Logic Programming: Techniques and Applications. Ellis Horwood, New York (1994)
16. Jakkula, V., Cook, D.: Anomaly detection using temporal data mining in a smart home environment. Methods of Information in Medicine (2008)

Design of Novel Feeding Robot for Korean Food

Won-Kyung Song[1], Jongbae Kim[1], Kwang-Ok An[1], In-Ho Lee[1], Won-Jin Song[1], Bum-Suk Lee[2], Sung-Il Hwang[2], Mi-Ok Son[2], and Eun-Chang Lee[3]

[1] Research Institute, National Rehabilitation Center, 520, Suyu5-dong, Gangbuk-gu, Seoul, 142-884, Korea
wksong@nrc.go.kr, jbkim@nrc.go.kr, anko04@korea.kr, lio3596@korea.kr, swjli@naver.com

[2] National Rehabilitation Hospital, National Rehabilitation Center, 520, Suyu5-dong, Gangbuk-gu, Seoul, 142-884, Korea
iambs@nrc.go.kr, nrchsi@nrc.go.kr, sonmiok33@yahoo.co.kr

[3] DesignTV, 1 Fl. 451-5 Dogok-dong, Gangnam-gu, Seoul, 135-855, Korea
thedesigntv@gmail.com

Abstract. During mealtime, a feeding robot allows a person with upper limbs disability to enjoy chosen food with desired time intervals. Although many feeding machines are developed and commercialized over the world, Korean consumers are still hard to find a feeding robot that can handle the Korean food with boiled rice. In order to handle those kinds of food, we design a novel feeding robotic system that consists of two robotic arms: one is a food grasping robotic arm, and the other is a food transferring robotic arm. We expect that the proposed feeding robot could provide easy handling the Korean food with general bowls. In addition, when one caregiver supports the multiple persons, one part of feeding robots, i.e., a transferring robot, could be effectively applied in facilities or hospitals.

Keywords: Feeding Robot, Assistive Robot, Dual-Arm, Eating.

1 Introduction

Improving independence of growing weaker members of a society is one of crucial issues for the quality of life. Specifically, the disabled people who officially registered in Korea are already over two million, i.e., 4.5 per cent of total Korean population, due to illnesses, injuries, and natural aging processes [1]. More than one third of the disabled people are the elderly persons. In addition, the elderly people in Korea are over 10 per cent due to decreasing the birthrate and lengthening the span of their life. Effective caregiving is strongly required within restricted resources. An assistive robot could be one of solutions to tackle that problem in the activities of daily livings.

A caregiver should physically contact the disabled in several caregiving tasks such as changing their clothes, repositioning their posture, transferring, having a meal, bathing, and rehabilitation. These tasks are well known tasks for activities of daily living. Among these activities, having a meal is one of basic activities and this task could be replaced with an available technology if someone prepares a meal for a user.

Y. Lee et al. (Eds.): ICOST 2010, LNCS 6159, pp. 152–159, 2010.

Various assistive robots have been developed since late 1980s. Handy 1 [2] is an assistive robot for the daily activities like eating, drinking, washing, shaving, teeth cleaning and applying make-up. Handy 1 consists of a five DOF (degrees of freedom) robot, a gripper and a tray unit. The major function of Handy 1 is eating. Handy 1 allows a user to select food from any part of the tray. A cup is attached in order to drink water with their meal. The walled columns of a food dish make an important role to scoop the food on the dish.

Winsford feeder [3, 4] is a mechanical system for the self-feeding. Winsford feeder uses a mechanical pusher to fill a spoon and a pivoting arm to raise the spoon to a user's mouth, i.e., a preset position. A rotation of the plate places more food in front of the pusher. The user can choose two input devices: a chin switch and a rocker switch.

Neater Eater [5] has two types: a manual operation type and an automatic operation type. Neater Eater consists of the two degrees of freedom arm and one dish. Couples of foods could be mixed on the one dish. The manual type that has damping factor could be used to suppress the tremor of upper limbs while a user eats food.

My Spoon [6] is suitable to deal with Japanese food. My Spoon consists of a 5-DOF manipulator and a gripper with a meal tray. The meal tray has four rectangular cells. My Spoon combines several preprogrammed motions: automatic operation, semi-automatic operation, and manual operation. The semi-automatic operation allows a user to choose food. The manual operation can change a grasping position on the food as well. The input device could be selected among the chin joystick, the reinforcement joystick, and the switch. The end-effector of a robotic arm has one spoon and one fork that make the grasping motion. While the robot grasps food, the gap between a spoon and a fork changes and thus the end-effector grasps the food. Then, the robot moves to the preset position, and the fork that is located on the spoon moves backward to provide a user with food on a spoon.

Meal Buddy [3] uses a three-DOF robotic arm and three bowls which can be mounted on a board by magnetic attraction. After this system scoops the food, the robotic arm scrapes the surplus food off the spoon by the rod on bowls.

Mealtime Partner Dining System [7] locates in front of the user's mouth. Three bowls can rotate around the user's mouth. The spoon picks up the food, and then moves the preset location with short travelling distance. This system reduces the slip chance of wet food because the spoon's bottom wipes out after scooping. The user does not need to lean toward the feeder because the system locates in front of a user's mouth.

The food has a bite size in common. However, scooping sticky boiled rice is not an easy task. Most of feeding systems are scooping the food with a spoon, and those systems are not suitable to treat boiled short-grain rice. My Spoon has the grasping function to pick up food. However this system is hard to serve rice due to fixed grasping strength of a gripper.

The feeding robot allows a user to enjoy dishes independently during mealtime. At first, the feeding robot needs to prepare the dishes through a caregiver. After preparing the dishes, a user and a caregiver can directly solve following problems via a feeding robot.

- What does a user want to eat?
- When does a user want to eat?

The user can independently choose dishes and select a serving time of dishes.

In this paper, we present the requirements of a feeding robot for Korea food. Then, we propose the novel feeding robot for Korean dishes especially boiled rice. In Section 2, we will mention the requirements of a feeding robot for Korean food. The specific design results will be presented in Section 3. Finally, we will make the conclusion in Section 4.

2 Requirements of a Feeding Robot for Korean Food

The major users of a feeding robot are persons with upper limbs disability such as people with C4 (cervical 4) complete spinal cord injury, cerebral palsy, and muscle diseases who cannot move their shoulder. Those users are not large. However, if we include the number of senior citizens who have difficulties in the motor function of upper limbs, the overall population of target users will be growing in the near future.

We survey the requirements of a feeding robot through a focus group. The focus group includes people with spinal cord injury and a person with cerebral palsy. In addition, we collect the opinions of occupational therapists and medical doctors. We discuss the requirements of feeding robots in the group meetings and interviews. Their opinions are as follows.

First of all, a user can control the feeding interval for desired food. In case of care giving, one of common problems is hard to control the feeding interval. The people with spinal cord injury can talk quickly when the feeding interval is too short. However, the people with cerebral palsy are difficult to represent their intention quickly such as short talking.

Second, the specialists and the user candidates believe that the feeding systems for western style food are not suitable for Korean food. Korean food basically consists of boiled rice, soup, and side dishes like kimchi. The general procedure of having a meal is as follows: at first a user eats one of side dishes, and then eats boiled rice. Or someone eats boiled rice, and then eats one of side dishes. Those steps perform repetitively during mealtime. In comparison with foreign boiled rice, the Korean boiled rice hold together very well after cooking. One of problems is handling the sticky boiled rice. In addition, the Korean soup includes meat, noodles, and various vegetables, and thus existing feeding robots are hard to handle Korean foods.

Third, a feeding robot could be applied to private homes and facilities. In view of an economical point, a feeding robot is effective in facilities that have many persons with upper limbs disability. Those kinds of facilities do not have enough caregivers for feeding. The feeding is one of heavy time consuming tasks. Thus a robot reduces the burden of caregiving for feeding. On the contrary, a feeding robot could be applied in the ordinary home in order to improve the quality of life of consumers. The member of a family can face each other and freely enjoy talking. The other members of the family can go out without the burden of feeding during couples of hours.

Next, the location of bowls or a tray is one of important factors. According to Korean culture, the location of bowls or a tray is strongly related in the dignity of a person. Some senior user candidates hate the bowls rightly in front of a mouth and they prefer to eat the food like ordinary persons. Thus we mainly use a tabletop tray. However, if the bowls are located in front of a user's mouth, we are easy to make a simple structured feeding system.

Other comments of user candidates and specialists are as follows: simple machines that can serve simple dishes with water are required. When a caregiver goes out for a while, a user needs to eat corn flakes with milk through a machine. The water service machine should be located aside a user's body. The cover's meal tray is required in order to prevent dust contamination. The price should be reasonable. For example, the price should be between US$1800~2700. The feeding robot should deal with noodles. The feeding robot could consider the posture of a user because some persons recline on a wheelchair. A feeding robot should be lightweight.

On the basis of requirements, the system that supports the activities of daily living depends on a user's culture and environments. Especially Korean food consists of several dishes: rice dishes, meat & poultry dishes, stew & soup-based dishes, and seafood dishes. The Korean food is based on the rice. How to handle boiled rice is an important problem. In general, the rice is sticky, and thus a user is difficult to pick up the rice. Sometime, a user is difficult to release the scooped boiled rice.

We should choose how to handle rice. First, the rice is naturally loaded in a bowl or a tray. In this case, rice has no special shape, and is similar with rice of a general meal. Second, the caregiver prepares rice as several lumps of rice. The lump of rice has a bitable size in a mouth. By the focus group interview, we decide to use rice without reshaping in a bowl or a tray. The user candidates said that the complex preparing process of rice makes a caregiver or a user avoid using the assistive feeding system. Thus we put boiled rice in a bowl for a feeding robot generally.

We concentrate on the rice handling. We disregarded the soup into the bowl at first version. We pour water or soup in cups. We will handle the Korean soup in a next version's design. Instead of handling a Korean styled soup, we will provide the cup with a straw for intake water or soup.

Technically, we take into account four candidates of a feeding robot in order to grip and release boiled rice effectively. First, couples of bowls are located in front of a user's mouth, and the food is presented by the spoon with short travelling. For example, if the number of bowls is three, one bowl has rice and two bowls have side dishes. However, two side dishes are not enough to enjoy the food. In general, Korean persons eat three or four side dishes with boiled rice at a time. So we need the four or five bowls.

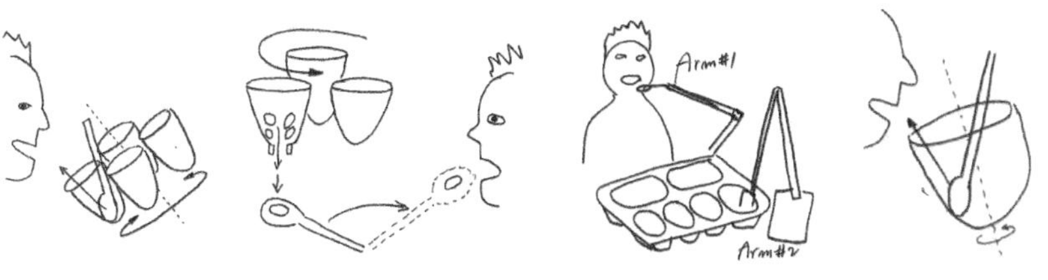

Fig. 1. Design concepts of a feeding robot

Second, the bowls are located in upper front of a user's mouth, and then the food drop from the bottom of a bowl. The food is located in the spoon by dropping, and then the spoon approaches a user's mouth. This method needs the mechanism of food dropping on the spoon. This method could be suitable for a bite-sized rice cake.

Third, the system with a food tray is located on a table. The robotic arm picks up food, and then the robotic arm moves the food to a user's mouth. These tasks are divided into two tasks: one is picking up food and the other is moving the food to a user's mouth. Two arms can be used to perform above two tasks, respectively. A user candidate talks about the easy installation of the feeding robots, especially a dual-arm manipulator, because caregivers could be senior people and are not familiar with brand-new machines.

Finally, one bowl is located in front of a user's mouth. The mixed food with rice is loaded in that bowl. Some users do not like the mixed food even though they prefer a simple feeding system.

We decide the third candidate that is located on a table in accordance with opinions of specialists and user candidates.

3 Design of Feeding Robot

We design a simple robotic system that has a dual-arm manipulator in order to handle Korean food like boiled rice with an ordinary food container effectively. Arm #1 transfers the food by a spoon from nearby a container to a user's mouth. Arm #2 picks up the food on a container and then loads up the spoon of Arm #1 with the food. If two arms have different roles, the end-effectors of two arms can be effectively designed. That is, the end-effector of Arm #1 has a spoon and the end-effector of Arm #2 has the gripper to pick up food. For the picking up the food, we can use an odd or sharp shaped gripper because that gripper does not approach nearby a user's mouth.

The two arms with two different end-effectors mimic Korean caregivers' behavior. In the cultural point of view, Korean uses a spoon and chopsticks during mealtime. The Korean caregivers usually pick up food with chopsticks, and then put food on a spoon in order to serve food to users such as children and patients. In the designed system, the gripper of Arm #2 and the spoon of Arm #1 make roles of chopsticks and a spoon, respectively. In that sense, the feeding system that has two arms stems from those feeding procedures.

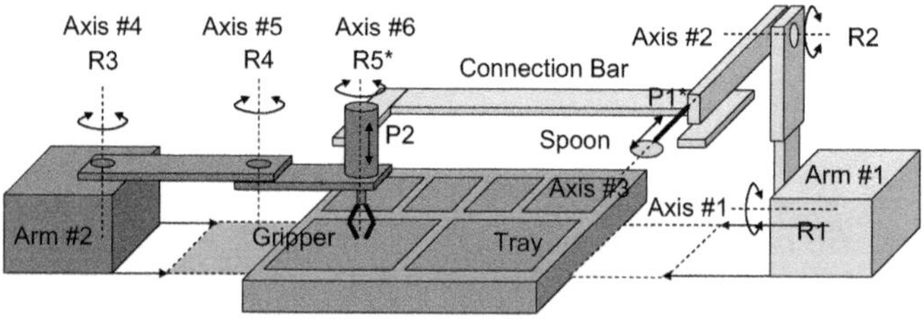

Fig. 2. The concept of a feeding robot for Korean food. P1 (Prismatic Joint #1) and R5 (Revolute Joint #5) are optionally applicable joints.

Arm #1 should have one or two degrees of freedom in order to transfer food on the spoon without changing an orientation of the spoon as shown in Fig. 2. If a revolute joint R1 connects to a revolute joint R2 through a belt, R1 and R2 have one degree of freedom. However, the prototype of Arm #1, we provide separated motors with R1 and R2. If Arm #1 does not use the belt between Axis #1 and Axis #2, we can change of the length between Axis #1 and Axis #2 manually and thus we can reduce the overall size of a system when a user is not in use. People with cerebral palsy are difficult to eat food on a spoon in front of their mouth. The feeding robot could add the additional prismatic joint P1 toward a user's mouth as shown in Fig. 2. Therefore, the robot effectively puts the food into their mouth.

Arm #2 should pick up food on a container, and two revolute joints and one prismatic joint are adopted for the effective motion along a food container. The revolute joint R5 could be added in order to control the gripper's rotation. The gripper that has a sharp tip is suitable to separate and grasp food.

In preliminary experiments on treating boiled rice, we observe that releasing rice is important like picking up rice. According to the temperature of boiled rice, the stickiness of rice is changing. The slightly cool rice is difficult to release rice from the gripper. In order to solve this problem, the feeding robot optionally put the gripper of Arm #2 in the water for a while. That process makes a layer of water on the gripper that can reduce the adhesive strength of rice. In that case, we can easily release sticky food as well.

The overall number of DOF could be four to seven excluding the gripper. A connection bar is applied between Arm #1 and Arm #2 because we need to connect electrical signals and fix the posture with respect to each other.

The feeding robot could use two kinds of containers. First of all, we could use the meal tray in the ordinary cafeteria. The tray could be located between Arm #1 and Arm #2. Second, we can use bowls that are usually used in a hospital. The bowls are hard to fix on the table when a robotic arm contacts with food in bowls. We can use a tray adaptor that can hold bowls in desired position. The tray adaptor removes the transferring food from original bowls to other trays. A caregiver only puts bowls in sockets of a tray adaptor. In order to position the lapboard on a bed in a hospital or a facility, Arm #1, a tray, and Arm #2 should be aligned in a line because of the restricted with of a lapboard.

In view of the practical application of a feeding system, a caregiver can support multiple users. At that time, a caregiver has a role of Arm #2 such as picking up and releasing food. Under the proposed concept, one caregiver can support couples of users by using Arm #1 that can deliver the food from the table to a user's mouth. The caregiver picks up the food on a dish and then loads the food on the spoon of Arm #1. Users need several tens of seconds in order to chew the served food. During one user is chewing the food, the caregiver can provide other user's spoon with food.

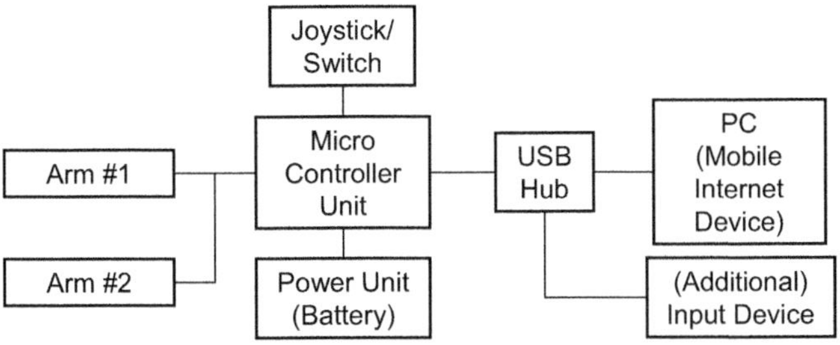

Fig. 3. Block diagram of feeding robot

The feeding robot uses a microcontroller unit to control the Arm #1 and Arm #2 as shown in Fig. 3. We add one small-sized PC with a touch screen in order to get the entertainment and to test various kinds of user interfaces. During mealtime, a user can enjoy the multimedia such as a movie or music. In addition, the small sized PC has a Windows operation system, and we can effectively add assistive devices for human computer interaction, i.e., switch, joystick, and bio-signal interface devices.

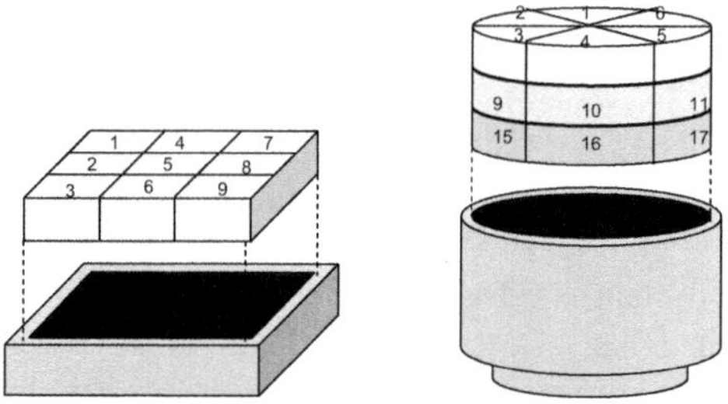

Fig. 4. The definition of grasping volume in containers

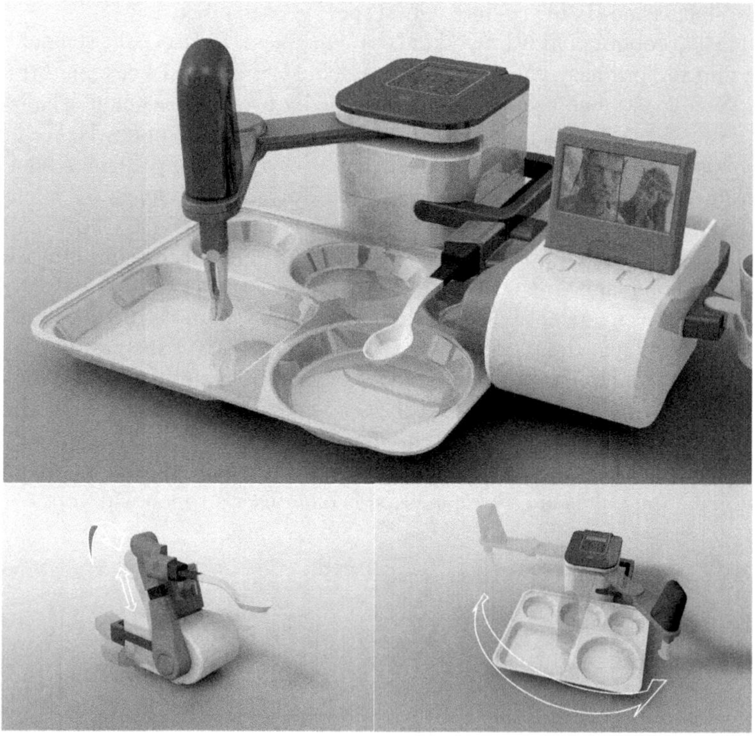

Fig. 5. Designed feeding robot for Korean food. Arm #1 (lower left-hand side figure) for transferring food and Arm #2 (lower right-hand side figure) for picking up and releasing food.

In the microcontroller unit, we allow a user or a caregiver to set the following items: an operation mode (automatic/manual), the shape and size of food containers, a mouth's location, a robot's speed, time to stay in front of a mouth, and so on. According to dishes, a user also selects the divided grasping region in each containers and the strength of a gripper of Arm #2. Our system will be open to select the above parameters. A user may make the parameters of various dishes and share with their colleagues through the internet. We hope that the user's community could exchange their own parameters for each cooking.

Grasping regions of boiled rice in a bowl could be specially defined in 3D space because a general bowl should have around 50 mm in height. The grasping volume of dishes could be defined as shown in Fig. 4. Our team is making the prototype of the proposed feeding robot now. Fig. 5 shows the estimated appearance of the system.

4 Concluding Remarks

Research Institute of NRC in Korea has been designed the novel feeding robot that suitably manipulates Korean dishes, e.g., sticky rice, in a general tray or a hospital's tableware. We are constructing the system now. According to the preliminary study, we observe that the basic operation works well through a dual-arm manipulator that has two end-effectors. We will make in experiments on the basis of the novel design soon and then analyze usability of the system. We will customize the system through users' evaluation. In addition, cost-effective user interface devices will be considered.

Acknowledgments. This Research was supported by a grant (code #10-A-01) from Research Institute, National Rehabilitation Center, Korea. The authors acknowledge the input of consumers, Mr. Hongki Kim and Mr. Kwangsup Lee, and specialists of physical medicine and rehabilitation in Korea National Rehabilitation Center in this study.

References

1. Survey & Statistics Team: 2009 Disability Statistics. Employment Development Institute, Korea (2009)
2. Topping, M.J., Smith, J.K.: The Development of HANDY 1, a Robotic System to Assist the severly disabled. In: International Conference on Rehabilitation Robotics (1999)
3. Sammons Preston, http://www.sammonspreston.com/
4. Hermann, R.P., Phalangas, A.C., Mahoney, R.M., Alexander, M.A.: Powered Feeding Devices: An Evaluation of Three Models. Arch. Phys. Med. Rehabil. 80, 1237–1242 (1999)
5. Neater Solutions Ltd., http://www.neater.co.uk/
6. Soyama, R., Ishii, S., Fukase, A.: The Development of Mealassistance Robot 'MySpoon. In: International Conference on Rehabilitation Robotics, Daejeon, Korea, pp. 88–91 (2003)
7. Mealtime Partners, http://www.mealtimepartners.com

Mild Dementia Care at Home – Integrating Activity Monitoring, User Interface Plasticity and Scenario Verification

Jit Biswas[1], Mounir Mokhtari[2], Jin Song Dong[3], and Philip Yap[4]

[1] Institute for Infocomm Research, Networking Protocols Department, Singapore
biswas@i2r.a-star.edu.sg
[2] CNRS-IPAL/Institut TELECOM & Institute for Infocomm Research, Singapore
Mounir.Mokhtari@it-sudparis.eu
[3] School of Computing, National University of Singapore, Singapore
dongjs@comp.nus.edu.sg
[4] Department of Geriatric Medicine, Alexandra Hospital, Singapore
Philip_Yap@Alexhosp.com.sg

Abstract. We discuss an integrated approach towards building systems for monitoring and assisting people with mild dementia in their homes. Our approach differs from existing approaches in three ways. First we improve context acquisition and understanding with the concept of micro-context that takes us beyond existing notions of location and temporal context; second, we incorporate plasticity concept into the human computer interface, in order to provide a natural interaction way and accommodative interface to the user; third we target robust and reliable systems that are easy to scale and deploy in diverse end-user settings, through the use of formal model building tools to specify and verify systems at key stages from requirements generation all the way to deployment and user statistics gathering. In order to address real-life end user requirements we are working closely with geriatric doctors and their staff, so as to get inputs as to precise challenges in caring for mild dementia patients, and how systems targeted at holistic, personalized assistance and care-giving can be built with a view towards scaled up deployment in diverse settings. The main contribution of this paper is an approach for system building that incorporates activity monitoring, user interface plasticity and scenario verification targeting people with cognitive decline in regards to a Singapore initiative called A-Star Home 2015 Phase II. We expect our work to lead to a methodology for systematic development of monitoring and assistive systems for cognitive interventions for mild dementia patients at home. Although the integrated framework is still not completely realized, the three areas mentioned above have each yielded significant results on their own, and these are mentioned in the paper.

Keywords: Smart Environments, Activity Recognition, Human Computer Interface, Scenario Verification, System Deployment and Replication.

1 Introduction

Caring for the elderly requires a holistic approach towards the person, his psychosocial status and the dynamics of his connection with the world. From a quality of life

Y. Lee et al. (Eds.): ICOST 2010, LNCS 6159, pp. 160–170, 2010.

standpoint, the person's own home provides the best environment where all aspects of well being, including spiritual, emotional, social, psychological and physical aspects can be met [Bond 04], and it is widely acknowledged that the elderly should stay in their own homes as long as possible and premature institutionalized be avoided.

Our focus among the elderly is on mild dementia patients who are living in their own homes, often alone. Due to memory deficits and problems with attention and concentration, our target group of mild dementia patients are particularly vulnerable to a variety of problems while living alone at home. Our primary goal is to enable such persons, through assistive technologies, to maximize their physical and mental functions and to continue to engage in social networks, so that they can lead independent and purposeful lives.

Information and Communication Technologies (ICT) may be employed in a variety of ways in smart homes, for the purpose of caring for the elderly with mild dementia. Assistive technology may be employed to prevent accidents and mishaps, ensure safety, enable self care and support daily needs. These needs could be in the area of medication, food, locating objects, telephone etc. ICT is also able to carry out monitoring of activity and behaviour and intervention (through prompts and reminders) when needed and appropriate. The use of ICT in the home has its challenges. Signal interference from other household electronics, mapping exact location of persons / objects, excessive amount of data (as with certain modalities such as video), high numbers of variables leading to computational complexity in classification of events, privacy issues, and a confusion of false positives giving rise to systems that are not reliable and difficult to trust. In the area of prompting for reminders or intervention, the following questions are germane: What & when to prompt? How to prompt? (eg. live verbal, audio, digital TV, cell phone, etc.) How to input prompts? How to cope with ignored prompts?

Geriatricians consider the ADLs to be the very basic activities of daily living, namely grooming, toileting, bathing, eating one's meals by oneself, taking medication on time, and ambulation as the very basic activities which one needs to be able to perform if one is to live independently in his/her own home. Instrumental ADLs are slightly more advanced (such as tidying ones home, cooking, vacuuming and mopping the floor and the ability to do other simple tasks such as answering phone calls and unlocking/locking doors). The person with early cognitive impairment (levels 3 & 4 in Table 1), is usually able carry out ADLs and iADLs but is often handicapped by his poor memory and thus forgets to carry out these tasks or omits key steps vital to their safe rendering. Assistive technology that provides timely prompts and reminders will enable him to preserve his abilities and independence. The interaction with pervasive environment represents a difficult task mainly when targeting people with special needs (mild dementia). Indeed, the interaction should be done through a user-friendly interface by making it easier to access to the environment and benefit from assistance. Consequently, the User Interface should support not only user preferences but also the cognitive capabilities. At the same time, different surrounding computing platform and devices/sensors are considered as an additional source of heterogeneity.

Table 1. Level of cognitive decline and corresponding deficits

1	No cognitive decline	No subjective or objective deficits
2	Very mild cognitive decline	Some subjective complaints, no objective deficits
3	Mild cognitive decline	Mild working memory deficits (attention, concentration)
4	Moderate cognitive decline	Episodic memory deficits (memory of recent events)
5	Moderately severe cognitive decline	Explicit memory deficits (ability to accomplish usual tasks)
6	Severe cognitive decline	Severe memory deficits (which cause delusion)
7	Very severe cognitive decline	All verbal activities are lost

The main contribution of this paper is an approach for system building that incorporates activity monitoring, user interface plasticity and scenario verification. The remainder of the paper is structured as follows. Section 2 discusses our five step methodology for building recognition and assistive systems. Sections 2 and 3 discuss respectively, how activity recognition and User interface plasticity will address key issues and gaps in existing approaches for helping with mild dementia at home. In Section 5 we discuss scenario verification, and how we intend to develop reliable and robust systems of sensors and actuators based on a tool called PAT. We end with conclusions in Section 6.

2 Methodology

In our methodology there are three five basic steps.

1. **Requirements gathering,** through gathering of knowledge from doctors, care-givers and other sources who can provide important information about important scenarios with respect to the mild dementia patients' ADLs. Problems associated with mild dementia patients are well known to the medical community, and also to those doing research in assistive living for the elderly. We aim to capture requirements from doctors and care-givers and other professionals who are in constant touch with the elderly, in order to get a good idea of the real needs of activities of daily living and the instrumental activities of daily living, so that the outcome will greatly impact the end user community through the use of appropriate aids and interventions. Note that the end user might be the mild dementia patient, a family member, the doctor, the physio-therapist or the occupational-therapist.
2. **Scenario definition**, or the encoding of knowledge into scenarios for the plans. This step determines important targeted ADLs and the scenarios in which they occur. Since the actors in the system are human and machine, they must be modelled with care, in a manner that the critical issues in human machine interaction are modelled with precision and tested for soundness, correctness, operational efficiency, and other types of consistency checking and correctness.

Our approach is to use *model based systems* for specification and verification of the distributed system that performs activity recognition, context acquisition & understanding, activity recognition and provides appropriate HCI interfaces for prompts and alerts. Besides the obvious inclusion of the mild dementia patient as an actor, other actors in the system should be considered. Actors can be human or machine. Using our formal tools it is possible to represent a human / machine interface through communication and synchronization primitives and the behaviour of human/machine can be modelled as processes of the possible events. Often these are ignored during requirements specification and verification, thereby giving rise to potential glitches in the system.

3. **Specification and design of activity and plan recognition with scenario verification.** From cues in the knowledge capture stage, rules are framed. These rules specify spatio-temporal relationships between objects, activities, actors and their partial orderings. We allow alternative plans and interleaved plans wherever possible or expected. As a refinement of this step, sensors are brought in as actors into the scenario, and constraints that arise from sensor data acquisition, fusion and combination algorithms are also incorporated.
4. **Specification and design of assistive systems with scenario verification.** This step involves the intervention or feedback to the user by means of appropriate prompts and reminders. Alerts to care-givers and doctors and other human actors are also in handled here, making sure that alternatives are considered. It is important to have a system that is user friendly and tolerant of varying behavioural pattern. Prompts generated when they are not needed, can be a nuisance and can lead to user frustration and rejection.
5. **Iterative refinement** of steps 1 through 4 leading to performance improvement. Sensor produced data may be accurate and timely (i.e. the information quality is high), however two features may be so close together in their sensor produced values (because of restricted domain or because of close proximity of feature values). In this case alternate modalities or methods must be selected to recognize the activity in order to reduce uncertainty. We have found that appropriate rules may be framed in many cases, in order to discriminate between activities, given additional context information.

3 Activity Recognition through Improved Context Understanding

Current approaches that aim to automatically capture context from the environment or to classify residents' activities stop short at summary statements such as Mr Jones was "performing kitchen activity" between 7pm and 9pm or "performing dining room activity" between 8pm and 10pm. Summaries of this nature are minimally useful, and do not give doctors and caregivers much information about the health and well-being status of the elderly residents who are being monitored. Ideally an activity and behaviour monitoring system should be capable of reporting what was the precise activity that the resident was engaged in, how long that activity took, and how well (meaning assigning some kind of rating) the activity was performed. For behaviour monitoring (we take behaviour to be meaningful sequences of activities leading to some well defined goal), the reporting should essentially be the same, but with more semantics such as degrees of ease, degrees of prompting or help that had to be provided and so on.

Micro-context is a fragment of information about a user and the user's activity context that may be germane to a particular line of reasoning. By itself a piece of micro-context may make no sense whatsoever, however in the larger context of a smart space and the history of activities that have taken place (or are taking place) within that environment, micro-context often provides key information to enable proper inference and decision making. For example the orientation of a person's head may give us vital information about whether or not to present a visual prompt on a TV screen (as opposed to using an audio prompt). Similarly, the precise position of a person's hand gives us a piece of vital information to determine (with a high probability) that the person is drinking or eating his food, given the larger context that he is seated at the dining table and it is meal time. We have found that to build a reasoning system based purely on one sensing modality is much harder to do, than one based on a mix of sensing modalities, each presenting its micro-context in a manner that is understood at a high level. Note that micro-context information is useful for activity recognition as well as providing accurate assistance.

In our work, sensor information from a particular sensing modality is processed to obtain a set of features. The features are mapped into primitives through training algorithms, either in-situ or remotely. In our early work [Foo 06] we used various modalities of sensing to classify to high degree of accuracy, certain types of movements, such as agitated outward movements of a dementia patient. The micro context in this work consisted of highly accurate inferences on body position and leg or arm movement, obtained through pressure sensors, ultra-sound sensors and video camera. In another work [Tolstikov 08] we show how in the presence of uncertainty from two modalities, namely accelerometer (with noisy information) and RFID (with insufficient information), we are able to classify eating activity primitives with a high degree of certainty. Such activity primitives are the micro-context in this example, since they provide important information about the targeted behaviors or activities that are being analyzed. In more recent work we have built a plan recognition engine based on Discrete Finite Automata, [Phua 09a, Phua 09b] which employs an algorithm that matches strings made up of pre-assigned labels, where each label corresponds to a piece of micro-context gathered by a particular sensor. In this case there are several types of sensors in the smart space, ranging from reed switches and PIR sensors to features extracted based on known patterns of images sequences produced by a video camera, into appropriate micro-context labels. The system developed is however quite rigid and doesn't permit flexibility in event sequences or adaptive (plastic) user interfaces. Having obtained these successful results in the area of activity recognition we will now proceed to incorporate micro-context into the overall system that provides assistance and prompts to the elderly in a flexible manner.

4 User Interface Plasticity for Flexible Adaptation

The design of dynamic user interface represents an open issue which should be considered especially when focusing on pervasive environment. The term "plasticity" is inspired from the property of materials that expand and contract under natural constraints without breaking, thus preserving continuous usage. Applied to HCI, plasticity is the capacity of an interactive system to withstand variations of context of use while preserving usability.

User interface models propose abstractions to improve the comprehension and the manipulation of what a UI is. The real-world objects abstracted away in this case concern all manifestation of a UI in the real world i.e., UI appearance (i.e., *presentation model*) and behaviour (i.e., *dialog model*). Methodologies described in the literature vary according various dimensions:

- ✓ ***Coverage.*** Some methods concentrate on behavioural specification only (e.g., for property checking) and leave aside the problems related to UI appearance e.g., Petri Nets [Palanque 97] or Process Algebra. The integration of these methods with presentational aspects is still a hot research topic.
- ✓ ***Separation of concerns.*** Some methods do not make a clear distinction between dialog and presentation. For instance, ADEPT [Markopoulos 92] relies on the task model as only description of the dynamics of the system.
- ✓ ***Level of abstraction.*** UI models proposed in the literature show a great diversity in terms of levels of abstraction of their concept. Three levels of abstraction, and corresponding model, are mentioned in the literature: abstract UI model, concrete UI model and final UI (also called implementation or code level). Abstract and Concrete UI raises many interpretation issues: What is abstract? What is concrete? With respect to what?

A final UI is composed of two sub-levels: The rendering level concerns the way a piece of UI related code is rendered on the screen (or other interactive space) and made perceivable by a user. Note that this level may also cover physical devices enabling the interaction with the system. The code level is the implementation of the user interface. This implementation is achieved using a programming language.

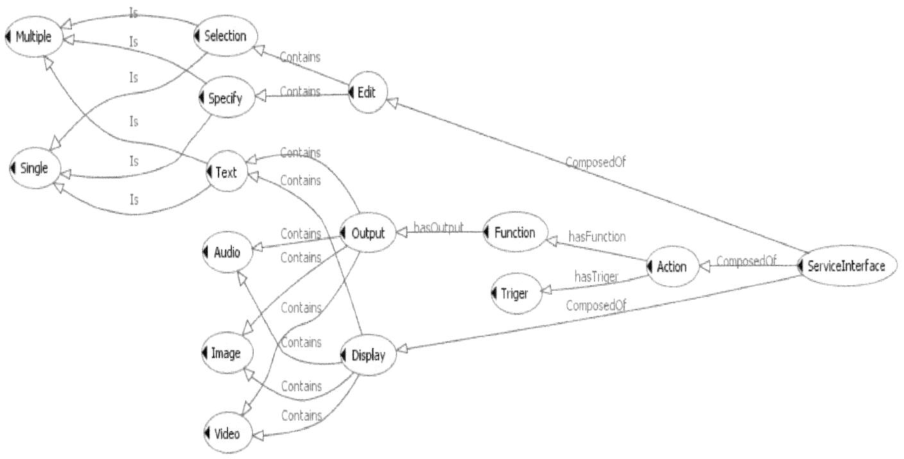

Fig. 1. Service Interface Ontology

i) Service Interface Ontology and Reasoning

An overview of the whole service Interface ontology is presented in Figure 1, which selects the Object properties between the various elements of the model. Each service has to instantiate the ontology to create its service interface. The ontology presented in the figure is considered as the ideal service interface which is composed of an Action, Display and Edit. In some cases service interfaces could be represented just as display with no corresponding action behind. This is usually the case for information services.

ii) System design and integration

In order to reach a multiplatform form concept, three different modalities have been considered for the design and implementation of abstracted user interface [Hariz 09] as shown in figure below (Figure 2):

1. **IPTV system**, allowing the user to interact with TV and receive different reminding events. A linux based set top box will be considered to implement OSGi Java bundles (service approach). This system has been developed in regard to Nuadu European Project [Nuadu 09] which involved about 25 end users (ageing people with and without cognitive decline) to validate the user interface content and interaction [Ghorbel 09]. Actually the system is under improvement in order to be deployed in a nursing home.
2. **Mobile device**, insuring the service continuity when the user in on the move or in different places at home. This work has been done through Cogknow European project which aimed at focusing on people with mild dementia [Cogknow 09]. Several field trials involving about 70 end – users has been performed. We are planning to extend this concept on open platform such as Android based Google phone in order to provide extended services (i.e. including indoor NFC technologies for location and outdoor GPS navigation system).

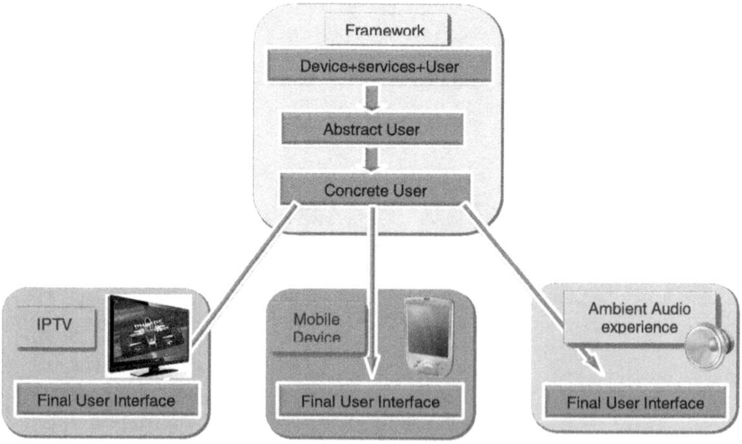

Fig. 2. User interface plasticity framework

3. **Ambient Audio experience** is an emerging issue, in order to provide pervasive service to specific users in the community. We developed an audio rendering reminder based on wireless speaker disseminated in the user environment. We are aiming now at extending this concept to context aware audio reminding system.

5 Evaluation and Validation

In order to validate user acceptability, several evaluations with end-users have been performed mainly in France at Geriatric hospital of Broca in Paris and a residence of ageing people in Kunheim (East of France). Investigation involved 70 aged persons and 25 experts (nurses and physiotherapists) [Hariz 09]. The study showed the interest of the users regarding the user interface on the TV (reminder, agenda, picture dialling, home control) and highlighted the complexity in using a mobile device. Another issue showed that nurse application on the mobile was welcome by the residence staff as it provides an efficient communication link with residents. An ongoing investigation is currently being undertaken in a residence of people with dementia through Alexandra Hospital in Singapore and preliminary results will be presented during the conference.

6 Scenario Verification – for Robust, Reliable Systems of Sensors and Actuators

Pervasive smart space systems are in general concurrent and real-time systems with smart sensors everywhere. Even though a smart space is not as mission critical as a jet airplane in war conditions, the set of criteria that determine its end-user acceptability are similar, and perhaps even more exacting. It must be reliable and robust otherwise patients and care-givers will stop using it after a few false alarms, it must be close to real-time (in order to catch user errors and react within a meaningful time bound), it must make use of a diversity of information coming from a large number of sources, i.e. it is a full fledged distributed system. The design of smart sensor based concurrent and real-time systems are difficult problems because of the increased complexity and evolved context changes. The principal validation methods for complex systems are simulation, testing, deductive verification, and model checking. Model checking [CGP99] is a method of automatically verifying concurrent systems. The process of model checking can be separated into system modelling, requirement specification and verification. It has a number of advantages over other traditional approaches. Model checking has been used successfully in practice to verify complex circuit design and communication protocols.

Recently at NUS we have developed a formal verification toolset PAT [SLDP09] and it supports an extensible framework which allows domain specific modules to be built for different applications. The formal PAT frame is illustrated as the following diagram (Fig 3):

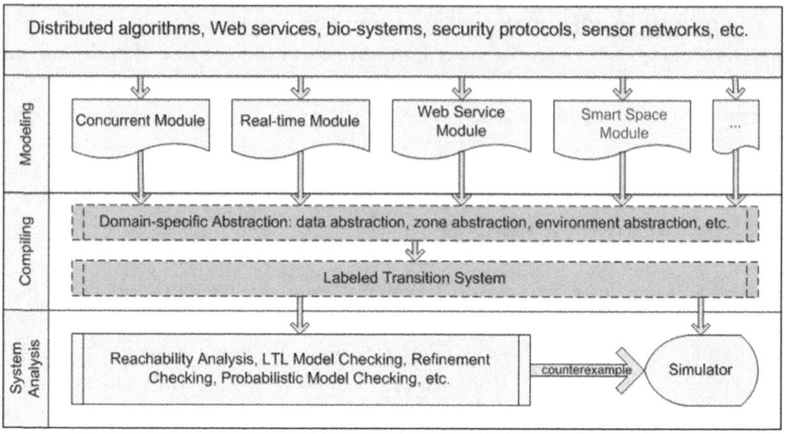

Fig. 3. PAT Architecture

PAT is useful to perform early resolution of requirements of distributed, scalable systems comprising man/ machine interfaces, sensors and actuators with timing constraints, communication and synchronization mechanisms and their use in order to capture realistic situations arising in complex man / machine systems. We intend to use PAT as a modelling tool for the modelling of various actors such as people, devices, wheelchairs, sensors, and virtual sensors and network gateways. We will also use PAT for model checking and verification.

We plan to build a specific module for the smart space system domain and the module may support design constructs that can directly model sensors and actuators. We believe this module can be built based on the Real-Time Module (RTM) that we have already developed [SLDZ09]. As an initial investigation we aim to apply RTM to design a timed event based reminder system that will help elderly with early cognitive impairment (levels 3 & 4) for activities, i.e., wake up, brush teeth, making phone calls, turn off stoves, taking medication, bring keys while going out.

In general, the timed reminding system can have

- Multiple reminders
- Reminders can interrupt or communicate with each other
- Reminders can be triggered at a specific time or by some events
- Reminders are associated with priorities

The screen capture (Fig 4) is the PAT tool with design window on the left hand side and verification/auto-simulation windows on the right hand side. The design model captures the behaviour of a work-in-progress timed reminding system.

In a particular context, i.e., medicine reminder, various individual requirements and constraints need to be captured in the design models, e.g.:

- Remind the elderly to take medicine 30 minutes after meal every day.
- Never prompt outside a certain time interval.
- Don't prompt if pill is already taken within the current time interval.
- Don't prompt if the participant is not at home.

- Don't prompt if the participant is sleeping.
- Don't prompt if participant is on the phone.
- Prompting will resume if the participant returns home before the specific time interval expires

There are cases that some reminding rules may lead to conflict scenarios. The model checking functions can automatically produce those conflict scenarios that may lead to undesirable status.

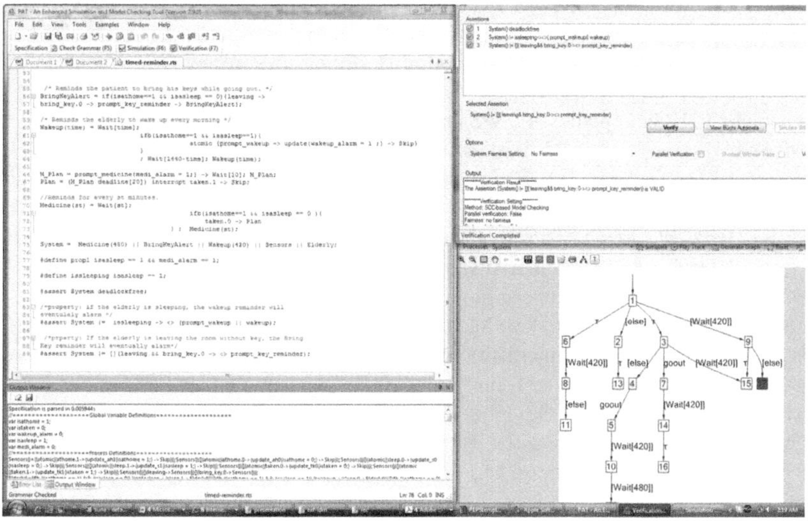

Fig. 4. PAT model of a timed and event based reminding system

7 Conclusions

We have presented a framework and an approach for system building that incorporates activity monitoring, user interface plasticity and scenario verification. Although an integrated framework is still not realized, the three areas mentioned have each yielded significant results, as reported in the paper. In our recently started project [AMUP10], we have embarked on bringing these three areas together into a common framework. It is expected that the use of formal methods for scenario verification, advanced flexible human computer interfaces for user interface plasticity and artificial intelligence for activity monitoring, will be important technical means in providing help to home-dwelling elderly with mild dementia, their caregivers and family members.

References

[Bond 04] Bond, J., Corner, L.: Quality of life and older people. Open University Press, McGraw Hill Education, England (2004)

[Foo 06] Foo, V., Qiu, Q., Biswas, J., Wai, A.A.P.: Fusion Considerations in Monitoring and Handling Agitation Behavior for Persons with Dementia. In: 9th International Conference on Information Fusion, ICIF 2006 (2006)

[Tolstikov 08] Tolstikov, A., Biswas, J., Tham, C.-K., Yap, P.: Eating Activity Primitives Detection - a Step Towards ADL Recognition. In: Healthcom 2008 (2008)

[Phua 09a] Phua, C., Biswas, J., Tolstikov, A., Foo, V., Huang, W., Jayachandran, M., Aung, A., Roy, P., Aloulou, H., Feki, M., Gioroux, S., Bouzouane, A., Bouchard, B.: Plan Recognition based on Sensor Produced Micro-Context for Eldercare. In: Proc. of RO-MAN 2009 Workshop on Context-Awareness in Smart environments: Background, Achievements, and Challenges, Japan (2009)

[Phua 09b] Phua, C., Foo, V., Biswas, J., Tolstikov, A., Aung, A., Maniyeri, J., Huang, W., That, M., Xu, D., Chu, A.: 2-Layer Erroneous-Plan Recognition for Dementia Patients in Smart Homes. In: Proceedings of Healthcom 2009, Sydney Australia, pp. 21–28 (2009)

[Palanque 97] Palanque, P.: Spécifications formelles et systèmes interactifs: Vers des systèmes fiables et utilisables. travail 'Habilitation à diriger des recherches. Technical report, Université de Toulouse 1 (1997)

[Markopoulos 92] Markopoulos, P., Wilson, S., Pycock, J., Johnson, P.: Adept - A task based design environment. In: 25th Hawaii International Conference on System Sciences, Conference Proceedings, vol. II, pp. 587–596. IEEE Computer Society Press, California (1992)

[Hariz 09] Hariz, M.: Mechanism for handling User Interface plasticity in Ambient Assistive Living. Ph.D. Thesis. Telecom SudParis/ University Pierre & Marie Curie (July 2009)

[Nuadu 09] NUADU ITEA European project, http://www.nuadu.org

[Ghorbel 09] Ghorbel, M., Arab, F., Mokhtari, M.: Assistive housing: Case study in a residence for elderly people. In: 2nd International Conference on Pervasive Computing Technologies for Healthcare 2008, 30 janvier – 1er février 2008, Tampere, Finland (2008)

[Cogknow 09] Helping people with mild dementia to navigate their day, http://www.cogknow.eu

[CGP99] Clarke, E.M., Grumberg, O., Peled, D.A.: Model Checking. Springer, Heidelberg (1999)

[SLDP09] Sun, J., Liu, Y., Dong, J.S., Pang, J.: PAT: Towards Flexible Verification under Fairness. In: Bouajjani, A., Maler, O. (eds.) CAV 2009. LNCS, vol. 5643, pp. 709–714. Springer, Heidelberg (2009)

[SLDZ09] Sun, J., Liu, Y., Dong, J.S., Zhang, X.: Verifying Stateful Timed CSP Using Implicit Clocks and Zone Abstraction. In: ICFEM 2009, pp. 581–600 (2009)

[AMUP10] Biswas, J., Mokhtari, M., Dong, J.S.: Activity Monitoring and UI Plasticity for supporting Ageing with mild Dementia at Home (AMUPADH), Home2015 Phase II Project, A*STAR Singapore

Behavior-Based Needs of Older Adults Concerning Aging-Friendly Digital Home Applications Using a Web-Based Survey

Hyunjoo Kwon, Yeunsook Lee*, and Soojin Lee

Dept. of Housing and Interior Design, Yonsei University,
134 Shinchon-dong, Seodaimoon-gu, Seoul, 120-749, Korea, Republic of

Abstract. With undergoing a stunning demographic transformation, a growing problem is how to support the elderly population who want to continue living independently as opposed to moving to an institutional care setting. Globally, the increasing number and proportion of frail and elderly adults with limitations in mobility, dexterity and mental capacity who are living in their own homes or desiring to live independently is a well- recognized social fact, which has provided clues to the needs and values for seniors to live in aging-friendly digital homes. The purpose of this study is to ascertain the needs of older adults in terms of the items of digital home applications supporting their daily living activities through a web-based questionnaire survey. It also empowers end users to make informed choices as they see their concerns and suggestions being addressed through the web-based survey.

Keywords: aging in place, digital home, smart home, older adults, web-based survey.

1 Introduction

Aging is the social factor shaping the future of the vast majority of countries today. With life expectancy rising and birth-rates falling to record lows, South Korea is about to undergo a stunning demographic transformation. According to the latest government projections, 38 percent of its population will be defined as elderly by 2050. It will be contending with Japan, Italy, and Spain as the oldest country on earth (Korean Statistical Information Service, 2006).

A significant concern as people grow older is that they may have to leave their homes. Traditionally, as people age and their health deteriorates, they may be forced to move from their homes and into assisted living facilities and, as they become more frail, into nursing homes. However, older adults want to remain at home as long as possible; they fear moving to a nursing home (Marek and Rantz 2000; Rantz et al., 2005). Attention is growing on finding ways to support elderly people who want to continue living independently in their homes (Ball et al. 2004).

The term "aging in place" has traditionally referred to individuals growing old in their own homes with an emphasis on modification of the home environment to

* Corresponding author

Y. Lee et al. (Eds.): ICOST 2010, LNCS 6159, pp. 171–177, 2010.

compensate for the limitations associated with aging (Pynoos 1993). According to the Korean Statistical Information Service (2005), 85.5% of older adults want to age-in-place while receiving care, and for as long as possible. With aging, we become less able to perform ADL (Activities of Daily Living) at the optimal levels we once did. ADLs are personal maintenance tasks performed daily, such as eating, getting in and out of bed, bathing, dressing, going to the toilet, and getting around indoors (Katz & Akpom, 1976). As decreased mobility and cognitive impairments among the elderly lead to functional decline, the house environment is being asked to perform an increasingly important role in the provision of health and social care to frail older adults (Cheek et al., 2005).

Increasing numbers of frail and elderly people desiring to age in place have provided clues to the needs and values essential for effective digital homes. Digital home technology can be defined as "a collective term for information and communication technology in homes where components communicate through a local network." It may further be defined as "using basic and assistive devices to build an environment in which many features in the home are automated and where devices can communicate with each other"(Cheek, et al., 2005). However, most initiatives are primarily demonstrations of technological possibilities. Much work still needs to be done in addressing the potential end-users' needs and expectations.

The purpose of this study is to grasp the older adults' needs and preferences for the items of digital home applications supporting their daily living activities.

2 Methods

2.1 Data Collection

A web-based survey was selected to carry out the empirical research. Purposive sampling was used to select 80 respondents between 40 and 80 years old who have experience using computers and mobile phones, and who are expected to be the potential consumers of digital home. Web-based questionnaires were developed not only to provide more information to respondents, but also to communicate effectively with visual tools, which are rarely found in off-line questionnaires.

The survey was conducted between April 1, 2008 and April 15, 2008. Collected data were analyzed by SPSS with the Win 12.0 statistics program package.

2.2 Web Survey Compositions

The survey includes demographic and socioeconomic features, residential experience and the needs of aging-friendly digital home items supporting ADL and IADL (Instrumental Activities of Daily Living).

2.2.1 ADL and IADL Domains

To measure the level of functioning, social workers generally assess the types of activities that older people are able to complete on their own (Rogers, 2006). These activities fall into two general categories: 1) activities of daily living (ADL), and 2) instrumental activities of daily living (IADL). Based on the performance abilities of senior adults performing these activities, older people may determine whether they are able to live independently in their current houses or have to move to extended care facilities. In this study, twelve essential ADL and IADL domains for older adults' independent living are selected: transferring, going to the toilet, face washing, bathing and showering, eating, food preparation, dressing, laundry, housekeeping, operation of home appliances, responsibility for own medications, and ability to use the telephone. Based on relevance, the activity domains were classified into the types of rooms to be developed in the web survey questionnaire form. The types of rooms are the entrance, living room, bedroom, bathroom, kitchen and dining room, and utility/laundry room.

2.2.2 Aging-Fiendly Digital Home Items

Aging-friendly digital homes for older adults might be equipped not only with technologies, but also with the design features of the home environments to support ADL and IADL for the older adults. Forty seven digital home items were selected, considering the older adults' decline in several physical attributes: muscular strength,

Table 1. Digital home items in home areas

Entrance
no-step and flush thresholds, non-slippery floors, 34"-36" wide doors, lever door handles, motion sensor lights, and fingerprint door locks
Living Room
easy window lock, lift chair, picture button telephone, motion sensor concentrated lighting, and robot vacuum
Bedroom
light switches with lighting, large and simple thermostats, window grips, organized storage, adjustable-height hangers, motion sensor lights, home appliance remote control, and voice activated lighting
Bathroom
raised toilet seat with grab bars, large toilet flush button, bidet, simple and easy bidet control buttons, 36" high counter tops, single lever handle on faucets, basin with grab bars, tilt mirror, mirror with lighting, magnifying mirror, bath tub chair, bath tub and shower with grab bars, bathtub with non-slippery material, shower chair, intelligent emergency service, intelligent bath tub, and health checker
Kitchen and Dining Room
sink with grab bars, handcart, pedal faucets, range with large buttons, easy clean flooring, easy clean sink, refuse compressor, sink chair, sliding drawers, adjustable-height sink, spotlight on sink area, mirror under cabinet ceiling, C-type cabinet handle, counter top sill, automatic gas shut-off valve, smart refrigerator, automatic ventilation fan, and medication timer
Laundry Room
diagonal washer and dryer, smart washer and dryer, and home appliance faultfinder

bone articulation, vision, hearing, and tactual sense. Selection of the items was made by literature reviews,[1] field studies,[2] and website information. Those items classified into the types of rooms are as shown in Table 1 and Table 2.

Table 2. Examples of digital home items in entrance

Behaviors	Design items	Images
Transferring	**Motion sensor light** Turning a light on and off automatically with recognition of motion not operating a switch Source : Doosan Apartment. (2008). Korea©	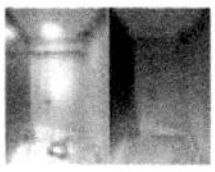
Operation	**Fingerprint door locks** Electronic biometric access without keys Source: Living Tomorrow. (2007).Belgium©	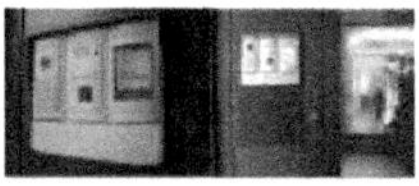
Shopping	**Smart home delivery box** Receiving and keeping delivery safely with computer systems Source: Living Tomorrow. (2007).Belgium©	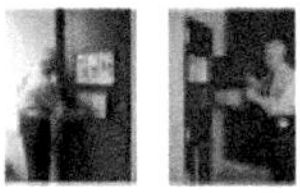

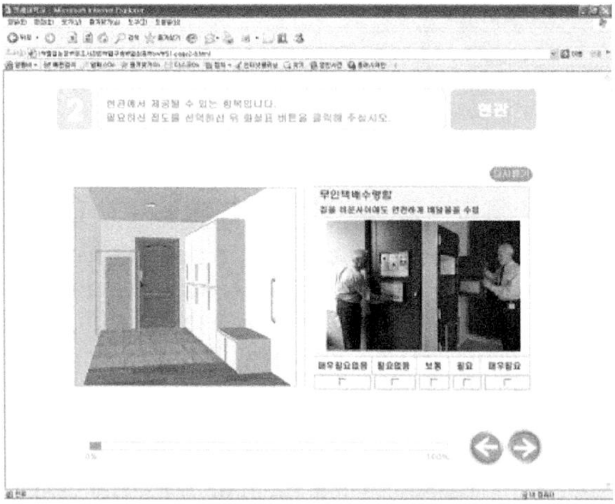

Fig. 1. Web survey questionnaire example in entrance

[1] Kwon, 2008; KNHC, 2000; Lee, 1994; Song, 2006.
[2] Smart Medical Home in University of Rochester, Aware Home in Georgia Tech, Living Tomorrow in Belgium, Digital Home in Korea and ABC Houses in Japan.

2.3 Web Survey Implementation

After linking to the survey site using a web browser, respondents see a welcoming screen informing them of the purpose of the survey. After starting the survey, participants click through a series of questions with audio explanations concerning their individual backgrounds and their needs in terms of the aging- friendly digital home items. The digital home items are presented in the framework of the types of rooms with the relevant ADL and IADL.

Needs are rated on a five-point scale ranging from "very necessary" to "very unnecessary, with a neutral mid-point. One of the web survey questionnaires is shown as Figure 1.

3 Results

3.1 Socio-demographic Characteristics

Respondents' average age was 64.5 years old. The female to male ratio was one to one. While less than half of them (42.5%) perceived their health as very healthy or healthy, most other respondents (45.0%) evaluated it as fair. And, nearly 12.6% perceived it as unhealthy or very unhealthy. More than half of the respondents (60.1%) had a college degree or higher.

3.2 Living Arrangements and Residential Features

While one half of the respondents was living together with a spouse and children (47.5%), almost all of the other half (42.5%) showed independent forms of living arrangements; living with a spouse or alone. Two thirds of the respondents (62.5%) wanted to live independently in an unrestricted environment as they age, and 23.8% wanted to move to an institutional care setting later in their lives.

Average living expenses per month showed a wide distribution. More than two thirds of the respondents (72.5%) were living in apartments, which are currently the representative type of housing in Korea.

3.3 Attitude to Aging-Friendly Digital Homes

In general, most of the respondents (82.5%) showed a very positive or positive attitude toward the aging-friendly digital home items, with the willingness to apply digital technologies to their houses later in their lives.

3.4 Needs of Aging-Friendly Digital Home Items

The digital home items that rated more than 4.0 on a five-point scale are as follows.

3.4.1 Transferring

The respondents needed "Non-Slippery floors in the bathroom" the most (4.66), followed by "No-step in the bathroom" (4.38), "No-step in the bedroom" (4.34), and "Wide doorways" (4.28).

3.4.2 Operation

The respondents needed "Intelligent emergency service" (4.71) the most. "Home appliance faultfinder"(4.41) and "Easy-to-See, Easy-to-Use thermostats" were the next ones (4.33) needed most among the nine items.

3.4.3 Housekeeping

Among the three items, "Refuse compressor" (4.51) was rated highest and "Food waste dryer" (4.41) was the second highest.

3.4.4 Face Washing

With a low standard deviation (0.779), “basin with grab bars” was rated 4.03 on a five-point scale, showing a high level of need.

3.4.5 Dressing

The only item in this category, “Adjustable-height hanger” making up for limited muscular strength, was rated 4.43 on the scale.

3.4.6 Ability to Use the Telephone

"Picture button telephone" for declining eye sight and memory was rated 4.11 on the five-point scale.

3.4.7 Shopping

“Smart home delivery box” to receive and keep shopping items safely and conveniently for the emerging home shopping generation was rated 4.04.

3.4.8 Food Preparation

The demand for“Automatic gas shut-off valve”got the highest score of 4.61 among the seven items in this category, followed by adjustable-height sink (4.39), sink cabinet sill (4.16), smart refrigerator (4.13), spotlight on the sink area (4.04), and sliding drawers (4.01).

3.4.9 Responsibility for Own Medications

"Medication timer” service was rated 4.43 on the scale, reflecting a need of the older adults due to declining memory.

3.4.10 Laundry

"Adjustable-height laundry hanger" was rated 4.26, reflecting the need of older adults with limited muscular strength, and Korean living culture contributed to low dryer use.

4 Conclusion

Overall, the respondents had a positive attitude toward aging-friendly digital home technologies in general. As previously stated, their perceptions concerning the potential of the technologies were identified on the behavioural basis of ADL and IADL. Future studies may include older adults’ emotional and psychological needs concerning the effectiveness of smart home applications.

This study provides insight into older adults’ attitudes toward specific digital home items, and also captures their level of willingness to allow installation of such technologies. Additionally, this study suggests further inquiry into the benefits of such technologies, in terms of reaction rather than prevention presented in this study. Further evidence of the effectiveness of aging-friendly digital home application is required before issues of integration into standard practice can be explored and guidelines can be defined for digital home technology implementation.

Acknowledgments. This work was supported by the Korea Science and Engineering Foundation (KOSEF) grant funded by the Korea government (MEST) (No. R11-2008-098-00000-0).

References

1. Ball, M.M., Perkins, M.M., Whittington, F.J., Connell, B.R., Hollingsworth, C., King, S.V., Elrod, C.L., (...), Combs, B.L.: Managing Decline in Assisted Living: The Key to Aging in Place. Journals of Gerontology - Series B Psychological Sciences and Social Sciences 59(4), 202–212 (2004)
2. Cheek, P., Nikpour, L., Nowlin, H.D.: Aging Well with Smart Technology. Nursing Administration Quarterly 29(4), 329–338 (2005)
3. Johnson, R.A.: Helping Older Adults Adjust to Relocation: Nursing Interventions and Issues. In: Swanson, L., Tripp-Riemer, T. (eds.) Transitions in the Older Adult, pp. 52–72. Springer, New York (1999)
4. Katz, S., Akpom, C.A.: A Measure of Primary Sociobiological Functions. International Journal of Health Services 6, 493–507 (1976)
5. Korea National Housing Corporation. Development on the Model of Intelligent Apartment Housing Corresponding to Residents' Characteristics. Korean National Housing Corporation Press, Seoul (2000)
6. Kwon, H.: Behavior-Based Design of Aging-Friendly Digital Home Using a Web-Based Survey. Unpublished master thesis. Yonsei University, Seoul, Korea (2008)
7. Lee, Y.: Aging Friendly Housing Design Guidelines. Yonsei University, Seoul (1996)
8. Manion, P.S., Rantz, M.J.: Relocation Stress Syndrome: A Comprehensive Plan for Long-term Care Admissions. Geriatric Nursing 16(3), 108–112 (1995)
9. Marek, K.D., Rantz, M.J.: Aging in Place: A New Model for Long Term Care. Nursing Administration Quarterly 24(3), 1–11 (2000)
10. Pynoos, J.: Strategies for Home Modification and Repair. In: Ageing in Place, Baywood, Amityville, NY, pp. 29–38 (1993)
11. Rantz, M.J., Marek, K.D., Aud, M.A., Tyrer, H.W., Skubic, M., Demiris, G., Hussam, A.A.: Technology and Nursing Collaboration to Help Older Adults Age in Place. Nursing Outlook 53(1), 40–45 (2005)
12. Rogers, A.: Human Behavior in the Social Environment. McGraw Hill, New York (2006)
13. Song, J.: Ubiquitous House Model Based on the Human Behavior. Unpublished Dissertation. Yonsei University, Seoul (2006)

Object Recognition and Ontology for Manipulation with an Assistant Robot

Hélène Vorobieva[1], Mariette Soury[2], Patrick Hède[1], Christophe Leroux[2], and Philippe Morignot[2]

[1] CEA, LIST, Vision and Content Engineering Laboratory,
18 route du Panorama, BP6
F-92265 Fontenay-aux-Roses, France
[2] CEA, LIST, Interactive Robotics Laboratory,
18 route du Panorama, BP6
F-92265 Fontenay-aux-Roses, France
{helene.vorobieva,mariette.soury,patrick.hede,
christophe.leroux,philippe.morignot}@cea.fr

Abstract. This article presents a service robotic system for people loosing their autonomy developed at CEA LIST. In the past on SAM robot, we have developed a method for automatic manipulation and object grasping using visual servoing. This method is too stereotyped to correctly grasp objects with complex geometry or to assign particular use to the manipulated object. In this article, we present a new study to adapt the grasping and the usage of an object designed by the user. Our method uses vision object recognition (CBIR) and an ontology for robotic manipulation. This recognition is implemented as a Web Service. It relies on passive vision and does not use a geometric model for grasping. The implementation of this method enables us to automatically search objects in the surrounding areas and to play cognitive and physical stimulation games with the user.

Keywords: cognitive robotics, service robotics, manipulation, grasping, handicap, quadriplegia, elderly people, loss of autonomy, object recognition, ontology, Web Service, interoperability, object search, stimulation games.

1 Introduction

People loosing their autonomy (disabled, elderly persons) and needing assistance in their everyday life generally resort to caretakers. Nevertheless, some easy and frequent tasks could be done by a service robot in order to give more freedom and autonomy to those people. Among those tasks, there are grasping and manipulation of everyday life objects. Even if a lot of methods exist for grasping, they are generally stereotyped and without a favored and adapted posterior use of the object.

However, we would like for example to be able to ask the robot to bring something to drink, supposing that the drink is in a cup. The robot should then recognize a cup among other objects, associate the cup to the action "give a drink" and grasp it securely (by the side opposite to the handle).

Y. Lee et al. (Eds.): ICOST 2010, LNCS 6159, pp. 178–185, 2010.

1.1 Previous Works

Here we shortly describe some main past contributions.

Grasping knowing the place of the object or with controlled environment. It can be where the position of each object is *a priori* known (projects RAID [1], DEVAR [2], Master [3]). Environment can also be equipped with intelligent systems such as intelligent tables [4]. Those tactile tables, covered by a sort of artificial skin, allow localization of objects of more than 5 grams. Those methods need a perfectly controlled and equipped environment which can be costly, difficult to generalize and can reduce freedom of robot's actions.

Grasping with use of 3D geometric model. A 3D model of object is needed. During the grasping, information from sensors, cameras or lasers is compared with the pre-established model to estimate the position of objects during tracking [5]. This method is used in the project CARE-O-BOT [6]. The development of the 3D model and the information matching during the grasping can be difficult, in particular with the presence of concave and convex regions in the object.

Grasping without model or object marking. The user can select an object on a graphic interface by drawing a bounding rectangle as we previously did [7]. Another example is the selection with a laser cursor for the service robot EL-E [8]. Those methods do not allow an adaptation of the grasp strategy or the later use of the object.

1.2 Contributions

Here we describe our contribution for object grasping. The method is detailed in section 2. Our method does not need any 3D geometric models even partial. For us, the model of an object is a small group of 2D images. Acquisition of those images does not need technical competences as is required to build 3D models. The objects do not have to be in the vision field of the user as it is the case with a designation of the object by a laser cursor.

Our recognition method uses image indexing and allows estimating the angle or point of view on the object regarding the position of the arm. Once this made, the object grasping strategy is obtained from an ontology, which also contains information on possible usage and type of objects. Unrecognized objects can be always grasped by our previous method [7]. A recognition Web Service using DPWS standard [9] was created for this method to assure interoperability with the services from partners of ITEA MIDAS project[1]. The objective of this European project is the design of a multimodal interface for assistance at home or during driving for people loosing their autonomy.

This recognition enabled us to develop an intuitive object selection to ease the use of the interface during object grasping and an object search program. It can also be used for cognitive and physical stimulation games with the user.

The next section presents the robot we are using for the development of the recognition and the interoperability resulting from our implementation. Section 3 deals with the details of object recognition and associated ontology. Our intuitive

[1] More details on http://www.itea2.org/public/project_leaflets/MIDAS_profile_oct-08.pdf

object selection is detailed in section 4 and section 5 presents the applications to object search and stimulation games.

2 Implementation on the Robot and Interoperability

This study takes place as part of European project ITEA MIDAS on assistance to people loosing their autonomy. Our team works on home assistance. The robot SAM [7] which we develop (Fig. 1) is meant to stimulate and help people in their everyday life. This means being able to understand the environment and being able to automate as much as possible actions to accomplish. In that respect grasping and manipulation of various objects become essential. Nevertheless the equipment of the robot should stay cheap and easy to use. We use a gripper with stereo camera (for the visual servoing), pressure sensors, optical barrier to detect when the object is in the gripper (Fig. 1).

An intuitive interface allows the user to send the robot to another room, to see its travel with a panoramic camera and then to select an object. This interface was tested during clinical assessment [10] which demonstrated its efficiency, ease of use and the satisfaction of the users towards this type of control.

The object recognition program was developed as a Web Service with a client server structure. When the user wants to select or search for an object, the client sends the current image to the network, the server receives and analyzes it and sends the result back on the network for the client. This method facilitates the interoperability with other software or home automation devices for home or driving assistance: there is no need to insert the whole recognition program, a client is sufficient.

For this Web Service, we resort on the DPWS architecture [9] (Device Profile for Web Service), a communication protocol based on SOAP-XML, which homogenizes the exchanges between the various services connected to the same network. This technology allows the "plug and play" of different services available from the network immediately after connection. DPWS is implemented in C++ and in Java, so programs written in different languages can communicate easily.

This Web Service is one of several with other already developed Web Services to control the robot (mobile platform, arm, user's interface) [7].

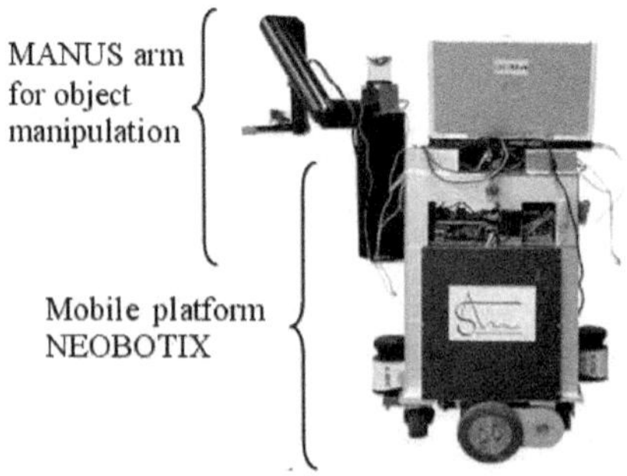

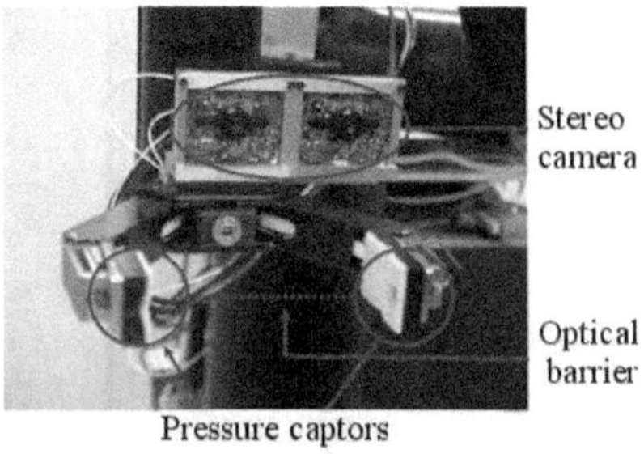

Fig. 1. Service robot SAM (*left*) and its gripper (*right*)

3 Object Recognition and Ontology

3.1 Learning and Recognition

To learn an object we need photos corresponding to different points of view on the object (Fig. 2). For each photo the interest points, or keypoints, are extracted using the software ViPR from Evolution Robotics [11] with the SIFT method [12] which relies on difference-of-Gaussian of nearby scales separated by a constant factor k:

$$DoG(x,y,\sigma) = \frac{1}{2\pi\sigma^2} e^{-(x^2+y^2)/(2\sigma^2)} - \frac{1}{2\pi k^2\sigma^2} e^{-(x^2+y^2)/(2k^2\sigma^2)} . \quad (1)$$

A point of view on the object is described by a vector of coordinates of the keypoints and their texture. The name of those photos is chosen to ease use in an ontology.

This database is easy to create and does not need specific competences. Indeed, the images (2D photos) can be done putting the object on a turntable like in [13] and taking photos of object's views with nearby camera. With a motorized turntable and automatic photo capture, new objects can be easily learned to complete the database.

During the recognition, ViPR extracts the keypoints from the image and compares their feature vectors with those of the database to find potential object matches [11]. Several objects can be identified in one image, including partially occulted objects, if there are at least 4 keypoints (Fig. 3). This recognition is robust to variations of luminosity and can be used in non uniform lightened places.

For this recognition, we first need to load the database (only once). Using our Web Service it takes 15,5s for a database of 72 images on a PC Intel Core 2 CPU 2,66 GHz 3,50 Go RAM. Next, the Web Service can recognize the objects (average 450ms).

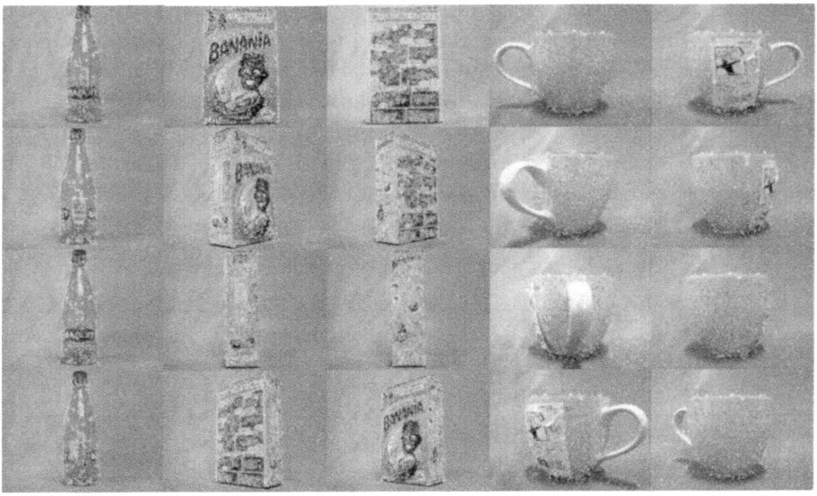

Fig. 2. Different points of view of some objects from the database and extracted keypoints. Plastic bottle (*left*), box of chocolate milk mix (*center*), cup (*right*).

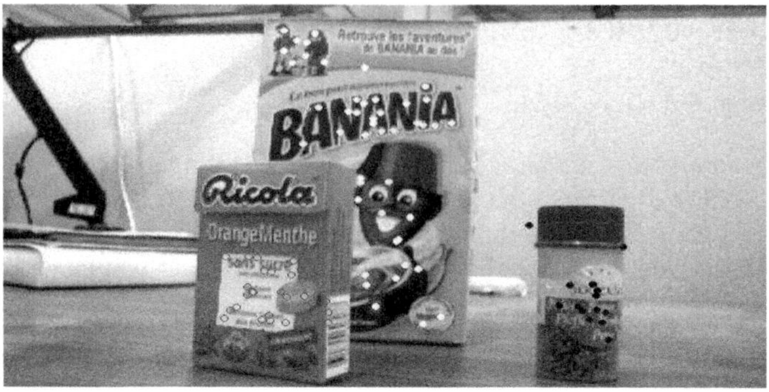

Fig. 3. Keypoints corresponding to different recognized objects: box of chocolate milk mix (*full white circles*), box of sweet (*empty circles*), pepper pot (*full black circles*).

3.2 Ontology

Ontology in computer science is a concept used for knowledge representation i.e. objects and concepts of a domain and the relations between them. It allows a level of abstraction of data models with a more semantic representation [14].

To find which grasping or object manipulation strategy to use, we create an ontology for robotics manipulation with XMLSpy. The ontology contains grasping strategies suited to each image or group of images from the database, according to the point of view on the object and its geometric structure (Table 1). It includes particularly the moves to make to position the gripper in an adapted place to grasp the object according to the morphology of the object and of the gripper (Fig 4). When the gripper has reached this place, it has only to move forward and do a blind grasp. All those moves are done after a visual servoing as in [7] in order to be always at the same distance from the object before the beginning of the motion from the strategy.

The ontology can also contain information about pressure to apply on the object during the grasping, about use of the objects: for example, the action "drink" can be associated to containers (cup, can), the concept "breakfast" – to coffee and cereals boxes, the place "bathroom" – to toothpaste (probable place where this object is). This information can be used for an oriented research of an object.

Table 1. Examples of grasp strategies in our ontology

Name of the strategy	Object's geometry	Possible objects	Angle, point of view
RevolutionSymetry	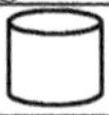	Can, bottle, glass	indifferent
RectangularCuboid000	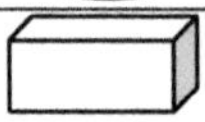	Box of pills, box of cereals	0° or 180°
RectangularCuboid045			45° or 225°
Cup000	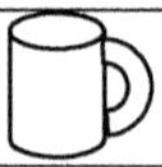	Cup	0°
Cup045			45°
Cup090			90°

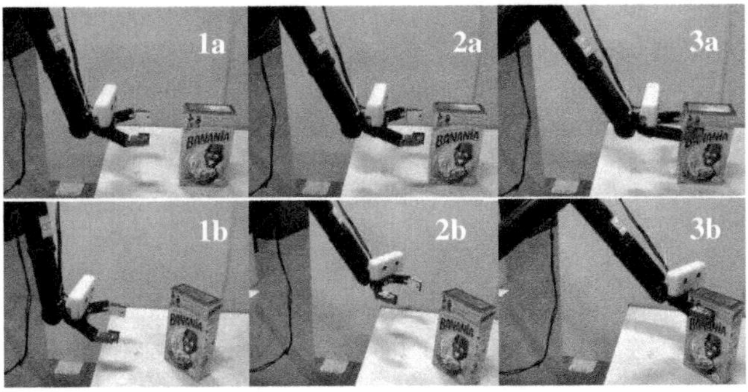

Fig. 4. Examples of grasp strategy: (*a*) RectangularCuboid090: box seen with an angle of 90°, the gripper moves straight forward; (*b*) RectangularCuboid045: box seen with an angle of 45°, moving of the arm in left direction, modification of orientation of the gripper before moving forward

4 Intuitive Object Selection

Before grasping an object, we use a visual servoing [7] to place the arm in front of the object. As explained before, this action is essential for the correct grasping. For this servoing we need to select the object in a bounding box. Previously, this selection was done in 2 mouse clicks which defined the opposite corners of a bounding box containing the object [7] [10]. This method requires only 2 clicks but for disabled persons every action can take a lot of time and effort: inaccurate clicks because of cognitive difficulties, physical difficulties which require specific equipment instead of mouse. So, when the object is known in the database, we want to reduce even more the number of actions for the object selection.

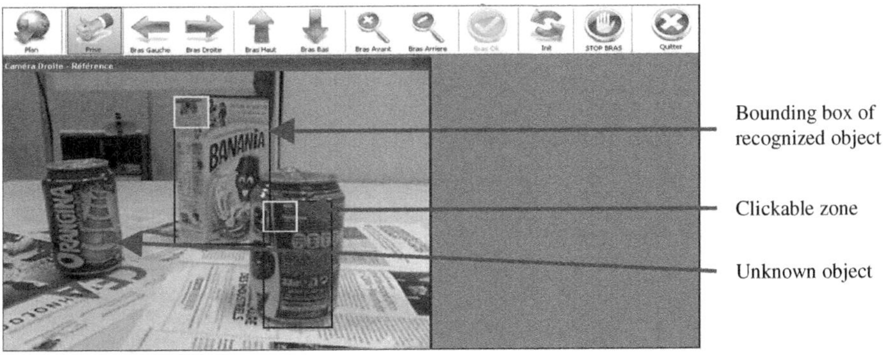

Fig. 5. Interface during object selection. Recognized objects are in bounding boxes (*blue*) and can be selected with a click in the clickable zone (*yellow*). Unrecognized object can be selected by two clicks.

When an object is recognized, we know the position of the recognized points of interest $P_{x,y}$ and define the bounding box thanks to those points. We noticed that those points reach rarely the edges of the object so we decided to enlarge the bounding box extremities with an empirically defined constant 'e':

- left top corner of the box [max(x_{min}-e,0),max(y_{min}-e,0)]
- right bottom corner of the box [min(x_{max}+e,width$_{image}$),min(y_{max}+e,height$_{image}$)]

When the user wants to choose an object in the scene, all the recognized objects are shown with their bounding box so the user only has to click in the desired bounding box. To prevent object box superposition, we decided to reduce the clickable zone for this selection (Fig. 5). If the object that the user wants to select is not recognized, he can define a bounding box by 2 clicks as it was done before. So when the user clicks on a clickable zone, the recognized object is selected, when the user clicks otherwise, this click defines one of the corners of a bounding box.

5 Applications to Object Search and User's Stimulation

Since selection of known objects in a bounding box is now automatic, we have implemented an object search in the environment. The user asks the robot to find an object (in a list of known objects) and the robot travels in the environment until he has found the object or has searched in all possible places. If the object is found, it can be automatically brought to the user. For example, we have assigned to each possible station (like tables) different positions of the arm to glance over all the surface of the station. We have tested our search program for one of those stations (120x100 cm). When the objects presents a lot of points of interest (big and textured objects), the research has a good success rate. This rate decreases with the number of detected points of interest (Table 2).

Assistance robotics can also be preventive or stimulating regarding cognitive or physical state of users. So with the object recognition, we can create stimulating games (for children or people with Alzheimer's disease).

For example the robot asks the user to show him one by one a set of known objects and places the arm every time in a different position. The stimulation is cognitive because the user has to find the right object and physical because the user has to reach the camera on the gripper in order to show the object and validate this task.

Table 2. Success search rate for different types of objects. Occultation decreases the number of interest points avalable for the recognition during object research.

Type of object		Big, textured	Big, little textured	Small, textured	Small, little textured
Success search	**No occultation**	86%	64%	68%	42%
	Occultation	71%	42%	29%	25%

6 Conclusion and Future Work

This article presented a new study on assistance for object grasping and manipulation. A 2D object recognition allows an adaptation (movement, pressure of grasping) of object grasping, but still allows grasping unknown objects. This vision method does not need geometric model of the object and is robust. Object learning is easy and can be done without robotics knowledge. All types of objects can be recognized if they have enough texture. Thanks to this recognition, we can grasp objects which could not be grasped before (such as box which width is bigger than gripper and seen full-frontal). The object selection by the user is eased and the robot can autonomously search objects. Cognitive and physical stimulation games can be implemented. The recognition allows the amelioration of the robot's environment knowledge and represents one more step toward intelligent and autonomous object manipulation.

We are currently working on the elaboration of new assistance scenarios and stimulation games. The ontology will be completed with an association of probable places for different objects to make the object search faster. Plan generation will soon give the possibility to user's assistants to define by themselves individualized scenarios. Clinical assessment of this method is planed in the ITEA MIDAS project.

References

1. Dallaway, J., Robin, S.: Raid -a vocational robotic workstation. In: IEEE ICORR. RU (1992)
2. Van der Loos, H.: Va/stanford rehabilitation robotics research and development program: Lessons learned in the application of robotics technology to the field of rehabilitation. IEEE Trans. on Neural Systems and Rehabilitation Engineering, 46–55 (1995)
3. Busnel, M., et al.: The robotized workstation "MASTER" for users with tetraplegia: Description and evaluation. Journ. of Rehabilitation Reseach &Development 36(3) (1999)
4. Volosyak, I., Ivlev, O., Gräser, A.: Rehabilitation Robot FRIEND II The General Concept and Current Implementation. In: Proc. of the 2005 IEEE ICORR, Chicago, IL, USA (2005)
5. Bourgeois, S., Naudet-Collette, S., Dhome, M.: Recalage d'un modèle CAO à partir de descripteurs locaux de contours. In: RFIA, Tours, France (2006)
6. Graf, B., Hans, M., Schraft, R.: Care-o-bot II development of a next generation robotic home assistant. Auton. Robots 16(2), 193–205 (2004)
7. Remazeilles, A., Leroux, C., Chalubert, G.: SAM: a robotic butler for handicapped people. In: IEEE RO-MAN, Munich, Germany (2008)
8. Jain, A., Kemp, C.C.: EL-E: An Assistive Mobile Manipulator that Autonomously Fetches Objects from Flat Surfaces. Autonomous Robots, Special Issue (2009)
9. Jammes, F., Mensch, A., Smit, H.: Service-oriented device communications using the devices profile for web services. In: AINA Work, Washington, USA, pp. 947–955 (2007)
10. Leroux, C., et al.: Robot grasping of unknown objects, description and validation of the function with quadriplegic people. In: IEEE ICORR, Noordwijk, Pays-Bas (2007)
11. Karlsson, N., et al.: Core technologies for service robotics. In: IROS (2004)
12. Lowe, D.G.: Object recognition from local scaleinvariant features. In: International Conference on Computer Vision, Corfu, Greece, pp. 1150–1157 (1999)
13. Nene, S.A., Nayar, S.K., Murase, H.: Columbia Object Image Library: COIL-20. Technical Report CUCS-005-96. Columbia University (1996)
14. Gruber, T.: Ontology. In: Liu, L., Tamer Özsu, M. (eds.) Encyclopedia of Database Systems. Springer, Heidelberg (2009)

Abnormality Detection for Improving Elder's Daily Life Independent

Ya-Xuan Hung[1,*], Chih-Yen Chiang[1], Steen J. Hsu[2], and Chia-Tai Chan[1]

[1] Institute of Biomedical Engineering National Yang-Ming University, Taipei, Taiwan
[2] Department of Information Management, Minghsin University of Science and Technology, Hsinchu, Taiwan
{snoopycindy,phinyen,ctchan}@bme.ym.edu.tw,
steenhsu@must.edu.tw

Abstract. Since the dramatic demographic change makes it inevitable that rapid aging of the population is an unprecedented phenomenon in Taiwan. A growing social problem is supporting older adults who want to live independently in their own homes. It needs a health assistance system to make them independent living up to a higher age. Recently, technological advancements have spurred various ideas and innovations to assist the elders living independently. In this paper, we proposed a homecare sensory system that uses RFID-based sensor networks to collect elder's daily activities and conducts the data into Hidden Markov model (HMM) and Support Vector Machines (SVMs) to estimate whether the elder's behavior is abnormal or not. Through detecting and distinguishing the abnormal behaviors of elder's daily activities, the system provides assistance on elder's independent living and improvement of aged quality of life.

Keywords: RFID HMM SVM abnormal activity.

1 Introduction

Since the U.S.A. population aged over 65 is growing rapidly and is going to over 14% of population in 2010 [1]. Similarly, it has reached 10.63% of Taiwan population in 2009 [2]. As transformed to aging society rapidly, the number of old persons who live alone is drastically increased. Therefore, how to support the elder who lives alone at home through information techniques has attracted a lot of researchers' interests. With the advances in modern medicine and technology, human life expectancy has increased significantly in the last century. Gerontechnology, the study of technology in improving daily functionality of the elderly, has developed rapidly these years [3]. One of the most important aspects of Gerontechnology is to ensure people independent living up to a higher age. Particularly, automatic detection of the elder's abnormal activities is one of the main concerns of the research.

* This work is supported in part by the National Science Council under Grant No. NSC 98-2221-E-159- 020.

Y. Lee et al. (Eds.): ICOST 2010, LNCS 6159, pp. 186–194, 2010.

Detecting abnormal activities of a remote homecare sensory system is an important issue in activity recognition. Medical professionals believe that one of the best ways to detect emerging medical conditions before they become critical is to look for changes in the activities of daily living (ADLs), instrumental ADLs (IADLs) [4], and enhanced ADLs (EADLs) [5]. If it is possible to develop computational systems that recognize such activities, automatic detection of the elder's abnormal activities at home will be greatly beneficial on indicating the declines in health. Due to the importance and challenging of the problem, several approaches have been proposed to learn the daily activities of individuals based on sensor readings, examples include Hidden Markov models (HMMs) [11] , dynamic Bayesian networks (DBNs)[13-15] and neural networks (NN)[18]. With the increasingly accessible sensor technology, automatic activity recognition is becoming a reality. By attaching different types of sensors on various objects, locations, and the human body, a user's activities can be tracked and monitored. The sensors we can use range from various wall-mounted sensors (e.g. reed switches [6, 7], motion detectors [8], cameras [9]) to all sorts of wearable (e.g. accelerometers [10], wrist worn RFID reader [11]). The various technologies differ from each other in terms of price, intrusiveness, ease to install and the type of data they output [12]. Due to the advantages of passive RFID, power free, cost effective, small size, it is convenient to monitor the activities of elders. If a safe and smart house can be deployed with a sensor network, the elders would have a better chance to live safely and independently.

In this paper, we incorporate Hidden Markov model with Support Vector Machines approach for daily abnormal activity detection using data from RFID sensor networks. The proposed homecare sensory system installs RFID antennas to the entrance of rooms in home, and passive tags are attached to users and objects. Recognizing daily activities based on the position information, i.e., stay time and frequency, of elders. By using the RFID-based sensor system, the homecare sensory system provides secure monitoring on identifying abnormal activities is demonstrated. As soon as abnormal events are detected, the system will sound an alarm for immediate attention.

The rest of the paper is organized as follows. In Section 2, we review previous work related to the abnormal activity detection problem. In Section 3, we present the proposed abnormality detection approach in detail. Using real data collected from a RFID-based sensor network, the experimental results validate the capabilities of our proposed algorithm are addressed in Section 4. Finally, we conclude the paper and discuss directions for future work in Section 5.

2 Related Works

Recently, activity recognition plays an important role in artificial intelligence and ubiquitous computing, partly due to the increasing availability of wireless sensor networks. In the past decade, various model-based approaches such as Hidden Markov models and dynamic Bayesian networks have been proposed to model and recognize users' activities.

Various models have been used in settings. Patterson et al. applied a dynamic Bayesian network to predict a traveler's location and current mode of transportation based on GPS readings in an urban environment [13-14]. Likewise, the work by Yin et al. adopted a DBN model to infer a user's indoor activities from sequences of signal-strength values in a wireless local area network (WLAN) environment [15].

Hidden Markov model was used to perform activity recognition at an object usage level using a wrist worn RFID reader [11]. Hierarchical hidden Markov model was used to perform activity recognition from video [9]. Lester et al. proposed a hybrid discriminative/generative approach to recognize human activities, in which useful features were first extracted to build an ensemble of static classifiers and HMMs were trained thereafter to recognize different activities [16]. In [17], the authors developed a two-layer hidden Markov model to estimate hospital-staff activities. Although most researches have dealt with the recognition of normal human activity, detecting a user's abnormal activities is interesting and challenging.

In the past, several approaches have been proposed to tackle the abnormality detection problem. T.Tam et al. developed a health monitoring system with machine vision and pattern analyses to track the occupant, learn his/her pattern of activity, and detect significant deviations that may be abnormal activities [19]. S.J. McKenna et al. used automated visual tracking and monitoring to support older people within their homes by analyzing their activity and raising the alarm when they fall [20-22]. These researches focus to detect the specific abnormal activities, such as fall. However, the abnormal behavior is not limited to fall.

Several approaches have been proposed to detect unusual events in video sequences. The work by Xiang and Gong applied DBN to model normal video patterns [23]. If the likelihood of being generated by normal models is less than a threshold, an activity is identified as abnormal. This approach is attractive due to its simplicity; however, an appropriate threshold is hard to determine in practice. T. Duong selected hidden semi-Markov models to represent a user's activities and perform abnormality detection [24]. However, this work only focused on detecting a more subtle form of abnormality, which is the abnormality only in the state duration but not in the state order.

Since the abnormal behavior detection is worth investigating in an aging society. In this paper, we propose a HMM approach training a normal life pattern to detect abnormality in the state sequence order and use SVM to classify the normal and abnormal behavior. Comparing with the traditional analytical methods, soft decision with learning function will reasonably shorten the time needed.

3 Material and Method

Since HMM is an essentially dynamic tool in handling the information with sequential characteristics. It can capture the features of behavior dynamically. And rigorous mathematical theories like the Viterbi algorithm and Baum-Welch algorithm are constructed to support HMM. In the other hand, SVM has shown outstanding performance in the limited samples. Compared to other machine learning techniques, it is capable of executive soft decision classification, soft decision with learning function, and time needed is reasonably short.

The proposed approach is able to effectively process the information with sequential characteristics and execute soft decision classification in the limited samples. Combining the advantages of HMM in handling sequential data and discriminative model of SVM, we propose an effective homecare sensory system to abnormal activity detection.

3.1 System Architecture

We design a two-phase classification model to achieve abnormal activity recognition, as shown in Fig. 1. In the preprocess phase, we apply HMM to extract the significant features from normal traces, where these feature vectors are then used to train an SVM classifier. In the detection phase, we use feature vectors in training an abnormal detection model to classify activities as normal or abnormal. We intentionally train the SVM so that it can identify normal activities with a higher likelihood, under the assumption that everything else is abnormal with a lower likelihood. We first briefly describe how to learn a normal activity model via HMM. Then, we present how to build abnormal activity detection model using SVM.

The normal activity model is trained using the information of normal activity by Baum-Welch algorithm. The normal activity model uses the input of test sequence to obtain hidden state sequence by Viterbi algorithm. Applying the standard forward algorithm, the log-likelihood is calculated by a hidden state sequence. Then, the data is preprocessed into vector-form consisting of log-likelihood and time-marked in each pair. After transforming the *N* training traces into a set of feature vectors, we train a SVM classifier based upon the vector space. The basic idea is to find a linear decision boundary to distinguish between normal and abnormal.

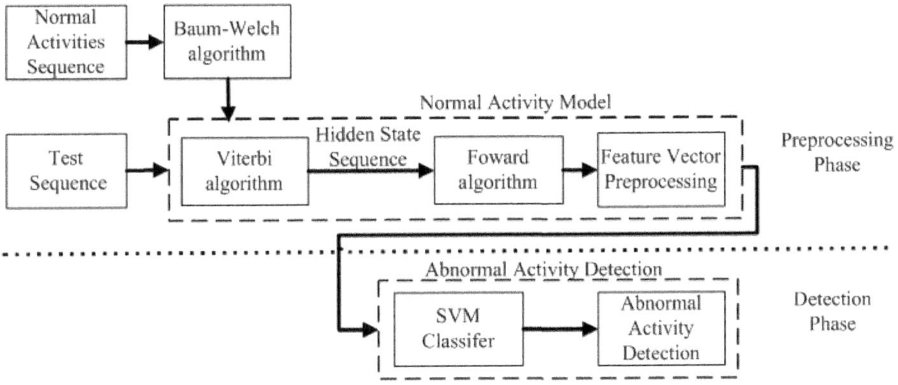

Fig. 1. System Architecture

4 Implementation

In our previous work, the intelligent reminder system combines with location tracking and scheduling, leading elders can take care of themselves. It has been demonstrated that RFID reminder system will bring about the convenience of elder life and enhance the quality of their life [25]. In this work, we adopted RFID reminder system to collect ADLs data. In order to evaluate the performance of our proposed algorithm, experiments were carried out on a real data set. Moreover, we use the Matlab HMM toolbox for processing daily activities data.

4.1 Data Collection

In our experimental environment, there are three RFID antennas deployed around our lab, one is outside and the others are in the labs, as shown in Fig.2. Each antenna's coverage is set nearly 5.79 meters long and 3.07 meters wide fitting the size of general space. The passive tags are attached to users. Once an antenna senses the passive tag, then homecare sensory system will records the positions of elders with timestamp for detecting the elders' activities. The experiment lasted over thirty days, 2 female and 3 male volunteers were recruited to assist the data collection. We collected these traces across multiple days (from Monday to Friday) in order to capture the day-to-day variations in the activities and sensor readings.

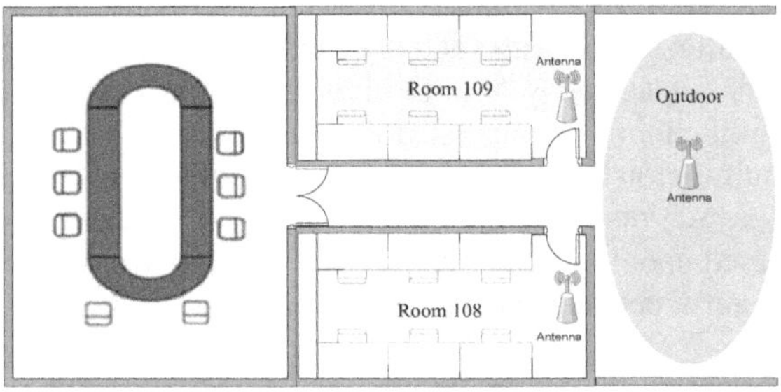

Fig. 2. The deployment of the detecting system in office environment

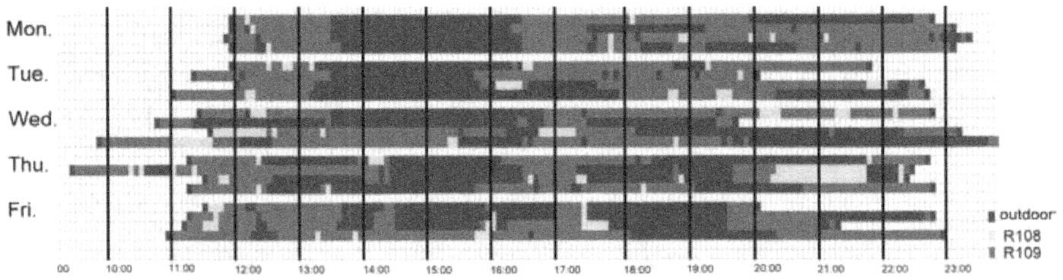

Fig. 3. Location maps of daily life. The red block represents outdoor; the yellow block is in room108; and the green block is in room109

4.2 Data Preprocessing

The collected traces over one month, from Monday to Friday are shown in Fig.3. Data preprocess procedure will sample location data to be a symbol every five minutes, and make location information of 1 hour (12 symbols) be an input sequence. By applying the standard forward algorithm, the log-likelihood of an input sequence is calculated. Then, the vector-form is generated as two-tuple [log-likelihood, time- marked] of variables of log-likelihood, and time-marked, respectively.

4.3 Results

For training a SVM, it needs to transform the training traces into a set of feature vectors. Since such traces are generated by a hidden mechanism associated with users' underlying activities, it is desirable to model such data using a generative model. In this work, the idea is to find a linear decision boundary to distinguish between normal and abnormal, as shown in Fig.4. The red dot under the linear decision boundary represents abnormal behavior; and the green triangle above the linear decision boundary represents normal behavior.

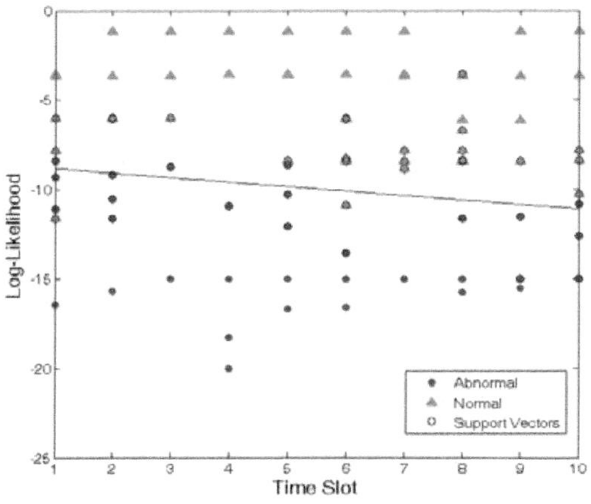

Fig. 4. The linear decision boundary of SVM classifier

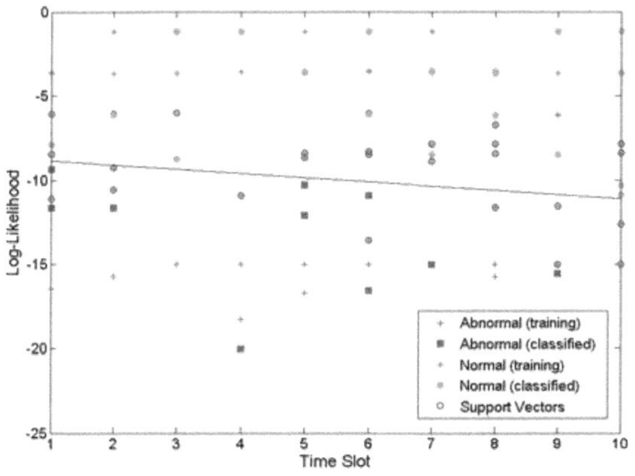

Fig. 5. The implementation of SVM classifier

The test sequence is inputted into the normal activity model to obtain hidden state sequence by using the Viterbi algorithm. The log-likelihood is calculated for each sequence. Then, the vector-form data is generated. After input the vector-form data into SVM classifier, it can distinguish between normal and abnormal behaviors, as shown in Fig.5. The pink square under the linear decision boundary represents abnormal behavior; and the blue circle above the linear decision boundary represents normal behavior.

5 Conclusion and Future Work

Automatic detection of abnormal activities of the elder who lives alone is one of the most important objectives of Gerontechnolgoy. We proposed homecare sensory system to discriminate elders' abnormal activities from normal activities. In this work, we develop an elder abnormality detection model based on SVM classifier to find a linear decision boundary to distinguish between normal and abnormal. This approach recognizes the abnormal behaviors of the elder's routine daily activities is able to assist the elders living independently and can be used to deliver adequate care on the urgent events.

This work contributes to the following topics. First, we present a sensor network setup that can be easily installed and used in different household environment. Second, we present an inexpensive and accurate method for real-time daily abnormal activity detection. Finally, we successfully combine the HMM and SVMs into abnormality detection system. Since the methods of HMM and SVMs have been widely used on abnormality detection system, this study attempts to integrate the advantages of two approaches. We make a series of experiments, the experimental results demonstrate that the combination of HMM and SVMs in abnormality detection system can effectively distinguish between normal and abnormal behavior.

In the future, we will aim at the direction of detecting abnormal activities from continuous user traces. This requires advance design of efficient segmentation and discrimination algorithm that can precisely partition the whole trace into consecutive segments and detect abnormal activities from these segments in an online manner. And we are going to explore more effective online inference algorithms in tackling the abnormal activity recognition to meet the need of real-world applications. Ideally, the system would be capable of adjusting the model in real-time as new data of activities become available.

References

1. World Health Organization, http://www.who.int/en/
2. Ministry of the Interior, http://www.moi.gov.tw/stat/
3. Bouma, H.: Gerontechnology: Making technology relevant for the elderly. In: Bouma, H., Graafmans, J.A.M. (eds.) Gerontechnology, pp. 1–5. IOS Press, Amsterdam (1992)
4. Lawton, M.P., Brody, E.M.: Assessment of older people: self-maintaining and instrumental activities of daily living. Gerontologist 9, 179–186 (1969)

5. Rogers, W.A., Meyer, B., Walker, N., Fisk, A.D.: Functional limitations to daily living tasks in the aged: a focus groups analysis. Human Factors 40, 111–125 (1998)
6. Tapia, E.M., Intille, S.S., Larson, K.: Activity recognition in the home using simple and ubiquitous sensors. In: Ferscha, A., Mattern, F. (eds.) PERVASIVE 2004. LNCS, vol. 3001, pp. 158–175. Springer, Heidelberg (2004)
7. Wilson, D., Atkeson, C.: Simultaneous tracking and activity recognition (star) using many anonymous binary sensors. In: Gellersen, H.-W., Want, R., Schmidt, A. (eds.) PERVASIVE 2005. LNCS, vol. 3468, pp. 62–79. Springer, Heidelberg (2005)
8. Living independently - quietcare system, `http://www.livingindependently.com`
9. Duong, T.V., Bui, H.H., Phung, D.Q., Venkatesh, S.: Activity recognition and abnormality detection with the switching hidden semi-markov model. In: CVPR 2005: Proceedings of the 2005 IEEE Computer Society Conference on Computer Vision and Pattern Recognition (CVPR 2005), Washington, DC, USA, vol. 1, pp. 838–845. IEEE Computer Society, Los Alamitos (2005)
10. Lester, J., Choudhury, T., Kern, N., Borriello, G., Hannaford, B.: A hybrid discriminative/generative approach for modeling human activities. In: IJCAI, pp. 766–772 (2005)
11. Patterson, D.J., Fox, D., Kautz, H.A., Philipose, M.: Fine-grained activity recognition by aggregating abstract object usage. In: ISWC, pp. 44–51. IEEE Computer Society, Los Alamitos (2005)
12. Schmidt, A.: Ubiquitous Computing – Computing in Context. PhD thesis, Lancaster University (2002)
13. Liao, L., Fox, D., Kautz, H.: Learning and Inferring Transportation Routines. In: Proc. 19th Nat'l Conf. Artificial Intelligence (AAAI 2004), July 2004, pp. 348–353 (2004)
14. Patterson, D.J., Liao, L., Fox, L., Kautz, H.: Inferring High-Level Behavior from Low-Level Sensors. In: Dey, A.K., Schmidt, A., McCarthy, J.F. (eds.) UbiComp 2003. LNCS, vol. 2864, pp. 73–89. Springer, Heidelberg (2003)
15. Yin, J., Chai, X., Yang, Q.: High-Level Goal Recognition in a Wireless LAN. In: Proc. 19th Nat'l Conf. in Artificial Intelligence (AAAI 2004), July 2004, pp. 578–584 (2004)
16. Rabiner, L.R.: A tutorial on hidden markov models and selected applications in speech recognition. Proceedings of the IEEE 77(2), 257–286 (1989)
17. Sánchez, D., Tentori, M., Favela, J.: Activity Recognition for the Smart Hospital. IEEE Intelligent Systems 23(2), 50–57 (2008)
18. Favela, J., et al.: Activity Recognition for Context-Aware Hospital Applications: Issues and Opportunities for the Deployment of Pervasive Networks. Mobile Networks and Applications 12(2-3), 155–171 (2007)
19. Bradley, A.P.: The Use of the Area under the ROC Curve in the Evaluation of Machine Learing Algorithms. Pattern Recognition 30, 1145–1159 (1997)
20. Breunig, M.M., Kriegel, H.P., Ng, R., Sander, J.: Identifying Density-Based Local Outliers. In: Proc. ACM SIGMOD Int'l Conf. Management of Data (SIGMOD 2000), May 2000, pp. 93–104 (2000)
21. Chan, P., Stolfo, S.: Toward Scalable Learning with Non Uniform Class and Cost Distributions. In: Proc. Fourth Int'l Conf. Knowledge Discovery and Data Mining (KDD 1998), August 1998, pp. 164–168 (1998)
22. Domingos, P.: Metacost: A General Method for Making Classifiers Cost-Sensitive. In: Proc. Fifth Int'l Conf. Knowledge Discovery and Data Mining (KDD 1999), August 1999, pp. 155–164 (1999)

23. Xiang, T., Gong, S.: Video Behaviour Profiling and Abnormality Detection without Manual Labeling. In: Proc. IEEE Int'l Conf. Computer Vision (ICCV 2005), October 2005, pp. 1238–1245 (2005)
24. Duong, T., Bui, H., Phung, D., Venkatesh, S.: Activity Recognition and Abnormality Detection with the Switching Hidden Semi-Markov Model. In: Proc. IEEE Int'l Conf. Computer Vision and Pattern Recognition (CVPR 2005), June 2005, pp. 838–845 (2005)
25. Huang, K.-T.: An Intelligent RFID System for Improving Elderly Daily Life Independent in Indoor Environment. In: Helal, S., Mitra, S., Wong, J., Chang, C.K., Mokhtari, M. (eds.) ICOST 2008. LNCS, vol. 5120, pp. 1–8. Springer, Heidelberg (2008)

AAL 4 ALL – A Matter of User Experience

Gerhard Leitner and Anton Josef Fercher

University of Klagenfurt,
9020 Klagenfurt, Austria
{Gerhard.Leitner,AntonJosef.Fercher}@uni-klu.ac.at

Abstract. Population over aging is at present a widely discussed and researched challenge that society will have to face in the future. Research on ambient assisted living (AAL) yields promising solutions to master those challenges and the IT industry meanwhile has identified AAL as an important future market. However, AAL solutions which are adequate for large portions of the population are still missing. When considering that population over aging will be a mass phenomenon, solutions have to be provided which are applicable for a majority of the population living in different environments and having different income levels and, most importantly, consider a broad range of usability and psychological aspects which influence the acceptance and usage of technology. In this paper we identify and discuss shortcomings of existing research activities and technological developments and present approaches overcoming these shortcomings on the basis of the concept of user experience.

Keywords: Ambient assisted living, aging in place, usability, user experience.

1 Introduction

Ambient assisted living (AAL) is a booming research area as well as a growing market sector. The reason is that the aged population is virtually standing at the gates of our societies [7,28]. Researchers intensively investigate and evaluate possibilities to face these challenges [5,9,12] because the future change in the ratio of employed to retired people will lead to scarcity of qualified nursing personnel as well as insufficient capacities in nursing homes and other care giving institutions. However, in many cases the most preferable alternative is probably to stay in the familiar environment because of several problems being connected to a relocation in age.

Information technology increasingly reaches out for our homes and seems to offer new possibilities enabling elderly to master their lives themselves longer than in the past. But when observing the situation critically, there are still a lot of hurdles to overcome until home automation technology can be smoothly integrated into arbitrary living environments and utilized by large portions of the elder population.

The IT industry impressively demonstrates the potential of cutting edge technology in show case projects (cf e.g. [16,17]). However, most of these show case systems are most probably not affordable for people with an average income. Besides the financial costs big installation efforts are incorporated to a retrofit of such high

Y. Lee et al. (Eds.): ICOST 2010, LNCS 6159, pp. 195–202, 2010.

end systems, as they are often based on wired technologies. Especially for elderly, the cost/benefit ratio is known to be important and influences the motivation to install and use new technology.

Although a lot of research has already been carried out in the field of smart home systems (cf. e.g. [1,13,29]), the results are rarely applicable to the living contexts and environments of most elderly people: evaluations are often carried out in artificial environments equipped with high-end information technology. Furthermore, the evaluations are based on observations of artificial groups of people living in the study environments for a limited time. Although the results gained so far are of great importance for the further development of AAL, conclusions for the applicability to everyday routines are difficult to draw.

Numerous systems with smart functionality congest the end consumer market which theoretically could be used for AAL tasks. Commonly, they are quite cheap in relation to the high end systems mentioned before, and often operate on wireless technology which eases installation into various environments. However, most of these systems do not offer holistically integrated solutions and thus additional remotes or other interaction devices are required to control them. Moreover, they are neither suitable for special groups of users as their interfaces are often based on controls like joysticks, toggle buttons, buttons with different modes or software menus based on hierarchical tree navigation, nor they are adaptable to actual and changing needs.

The factors influencing the potential success or failure of AAL technology the most are, however, psychological factors, but coincidentally those disregarded most in the development and research of assistive technology. In some cases they seem to represent a *"blatant technology push"* [5]. There is a broad range of influencing variables, e.g., changes in intelligence structure, technology acceptance and social relationships.

Apparently there are many aspects which influence success or failure of AAL, some of which already identified, discussed and considered in existing AAL solutions, many of them still not clearly defined or even not identified yet. A major task for future research will therefore be to establish a comprehensive framework including all relevant dimensions, categorizing and integrating research results already gained in the past and orientate research on AAL to aim on the completion of such a framework.

This paper is structured as follows: After providing an overview on related work, we propose the concept of user experience as the basis of the framework to be established and give examples for factors already identified in literature. Afterwards example approaches including field trials aiming on the completion of the factor framework are presented. The paper closes with a discussion and a description of future work.

2 Related Work

Ample literature on smart home research in general, and AAL related activities in particular is available [1,4,9,11,12,18]. Based on the quantity of related work it can be assumed that there is no lack of basic technology. However, up to now these basic technologies did not spread in the predicted degree, and a breakthrough of smart home technology failed to appear [18]. Reasons for this failure are subject of literature discussion.

One of the rather pragmatic reasons hindering success is the financial costs (cf e.g. [5,29] which still turn out to be considerably high. On the other hand, there are several possibilities to compensate the costs for smart technology, for example, the costs could be amortized by energy savings supported by smart technology and home based care could reduce costs for public health care systems [20]. Although being an important criterion, financial investments are of lower importance than quality of life [5]. When asked about their plans in old age, most respondents are more likely to invest in reconstructing in their own homes than moving to nursing institutions, to their relatives or to other locations [9,18].

However, financial resources can be assumed not being unlimited, therefore off-the-shelf instead of customized high end systems could be a practicable alternative, although these systems show several weaknesses, such as missing interoperability or a broad variety of incompatible interaction concepts. In 2004, Nielsen [21] spoke of the remote control anarchy which will exacerbate when smart home technology develops in the wrong direction. The preferred alternative are integrated systems supporting AAL rather than single purpose systems. They ideally support needs and functionality such as comfort functions, autonomy enhancement and emergency assistance [14] and they are flexible and adaptable to changing requirements [18]. To promote the development of such multipurpose systems, standards have to be defined to ensure interoperability of devices from different manufacturers which support different purposes and needs and are based on different technologies (e.g., different wireless and wired systems).

Other than in areas such as the automotive sector or computing networks (e.g., ISO/OSI) there is a lack of standards in smart home technology although, some initiatives for standardization in the smart home sector have been taken (cf. [1]) and several projects (e.g., Mavhome or Gatortech [2]) have employed promising open standards like OSGi [8].

One level above the technical requirements, factors being of importance in the context of AAL are related to interaction and usability. It is commonly agreed in literature that elderly people are less likely to adopt to new technology [18,19], are characterized by lower computer self-efficacy and are more likely to develop computer anxiety [12]. But even young people *"feel at the mercy of, instead of in control of technology"* [4]. One of the reasons for suboptimal usability can be identified in the high complexity of fully networked smart home systems [25], but also the motivation to deal with technical systems influences the interaction. Davidoff [4] brings it to the point: *"People don't want to control devices, they want to have more control of their lives"*. To overcome the resistance to use new technology, devices more customized for the target group have to be developed. Examples of alternative interaction mechanisms or devices are, e.g., the digital picture frame and similar systems discussed in [3,20,23]. Some projects even demonstrate pieces of furniture [27] or informative art [24] as alternative means of interaction.

In the discussion of usability mainly short-term handling aspects are considered, other relevant dimensions (e.g. learnability, adaption) often could not be regarded sufficiently because most projects – with some exceptions - are based on short term evaluation and observation under more or less artificial circumstances [18,25].

User needs, subjective and psychological aspects were also not considered sufficiently in the past [5,12,20], although many reasons for accepting or avoiding technology are of psychological nature and go far beyond the features of basic technology or the means of interaction. Psychological aspects are manifold and difficult to be considered exhaustively, however, some of them are frequently discussed in literature. For example, there are age related changes in intelligence structure. Whereas crystalline intelligence seems to remain relatively stable throughout life, fluid intelligence is reduced [29]. A possible side effect of this change is the reduced willingness of elderly to adapt to new technologies [19]. Another psychological aspect to be considered in designing technology mentioned by Ijsselstein et al.[12] is that mental models of interaction are based on the formative period of life and are characterized by the devices predominantly present in that period. According to this, the generation born before the 1960s is classified as the electro-mechanical generation and people born after the 1960s are members of the software generation. This perspective has parallels to the differentiation between digital natives and digital immigrants. Regarding AAL, the differentiation of user groups is important for two reasons. The first reason is that the group of elderly is heterogeneous in itself, the other – often neglected – reason is that other groups of users playing an important role in AAL, i.e. the relatives, are probably not representatives of the same category as the elderly.

The role of the anyway already important relatives will increasingly gain importance. Results of projects where relatives where involved show that they are grateful for any support they can get [5] and technology they can rely on supports their “peace of mind” [20].

2.1 The Concept of User Experience

A systematic approach seems to be necessary which ensures a comprehensive consideration of already classified as well as potential dimensions of relevance in the context of AAL.

The question occurs whether there is a concept which could serve as a basis for the resulting framework. As the discussion of related literature demonstrates, one of the factors considered important is usability. Although usability as defined in the ISO 9241-11, is a well structured concept regarding performance measures (efficiency, effectivity) it has weaknesses in the level of detail regarding psychological and personal factors (i.e. the dimension satisfaction, as defined in ISO 9241-11) which, also according to the related literature, are of high relevance in the context of AAL. A proposal for a framework based on HCI aspects is presented by Saizmaa and Kim [26]. However, this proposal is focused on Smart Home and does not sufficiently address psychological factors. Therefore we propose the notion of *user experience* (UX) as the basic concept of our framework. UX itself is a notion the definition of which has not reached consensus [15]. However, it covers psychological aspects in a more detailed manner and goes further than concepts dealing with interaction, such as usability (ISO 9241-11) or the technology acceptance model presented by Morris and Venkatesh [19]. We take the definition of UX from Hassenzahl and Tractinsky [15] as a preliminary basis, which states, that: User experience is...

"A consequence of a user's internal state (predispositions, expectations, needs, motivation, mood, etc.), the characteristics of the designed system (e.g. complexity, purpose, usability, functionality, etc.) and the context (or the environment) within which the interaction occurs (e.g. organisational/social setting, meaningfulness of the activity, voluntariness of use, etc.)"

3 Method

As a first step in the development of a framework of aspects relevant for AAL system usage, we observe the main factors internal state, characteristics of the designed system and context only, serving as examples for further discussion. Based on these main factors we illustrate our approach to build the framework in our future work.

Although system characteristics can be seen as the factor considered most likely in past AAL research, further engagement in this dimension is necessary to establish a solid basis which provides the robustness and flexibility for further evaluation of the other UX factors (internal state and context). As discussed in the preceding sections there are some aspects related to system characteristics which have hindered the acceptance of AAL technology, such as high costs, difficulty to retrofit and missing compatibility. We therefore chose a relatively inexpensive off-the-shelf system based on radio communication comparable to systems meeting the X10 standard (cf. e.g. [8]) for our initial evaluation purposes. A layered software platform [8] supporting smart home functionality based on OSGi was developed which provides a high level of adaptability to further research activities.

During initial field trials the basic system was installed on two locations: in a laboratory located on the university campus and in a family house which is occupied by a member of the research team, his wife and two children (6 and 9 years). A prerequisite has been that the base system could be installed in parallel to the existing wiring and controls to ensure that familiar devices and controls still can be operated in a familiar way, even if the added components stop working. Different analyses were performed, the first was a usability inspection, focusing on the usability and utility of the system from the administrator/maintainer point of view. The findings were combined with the observational data that were gained by observing and interviewing the other family members and users of the laboratory. The third analysis was based on the investigation of a log file generated by the standard software shipped with the system.

The results gained in the family house show that the system in its original form is not suitable for operation by average consumers especially in case of malfunction because of several reasons, ranging from simple (batteries of remote control empty) to complex (central unit has lost configuration or connectivity). The GUI interface and a reduced web interface provided by the system, were not used by other family members than the colleague himself. In relation to UX the basic problem is located in system characteristics (low costs but also low reliability). Thus, the hardware controls, e.g. the remote, were used frequently. Some of the functions of the system were appreciated, e.g. macros for controlling the roller blinds, whereas others were avoided. For example, the control of radiators via remote thermostats was not used voluntarily because this did not fit in the mental model of the users. Another finding was that the installation of the system influenced trust on the house`s security. Because of malfunction, the garage door operated accidentally, which caused family members to keep a wary eye on the locking of doors, which was not a big issue before installation. In relation to UX it seems that internal factors (e.g. motivation to use functions which enhance comfort) can outweigh technical problems when the basic function is considered useful however, in the case of security, trust has a higher relevance than technology.

In the laboratory interferences with other smart systems installed were responsible that some functions did not work properly. This led to a kind of magic thinking among the colleagues (mainly psychologists, involved in other projects) the laboratory was shared with. When they were not able to switch e.g. lights in the intended way they blamed themselves rather than the (actually malfunctioning) smart home technology. In relation to UX, internal factors (not being able to perform the intended task) seemed to have a higher importance than contextual factors (the malfunctioning system).

Based on the early results which were tendentially promising, another field trial focusing on AAL has been performed. A set of components was installed in a family house occupied by a seventy years old woman. On the basis of motion sensors, placed on neuralgic locations in the house scenarios simulating alarm situations (e.g. by estimating the computational probability of falls) were evaluated. The installation was configured in such a way that it was not necessary for the woman to explicitly interact with the system. One of the most interesting outcomes was that although the woman was informed that the system is not capable of serving as an emergency system yet, she expressed the feeling of safety when the infrared lights of the motion sensors “confirmed” her presence. In relation to UX different factors are involved. Obviously the feedback of the devices (system characteristic) worked well for the user because no direct interaction was necessary, which led to the development of positive feelings (internal state).

4 Discussion and Conclusion

The results we gained from these small field trials are – in relation to the duration of the trials and the complexity of the basis setup - very promising. A lot of insights on usability (e.g. usage avoidance in the family house, self blaming users) as well as psychological factors (e.g. magical thinking, influence of trust, feeling of safety) could be gained.

The next steps in our approach are focused on the project *Casa Vecchia* which is consisting of a longitudinal field study which will start in the next couple of months. In this study, 20 households of elderly people will be equipped with a set of smart home technology. The participants will be motivated to actively use this system for research purposes but it is not expected to impair daily routines too much since the infrastructure the persons are used to will still work in the accustomed way. The field study will last for the next three years and will directly involve relatives to consider, e.g., the UX aspect of social context. Relatives will also interact with the system, although with different tasks and devices than the elderly. The main device for the elderly either will be a system masked as a digital picture frame (as used in [3,20,23]), hiding an embedded PC with touch screen functionality. The basic interface concept will be informative art, employed to provide information and interaction mechanisms, but hiding potentially frightening computer technology.

The main goal of the study is to collect a broad spectrum of influencing variables relevant in the context of AAL. Because of its longitudinal character, the factors disregarded in earlier AAL research related to the UX dimensions internal state and contextual conditions can be thoroughly investigated. Besides the evaluation of usage patterns (based on log analysis) participants will be asked to keep dairies, will be frequently interviewed and motivated to give as much on information as possible related to the role of technology in their lives, their opinions on the further development of AAL technology etc. The goal of the project is to jump a great leap forward in the understanding of success factors as well as factors responsible for the failure of technology by finding as many missing pieces of the jigsaw of UX in the context of AAL as possible.

Acknowledgments. We are grateful to Austrian Research Promotion Agency (FFG) for the funding of *Casa Vecchia* (project nr. 825889) within the program benefit.

References

1. BMBF/VDE-Innovationspartnerschaft, AAL: Interoperabilität von AAL Systemkomponenten, Teil 1: Stand der Technik, Vde-Verlag (2010)
2. Chan, M., Esteve, D., Escriba, C., Campo, E.: A review of smart homes - Present state and future challenges. Computer Methods and Programs in Biomedicine 91(1), 55–81 (2008)
3. Consolvo, S., Roessler, P., Shelton, B.E.: The CareNet Display: Lessons Learned from an In Home Evaluation of an Ambient Display. In: Davies, N., Mynatt, E.D., Siio, I. (eds.) UbiComp 2004. LNCS, vol. 3205, pp. 1–17. Springer, Heidelberg (2004)
4. Davidoff, S., Lee, M.K., Yiu, C., Zimmerman, J., Dey, A.K.: Principles of smart home control. In: Dourish, P., Friday, A. (eds.) UbiComp 2006. LNCS, vol. 4206, pp. 19–34. Springer, Heidelberg (2006)
5. Dewsbery, G.: The Social and Psychological Aspects of Smart Home Technology within the Care Sector (2001)
6. Dishman, E.: Inventing Wellness Systems for Aging in Place. IEEE Computer 37(5), 34–41 (2004)
7. Evans, R.G., McGrail, K.M., Morgan, S.G., Barer, M.L., Hertzman, C.: APOCALYPSE NO: Population Aging and the Future of Health Care Systems. In: Social and Economic Dimensions of an Aging Population Research Papers 59, McMaster University (2001)
8. Felsing, D.: Eine erweiterbare Smart Home Plattform auf Basis des FS20 Systems. Diploma Thesis, University of Klagenfurt (2010)

9. Georgieff, P.: Ambient Assisted Living. Marktpotenziale IT-unterstützter Pflege für ein selbstbestimmtes Altern, FAZIT Forschungsbericht Nr. 17, Stuttgart: MFG Stiftung Baden-Württemberg (2008)
10. Hirsch, T., Forlizzi, J., Hyder, E., Goetz, J., Kurtz, C., Stroback, J.: The ELDer project: social, emotional, and environmental factors in the design of eldercare technologies. In: Proceedings on the 2000 Conference on Universal Usability, pp. 72–79 (2000)
11. Intille, S.: Designing a Home of the Future. IEEE Pervasive Comp. 1(2), 76–82 (2002)
12. Ijsselsteijn, W.I., Nap, H.H., De Kort, Y., Poels, K.: Digital game design for elderly users. In: Proceedings of the conference on Future Play in Toronto, Canada, pp. 17–22 (2007)
13. Jiang, L., Liu, D.-Y., Yang, B.: Smart home research. In: Proceedings of the International Conference on Machine Learning and Cybernetics, vol. 2, pp. 659–663 (2004)
14. Kleinberger, T., Becker, M., Ras, E., Holzinger, A., Müller, P.: Ambient Intelligence in Assisted Living: Enable Elderly People to Handle Future Interfaces. In: Stephanidis, C. (ed.) UAHCI 2007 (Part II). LNCS, vol. 4555, pp. 103–112. Springer, Heidelberg (2007)
15. Law, E.L.-C., Roto, V., Vermeeren, A.P.O.S., Kort, J., Hassenzahl, M.: SIG on Towards a shared definition of user experience. In: Proc. of CH 2008I, pp. 2395–2398 (2008)
16. Living Tomorrow Brussels, http://www.livingtomorrow.be/
17. Microsoft Home of the Future, http://www.engadget.com/2009/05/14/video-microsofts-future-home-actually-makes-your-computer-a-bi/
18. Meyer, S., Schulze, E.: Smarthome für ältere Menschen. Handbuch für die Praxis (2008), http://www.agestiftung.ch/uploads/media/Smart_Home.pdf
19. Morris, M.G., Venkatesh, V.: Age differences in technology adoption decisions: Implications for a changing workforce. Personnel. Psych. 53, 375–403 (2000)
20. Mynatt, E.D., Rowan, J., Craighill, S., Jacobs, A.: Digital family portraits: supporting peace of mind for extended family members. In: Proceedings of CHI 2001, pp. 333–340 (2001)
21. Nielsen, J.: Remote Control Anarchy. Alertbox, June 7 (2004)
22. Norgall, T.: Fit und selbstständig im Alter durch Technik. Bundesgesundheitsblatt - Gesundheitsforschung - Gesundheitsschutz 52(3), 297–305 (2009)
23. Panek, P., Zagler, W.: Partizipative Entwicklung und Erprobung von AAL Technologien im Living Lab Schwechat. In: Proceedings of 1st VDE AAL congress, pp. 121–125 (2008)
24. Redström, J., Skog, T., Hallnäs, L.: Informative Art: Using Amplied Artworks as Information Displays. In: Proceedings of DARE 2000, pp. 103–114 (2000)
25. Ringbauer, B., Heidmann, F., Biesterfeldt, J.: When a House Controls its Master - Universal Design for Smart Living Environments. In: Proceedings of HCI International, vol. 1, pp. 1228–1232 (2003)
26. Saizmaa, T., Kim, H.C.: A Holistic Understanding of HCI Perspectives on Smart Home. In: Proceedings of the Fourth International Conference on Networked Computing and Advanced Information Management, vol. 2, pp. 59–65 (2008)
27. Siio, I., Rowan, J., Mynatt, E.: Peek-a-drawer: communication by furniture. In: CHI 2002 Extended Abstracts, pp. 582–583 (2002)
28. Steg, H., Strese, H., Loroff, C., Hull, J., Schmidt, S.: Europe is Facing a Demographic Challenge, Ambient assisted Living offers Solutions. Report: Frankfurt, Verband der Elektrotechnik, Elektronik, Informationstechnik (2006)
29. Stuart-Hamilton, I.: The Psychology of Ageing: An Introduction, 4th edn. Jessica Kingsley Publications (2006)
30. Yamazaki, T.: Beyond the smart home. In: Proceedings of the International Conference on Hybrid Information Technology (ICHIT), pp. 350–355 (2006)

Creating Digital Life Stories through Activity Recognition with Image Filtering

Basel Kikhia, Johan E. Bengtsson, Kåre Synnes, Zaheer ul Hussain Sani, and Josef Hallberg

Luleå University of Technology, Sweden
Department of Computer Science & Electrical Engineering
{Basel.Kikhia,Johan.E.Bengtsson,Kare.Synnes,
Josef.Hallberg}@ltu.se,
zaheer@memorylane.nu

Abstract. This paper presents two algorithms that enables the MemoryLane system to support persons with mild dementia through creation of digital life stories. The MemoryLane system consists of a Logging Kit that captures context and image data, and a Review Client that recognizes activities and enables review of the captured data. The image filtering algorithm is based on image characteristics such as brightness, blurriness and similarity, and is a central component of the Logging Kit. The activity recognition algorithm is based on the captured contextual data together with concepts of persons and places. The initial results indicate that the MemoryLane system is technically feasible and that activity-based creation of digital life stories for persons with mild dementia is possible.

Keywords: life logging, life story, memory assistance, activity recognition, image filtering.

1 Introduction

The idea of creating digital life stories goes back to 1945 when Vannevar Bush envisioned "a device in which an individual stores all his books, records, and communications, and which is mechanized so that it may be consulted with exceeding speed and flexibility" [1]. In order to fulfill this vision, life should be logged and clustered in manageable shots/activities [7], so it will be available for reminiscence and later retrieval.

Reviewing images and written diaries are the most obvious examples for stimulating memory with past activities [15]. To support this stimulation through a digital tool, images should be collected during the day then clustered into activities. Therefore, activity recognition is the key component for achieving digital life stories. Moreover, clustering life into activities supports the idea of having a written diary in a digital format. It is also important to filter out images that do not give meaningful information rather than overloading the user with too many images to review.

Y. Lee et al. (Eds.): ICOST 2010, LNCS 6159, pp. 203–210, 2010.

This paper discusses challenges in implementing activity recognition with image filtering, and it presents techniques that have been implemented in a tool and field tested by 4 researchers and 4 users suffering from mild dementia. The tool logs personal context and content of a person, then recognizes a sequence of activities based on the visited places and persons met - a digital life story, and finally allows the user to review and adjust the activities and related images, as a reminiscence process and to ensure suitable quality for later context-dependent retrieval. The research questions discussed in this paper are:

1. How can the number of images presented to the user in a life logging system be minimized using filtering techniques?
2. How can activities be automatically recognized based on context data, prior knowledge of places and persons, and a minimal set of equipment?

The rest of this paper is organized as follows: In Section 2, state-of-the-art related work is presented. Section 3 discusses the Logging Kit, presenting image filtering techniques to be embedded within the system, that drastically reduces the number of images for the user to review. Section 4 discusses the Review Client, and it presents the activity recognition techniques and the learning mechanism for increasing the system's understanding of known persons and places. The research questions are directly addressed in section 5, while section 6 concludes the paper and presents future work.

2 Related Work

Several techniques have been proposed for an efficient method in recognizing activities. For instance, using context to search parts of the recorded video [12], use of a wearable camera for capturing video and a sensor of brain waves [11], face detection and low level analysis of images [9].

Annotating images with contextual data has been explored by several studies. For instance, authors in [13] annotate an image with the location where it was taken, using a GPS device, and relating digital camera images to locations based on time. Most of the previous work have been using multiple devices and sensors, which results in having many sources of data for building knowledge into the system. Intensive studies have recently been done by using a wearable digital camera called SenseCam [4] [5] [8] [15], that periodically captures fish-eye lens images without user intervention. Onboard sensors in SenseCam are used to trigger additional image capture [15]. SenseCam reduces the need for equipment for a life logging system because of the built-in sensors. Authors in [4] used low-level features of SenseCam images to define high level semantic concepts such as eating, road, sky, office, etc. 27 semantic concepts have been evaluated for their relevance in accurate activity detection. This work provides significant knowledge about how content-based retrieval could be used to support clustering a day into activities. MPEG-7 and SURF have been used in combination with SenseCam device in [5]. The sensor readings were fused and normalized to improve the representation of events. Evaluation showed the possibility of retrieving similar events over a longer time span. For instance, the user can retrieve all the events when she was sitting in a restaurant. The studies in [4] and [5] concentrated on using content-based retrieval to support event segmentation. In [8] the feasibility of using GPS data and Bluetooth MAC addresses to improve retrieval of similar events was successfully tested.

In MemoryLane, we have emulated some of SenseCam functionality by developing software for the Microsoft Windows based mobile device "HTC Touch Cruise". This device has been used as a logging device worn around the neck to automatically capture images, Bluetooth MAC addresses and GPS data. The captured data are then transferred to a personal computer, where images are filtered automatically. We also extend previous work by introducing a Review Client, that clusters the collected data into activities with identified places and persons that can be adjusted by the user, to semi-automatically form digital life stories.

3 Logging Kit

The Logging Kit consists of two parts: MobileLogger and LogSync. MobileLogger runs in the logging device, and it periodically logs GPS, Bluetooth MAC addresses, and Image data. LogSync is a computer application that transfers the logs from the logging device when it is connected to the computer. It also filters the images while transferring.

The logging device was also given some add-on features; a temporary camera deactivator button and a manual shutter. The camera deactivation button disables image capturing for seven minutes, while playing a configurable voice message "camera deactivated". The manual shutter button captures an extra image while playing a shutter sound. GPS data and Bluetooth MAC addresses are logged and appended into separate XML files that are used later on for analyzing the day and clustering it into activities.

The set of images is reduced by applying filters for dark and blurry images, and for eliminating sequences of similar images, then the remaining images after filtering are rotated as necessary to compensate for camera orientation.

Dark images

Dark images frequently occur when something obscures the camera lens, or due to low environmental lighting. To filter out dark images, LogSync computes the HSB (Hue, Saturation, Brightness) values of all pixels in an image. The image is considered too dark when the average brightness value is less than a threshold value of 0.2. The threshold value has been chosen based on observation, and it showed positive results in eliminating dark images. Preliminary user feedback confirms the effectiveness of the brightness filter.

Blurry images

Images captured can be blurry due to many factors, for example movement of objects in view, or movement of the camera itself while capturing. Lower camera resolution and movement of the person who is wearing the logging device results in more blurry images. Blurriness caused by movement is known as motion blur [14] or linear blur [3], and there are many techniques to identify and improve images suffering from these defects [14]. Our approach is to identify blurry images and filter them out without attempting to improve them. This ensures that only non-blurry images are presented to the user, and it also saves processing time.

Motion blur that is caused by horizontal movement of objects can be applied to a non-blurry image by implementing Gaussian blur [2] horizontally. It has been observed that when applying a small amount of Gaussian blur horizontally on an already horizontally blurry image, the image will change slightly. While applying the same amount of Gaussian blur horizontally on a non-blurry image will change the image significantly. Therefore, the adopted approach is to apply little horizontal blur on an image and compare the result with the original. The comparison method described later to check similarity is used here. If the computed similarity is equal or more than 99.7 percent, the image is considered as blurry. The users during the field test complained about having few images by the end of the day, so the value 99.7 should be reduced to make the system results in much more images.

In Fig. 1 below, image (a) is originally captured by the logging device. A small amount of horizontal blur is applied on it, changing it only slightly (image (b)). When applying a small amount of horizontal blur on image (c), the result was image (d). Checking the similarity of (c) and (d) showed a result less then 99.7, so (c) is defined as a non-blurry image, while (a) would be automatically discarded as blurry image.

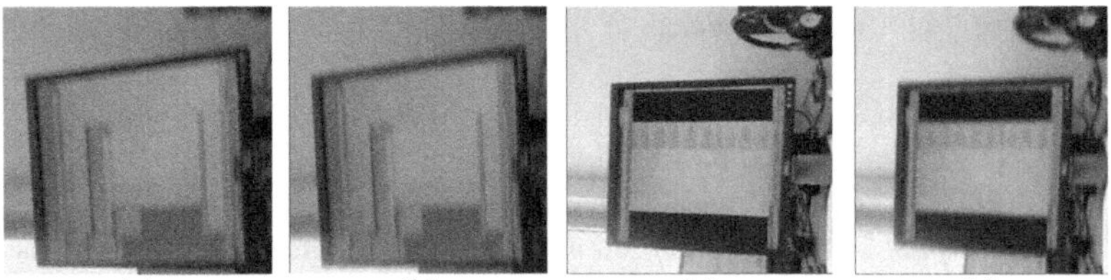

(a) (b) (c) (d)

Fig. 1. (a) Blurry image (b) Same image "a" after applying a small amount of horizontal blur. (c) Non-blurry image (d) Same image "c" after applying a small amount of horizontal blur

Similar images

An activity can have long sequences of similar images. Therefore, efficient methods to check for image similarity are called for. To compare two images, LogSync compares their grayscale form using the MAE (Mean Absolute Error) method which is computationally cheap [10]. Images are considered similar if the MAE value is at least 90 percent.

Groups of similar images are identified with the same group ID, and this is appended into an XML file. The first transferred image is given a "0" similarity percentage (no previous image to compare with). The similarity check is then applied on each pair of consecutive images, and the similarity values are appended into the XML file. If the similarity is less than 90 percent, a new group ID will be assigned to the transferred image. The system will assign the middle image of each group as a representative image of the group. The test during implementation showed that 90 percent is a reasonable value to define similarity between 2 images.

In Fig. 2, images are taken during an activity and checked for similarity. Images "b", "c", and "d" are identified similar to "a".

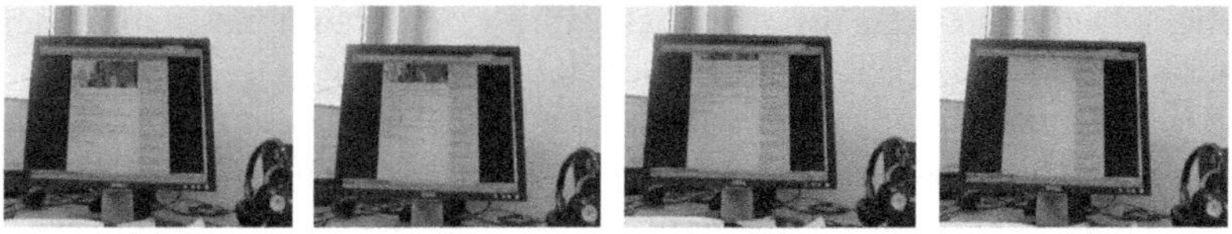

(a) (b) (c) (d)

Fig. 2. Images captured during an activity and identified as similar

4 Review Client

The Review Client typically runs on a touch screen computer at home. It analyzes the transferred logs in order to cluster them into activities (based on context data), relates content data (images) to those activities, and presents the day to the user as a sequence of activities in chronological order. GPS coordinates are used to detect places, while Bluetooth MAC addresses of nearby mobile devices are used to detect presence of persons. The Review Client basically creates digital life stories describing the life of a person based on visited places and persons met.

4.1 Detecting Context

The Review Client is limited by the resolution of the images captured by the logging device, for example creating difficulties in detecting the presence of faces. It is mentioned in [13] that using Bluetooth detection with face detection can improve the detection of persons' presence, but this relies on high quality images. Instead Bluetooth MAC addresses is the only source used to detect the presence of persons. The Bluetooth MAC addresses of mobile devices of known persons were added manually to the system.

Known places were defined using polygons based on GPS coordinates. Some places are contained by other places. For example, a city can contain a neighborhood that contains a shopping mall. In case of overlapping, the system takes the sub-place to give more accuracy about the user location. Partially overlapping places were not evaluated. There are many sources that cause GPS position error such as few satellites, atmospheric delay, receiver noise and receiver clock errors [6]. During field testing, GPS errors occurred when the logging device was indoors with few detected satellites. The field test showed that places should be defined wider to combat GPS errors, and GPS data based on few satellites should be ignored.

4.2 Analyzing Logs

After transferring the logs from the logging device, the Review Client analyzes the GPS data to identify the known places that the user visited during the day. It also analyzes the Bluetooth data to identify the known persons that the user met. After identifying the places and persons, the Review Client searches for time-based correlation resulting in activities "In a Place", "With a person", or "In a place with a Person". In our first implementation, each distinct set of present persons is considered to belong to an activity. For instance, if the user spends time with Carlos and Johan, then Eva joined them later, two activities with two different times will be generated "With Carlos and Johan" and "With Carlos, Johan, and Eva".

The activity recognition algorithm identifies a single place (or no known place) for an activity, meaning that walking with Johan, for example, from Home to University will be shown as three different activities "Home with Johan", "With Johan (on the way between home and university)" and "University with Johan". While the previous example could be shown as "Home and University with Johan", the priority was given to cluster activities based on places visited rather than on persons met. This means that the Review Client takes all the visited places as a main source to define activities, then relates all known persons who were present in those places during the visit, and finally considers situations when known persons where met in unknown places.

After clustering activities, the Review Client adds the captured images to the activities that coincide with the time when the images were captured. The Review Client presents the activities of the day in chronological order. A subject heading of each activity is generated automatically based on detected context data during the activity (places and persons), and the middle image taken during an activity is proposed as the representative image for the activity. Activities will thus be automatically annotated with information about subject, representative image, place, persons, and captured images.

4.3 Adjusting Activities

When reviewing the activities of the day, the user can adjust context and content data or even discard unwanted activities. This will empower the user and improve the accuracy of the saved activities. For instance, the user can change context data, or skip some of the images taken during an activity.

It is also possible to add new context data to the system. In case of adding a new place, the user has to choose an image for that place and enter some relevant information, then the Review Client will search for the closest detected GPS location when that image was captured. Based on that GPS location, a polygon will be created around this point, and the place will become a known place. Adding persons is done in a similar way by choosing an image and entering relevant information for that person. When adding a person, the right Bluetooth MAC address for that person is typically not well-defined since many devices not related to that person could have been detected at that time. A newly added place will therefore be detected if the user visits it again, while a new added person will not be detected if the user meets this person again. However, new added persons and places will appear as known context data in the system, and the user can manually relate them to any activity.

5 Discussion

How can the number of images presented to the user in a life logging system be minimized using filtering techniques?

Brightness, blurriness, and similarity filters can be embedded within the life logging system to reduce the number of the images, see section 3. Those filters are implemented sequentially to avoid extra operations within the system. The brightness filter will be applied first, discarding all images that are too dark. A blurriness filter is then applied, keeping only images that are of good quality. The remaining images are then compared to each other sequentially and clustered in groups based on similarity, then the system picks up the middle image from each group.

Our implemented approach helps in eliminating bad quality images and avoids keeping similar images. The filters work unobtrusively during transfer of images from the logging device to a personal computer.

How can activities be automatically recognized based on context data, prior knowledge of places and persons, and a minimal set of equipment?

Relying solely on context data in recognizing activities enables use of a single logging device. A logging device that periodically logs GPS, Bluetooth MAC addresses, and images data enables identification of places, and persons' present. Digital life stories based on visited places and persons met with associated images might be used to support memories of past activities, or at least make possible to later retrieve of the captured data based on context.

Known places and known persons need to be configured into the system in order to automate the activity recognition, and to reduce intervention by the user side in creating the life story. Having places and sub-places helps specifying the exact place, while ensuring that recognized activities can always be associated at least with the current city. While a-priori knowledge of relevant places for the user is helpful, the system can learn new places as the user adds them relating them to images captured during the visit.

Automation and unobtrusiveness keeps the interaction between the user and the system simple and efficient. However, the Review Client also provides easy-to-use interfaces allowing the user to manually navigate, adjust or discard activities.

Field testing has yielded positive user feedback on the perceived usefulness of a limited implementation of such a system.

6 Conclusions and Future Work

The algorithms for image filtering and activity recognition has been implemented in a prototype system, that successfully captures context and content data and organizes it into activities forming digital life stories. Initial results indicate that the MemoryLane system is technically feasible and that activity-based creation of digital life stories for persons with mild dementia therefore is possible.

The next stage of our work is to improve the detection of persons' presence, relying not only on Bluetooth MAC addresses. Improvements to the clustering algorithm are also needed to increase the accuracy of the system, and to enable the system to automatically recognize new contextual data (places and persons).

Acknowledgments

This work was supported by the eHealth Innovation Centre (EIC) at Luleå University of Technology and the MemoryLane research project, co-funded by the European Regional Development Fund (Mål-2).

References

1. Bush, V.: As We May Think. The Atlantic Monthly 176(1), 101–108 (1945)
2. Waltz, F.M., Miller, J.W.V.: An efficient algorithm for Gaussian blur using finite-state machines. In: SPIE Conf. on Machine Vision Systems for Inspection and Metrology VII (1998)
3. Tong, H., Li, M., Zhang, H., Zhang, C.: Blur detection for digital images using wavelet transform. In: Proc. of IEEE. Int. Conf. on ICME (2004)
4. Byrne, D., Doherty, A.R., Snoek, C.G.M., Jones, G.F., Smeaton, A.F.: Validating the Detection of Everyday Concepts in Visual Lifelogs. In: SAMT 2008 – 3rd International Conference on Semantic and Digital Media Technologies, Koblenz, Germany, pp. 3–5 (2008)
5. Doherty, A.R., ÓConaire, C., Blighe, M., Smeaton, A.F., O'Connor, N.: Combining Image Descriptors to Effectively Retrieve Events from Visual Lifelogs. In: MIR 2008 – ACM International Conference on Multimedia Information Retrieval, Vancouver, Canada, pp. 30–31 (2008)
6. Langley, R.B.: The GPS Error Budget. Innovation Column in GPS World magazine, 51–56 (March 1997)
7. Lin, W.-H., Hauptmann, A.: Structuring continuous video recordings of everyday life using time-constrained clustering. In: Multimedia Content Analysis, Management, and Retrieval SPIE-IST Electronic Imaging (2006)
8. Byrne, D., Lavelle, B., Doherty, A.R., Jones, G.J.F., Smeaton, Ȧ.F.: Using Bluetooth & GPS Metadata to Measure Event Similarity in SenseCam Images. In: Centre for Digital Video Processing (CDVP) & Adaptive Information Cluster (AIC), p. 9. Dublin City University, Dublin (2007)
9. Doherty, A.R., Smeaton, A.F.: Combining Face Detection and Novelty to Identify Important Events in a Visual LifeLog. In: IEEE International Conference on Computer and Information Technology, Workshop on Image- and Video-based Pattern Analysis and Applications, Sydney, Australia (2008)
10. Lin, Y.C., Tai, S.C.: Fast Full-Search Block-Matching Algorithm for Motion-Compensated Video Compression. IEEE Transactions on Communications (1997)
11. Aizawa, K., Ishijima, K.-I., Shiina, M.: Summarizing Wearable Video. In: Proceedings of ICIP 2001, pp. 398–401. IEEE, Los Alamitos (2001)
12. Aizawa, K., Hori, T.: Context-based Video Retrieval System for the Life-log Applications. In: Proc. of MIR 2003, pp. 31–38. ACM, New York (2003)
13. Bisht, M., Swords, D., Quigley, A., Gaudin, B., Bennett, M.: Context-Coded Memories: Who, What, Where, When, Why?: Supporting Human Memory with Interactive Systems. In: Workshop at the British HCI International Conference (2007)
14. Ji, H., Liu, C.: Motion blur identification from image gradients. In: IEEE Conference on Computer Vision and Pattern Recognition. CVPR (2008)
15. Hodges, S., Williams, L., Berry, E., Izadi, S., Srinivasan, J., Butler, A., Smyth, G., Kapur, N., Wood, K.: SenseCam: A Retrospective Memory Aid. Microsoft Research, 7 JJ Thomson Avenue, Cambridge, CB3 0FB, UK (2006)

Vowel Formant Characterization of Jaw Movements and Tongue Displacement for Possible Use in the Articulation Training Support System for the Hearing Impaired

Muhammad Hilmi Arbain, Jin-Woo Jung*, Byung-Chul So, and Mun-Sang Kwak

Dept. of Computer Science and Engineering, Dongguk University,
3-26 Pil-Dong, Jung-gu, Seoul 100-715, Korea
jwjung@dongguk.edu

Abstract. Formants are useful components to be used in order to recognize some meaningful contents from any sound. By using formants, vowel sounds in a speech can be recorded and categorized as a reference in a speech training system for the hearing impaired. The recorded sound then can be analyzed and the sound's formant values can be obtained. By using PRAAT system, the vowel speech is recorded and up-to three values of formants were gained. These formant values from five vowels (A, E, I, O, U) from three subjects were analyzed and characterized as a reference for a speech training system. The results shows that pronounced vowels' characteristics can be distinguished but may defer a little from a person to another.

Keywords: Formant Analysis, PRAAT, Speech Training System, Hearing Impaired.

1 Introduction

In today's society, hearing impaired person could not do much of anything, since most activity requires all major human senses to work co-operatively. But in retrospect, hearing impaired person did not lose the ability to speak. Most of the hearing impaired person is incapable of speaking not because of the lack in vocal capabilities, but essentially the lack of training involving the pronunciation [1]. If a person couldn't hear what he says, then how can he say it?

There are, however, classes and therapy that provides training for the hearing disabled people. But these classes require extensive times and effort plus the number of class provided is not enough [4]. So, therefore, a system that enables to replace the expertise in the field is required to reduce the complication. The approach of using articulation training support system is preferred as a possible solution to this complication due to its reliability and user friendliness.

But almost all kinds of currently available articulation training support system are based upon the training of voice or speech only as a result, not based upon the

* Corresponding author.

Y. Lee et al. (Eds.): ICOST 2010, LNCS 6159, pp. 211–217, 2010.

training of how to make the voice or speech as a process [1]. Therefore, the need for an approach based on the process of articulation of the organs and mouth is needed to add the value of the already available system.

2 Overview of the Articulation Training Support System

The articulation training support system aims to help the hearing impaired users to be able to articulate vowels by training them in forming the right lip shape and the pronunciation of the vowel [1]. The training process of the articulation training support system consists of two parts like Fig. 1; first the user must watch the panel for the correct example of the articulation. Then, the user must imitate the shown example correctly. The basic operation of the system can be summarized into two cores which are the diagnostic step and the feedback step. In the diagnostic step, the system recognizes the user's lip shape and vocal organs state, while, in the feedback step, the system gives feedback to the user in order to rectify the problem.

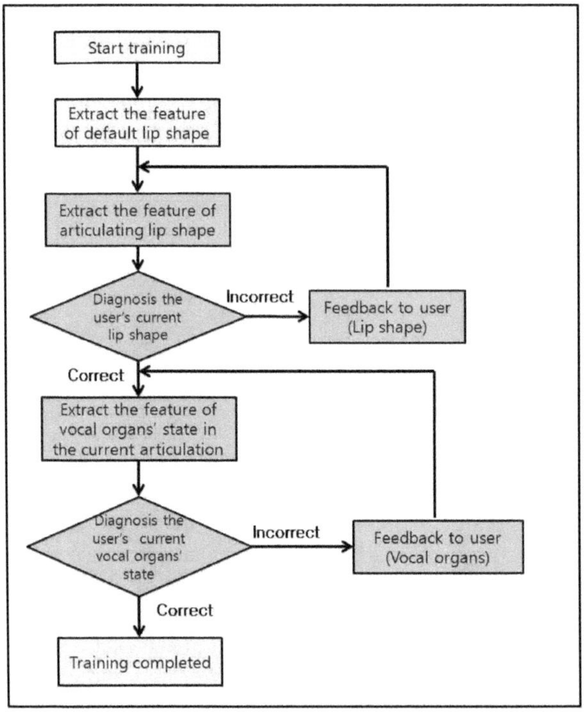

Fig. 1. Structure of the proposed articulation training support system

2.1 The Training for the Lip Shape

In order for the system to fully help the articulation of lip shape for the user correctly, the training process consists of four steps. First, the system gains the feature extraction for the non-articulating default lip shape as a reference. Then, the system extracts the current articulating lip shape from the user. After that, the system diagnoses the current lip articulation with the reference. And finally, the system gives feedbacks to the user using the diagnosed content of the previous step.

To gain the shape of the lip, the system uses the contour recognition method with four feature points (up, down, left, right) that bounded the lip. For finding the feature points, the system utilizes the color space transformation to HSV (hue, saturation, value). Then the image is enhanced using histogram equalization. To reduce any redundancy, binary transformation were done to get the rough shape of the lip. After that, the feature extraction of the lip shape was determined using corresponding vertical and horizontal lines to coordinate the threshold points. Points were then normalized and the diagnostic with the reference were done using ratio values. The feedbacks were given in terms of indicated locations of the proposed rectification via points and arrows.

2.2 Recognition for the Vocal Organs State

In addition to the lip shape recognition, the vocal organs state recognition is vital in the articulation. The recognition of the vocal organs state is done in there steps. The first step is to extract the current vocal state of the user, then the system will diagnose it with the reference, and then the system will gives it feedbacks to the user.

To extract the voice feature of the user, the system uses formant information in the recorded voice as the feature of the voice. The formant values were then processed by means of calculating the differences between the acquired formant values with the standard values using the standard deviation. After that, the feedbacks were then given to the user through text messages.

3 Problem in the Articulation Training Support System

The articulation training support system was tested and proved to have gained substantial results [1]. However, the sound recognition for the vocal organs state confirmation is not clearly defined in terms of the jaw movements and tongue displacements. The amount of jaw openings, either in ratio or exact value was not mentioned in the table. The referential position of the tongue was also not available. Table 1 shows the criterion formant for selecting feedback messages.

The problem arises when the feedback message is received; the user was told to "open" or "close" their jaw and to "move" their tongue, but the parameters were undefined. So how much of the openings and where the correct position of the tongue is not mentioned. The user needs to continuously try to repeat the actions until the correct feedback were received. It can be time-consuming and disturbing for users to repeatedly perform the acts several times.

3.1 Proposed Solution

In order to rectify this problem, a referential table or equation for the relationship needs to be constructed to provide assistance to the already given data. The table must

Table 1. Criterion for selecting feedback messages (CF: Criterion Formant)

Vocal organs		Too Low	Low	Correct	High	Too High
Jaw	Male	~ CF-93.3	CF-93.3 ~ Cf-62.2	CF-62.2 ~ CF +62.2	CF+62.2 ~ CF+93.3	CF+93.3 ~
	Female	~ CF-123.3	CF-123.3 ~ CF-82.2	CF-82.2 ~ CF+82.2	CF+82.2 ~ CF+123.3	CF+123.3 ~
Tongue	Male	~ CF-217.5	CF-217.5 ~ CF-145	CF-145 ~ CF+145	CF+145 ~ CF+217.5	CF+217.5 ~
	Female	~ CF-190.5	CF-190.5 ~ CF-127	CF-127 ~ CF+127	CF+127 ~ CF+190.5	CF+190.5 ~

provide the amount of jaw opening and tongue displacements that will enable users to understand how much or where the articulation supposed to be rectified. Since most humans have different sizes of lip and tongue, the value of the openings were to be represented in percentage form.

4 Method

In order to find a solution, some experiments were to be carried out to find the ratio of the openings and the displacements. The proposed articulation training support system and PRAAT system [5] were used in order to gather and synthesize the sounds up to three formants values. To make this experiment more organized in gathering and analyzing the raw data, the experiment is carried out in two stages. The first stage is the jaw opening formant evaluation, which gathers the formant of each vowel with instructed degree opening of the jaw. The second stage is the tongue displacements formant evaluation, which gathers the formant values of each vowel with instructed displacements of the tongue.

The venue of the experiments is the university laboratory with all windows and door closed and the environment was kept as quiet as possible when the experiment commence. The experiment was done in three separate sessions with each session lasts around 4 hours. Each person that undergoes the experiment took about 2 hours for each phase of the experiment. The total hours spent for the experiment is about 12 hours ranging in three separate days. No problems occurred during the time the experiment was conducted.

4.1 General Instructions

As a general rule, the subject of the experiment must stand in front of the proposed system at all times during the experiment. The visual of the mouth can be seen in the panel so that the subject can judge the correct position for the experiment. The subject then needed to pronounce the vowels A, E, I, O, U, to the microphone available clearly. If there are any disturbances in the system, the process needs to repeat for the current trial.

4.1.1 Formant Evaluation for Jaw Openings (Each Vowels)

For the first part of the experiment, the subject needs to pronounce the vowels with varying degree of openings of the jaw. Begin with fully opening of the jaw, after that normal openings, then decreasing to 2/3 of the opening, half of the opening, a quarter of the opening and finally with no openings (jaw is fully closed). Throughout the tests, the pronounced vowel sounds were recorded in the proposed system for each stages of the pronunciation.

4.1.2 Formant Evaluation for Tongue Displacements (Each Vowels)

For the second part of the experiment, the subject needs to pronounce the vowels with various positions of the tongue. Begin with the normal position of the tongue, then with the tongue is fully raised, followed by the tongue is not raised, and then the tongue is positioned to the front and after that to the rear of the mouth. Throughout the tests, the pronounced vowel sounds were recorded in the proposed system for each locations of the tongue.

5 Experimental Results

Based on Table 2 and Table 3, the formants values for each vowel are presented with three values of formant. The results shown are the average value of the experiments involving three male subjects, with five trials for each subject.

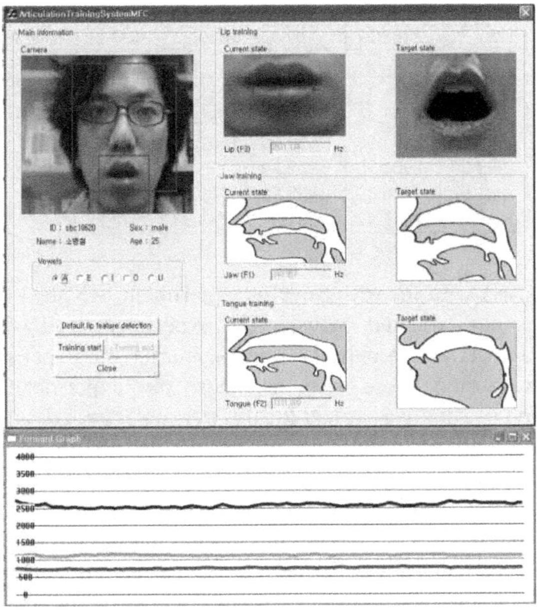

Fig. 2. Experiment with the proposed articulation training support system

Table 2. Average results for the jaw opening in up-to three values of formants (F1: 1st formant (Hz), F2: 2nd formant (Hz), F3: 3rd formant (Hz))

Jaw	100% Opening			Normal Opening			66.66% Opening		
Vowels	F1	F2	F3	F1	F2	F3	F1	F2	F3
A	739.00	1140.92	2734.28	715.67	1161.90	2688.96	673.94	1088.58	2593.80
E	664.67	1823.38	2570.08	577.23	1902.81	2619.77	552.94	1723.19	2507.37
I	388.64	2157.17	3105.12	325.03	2240.30	2989.35	333.74	2180.52	3003.28
O	482.15	747.23	2612.37	440.34	753.74	2648.86	414.94	739.71	2666.80
U	394.00	797.37	2432.67	372.07	823.72	2497.79	352.03	828.63	2568.30
Jaw	50%			25%			0%		
Vowels	F1	F2	F3	F1	F2	F3	F1	F2	F3
A	643.92	1071.71	2605.54	518.06	981.64	2520.64	598.38	1019.07	2481.94
E	542.22	1754.26	2469.53	516.00	1681.79	2358.64	545.88	1622.63	2308.04
I	320.61	2173.03	2732.26	298.84	2113.37	2716.80	364.80	2070.72	2641.45
O	431.36	844.65	2559.37	389.23	770.94	2567.65	418.67	932.86	2609.94
U	368.78	832.73	2687.75	342.05	829.42	2525.08	405.17	849.64	2545.96

Table 3. Average results for the tongue displacements in up-to three values of formants (F1: 1st formant (Hz), F2: 2nd formant (Hz), F3: 3rd formant (Hz))

Tongue	Down			Up			Normal		
Vowels	F1	F2	F3	F1	F2	F3	F1	F2	F3
A	720.78	1143.96	2685.56	676.56	1176.62	2547.71	713.40	1140.63	2604.83
E	643.24	1724.06	2493.05	633.36	1602.45	2499.88	582.79	1786.79	2501.64
I	345.02	2200.09	3086.55	367.93	2048.64	2849.18	327.25	2186.96	2916.11
O	435.91	774.03	2736.24	454.28	1029.68	2407.08	468.57	797.04	2649.16
U	373.15	1253.71	2768.27	389.92	1049.23	2427.29	358.36	901.16	2595.06
Tongue	Front			Rear					
Vowels	F1	F2	F3	F1	F2	F3			
A	768.88	1228.26	2571.46	700.40	1095.81	2616.00			
E	608.95	1769.47	2597.99	609.40	1661.21	2449.38			
I	352.13	1993.96	2901.98	322.39	2176.00	3014.49			
O	434.22	921.58	2636.35	425.51	708.82	2719.15			
U	384.61	1048.26	2562.42	361.37	793.33	2527.88			

In order to discuss with the result of this experiment, we need to consider that the result shown was not reflected only by the experiment itself. Furthermore, other factors can play into effect to either disrupt or clarify the experiment result. In any case, while disregarding these circumstances, the experiment result shown is generally portrayed of what was aimed for this particular experiment.

For the jaw articulation results, we can observe that the third formant is the most significant of the three recorded formants for the person identification. In each vowels pronounced by each test subject, the graph of the third formant differs from one another. This may prove usefulness in identifying characteristics in voice. However, the original aim of this study was to gain characteristics of formant in relation to the jaw-opening articulation. The first and second formant seems more or less the same from one test subject to another and could be useful in characterizing jaw articulation. The result of formant difference for the different jaw opening is like Table 2.

For the tongue displacement result, it is a little difficult to ascertain which formant value can gives the characteristics needed. Here, the first formant shows the least amount of difference for each vowel and does not undergo drastic changes from one test subject to another. But, the second and third formant can be considered as identical for each test subject in a test for each vowel and therefore can be determined as a characteristic point in our experiment. The result of formant difference for the different tongue displacements is like Table 3.

6 Concluding Remarks

By using formant analysis, vowel sounds in a speech can be categorized as a reference for the possible use in the proposed articulation training support system for the hearing impaired.

We have managed to gain the characterization of each vowel by representing them in formant values and measure them to gain a trend in each articulated vowel. However, certain aspect is still needed to be revised such as the standard of the opening in the jaw, since different people have different pose set of jaw. In addition, the setting of the experiment could play into effect for the experimental result. But nonetheless, the characteristics of articulation of vowels through jaw openings and tongue displacements were successfully gained and we found out that, characteristics are mostly identical to each person.

Acknowledgement

This work was partially supported by the Dongguk University Research Fund and the Korea Research Foundation Grant funded by the Korean Government.

References

1. Park, H.M., Jung, J.W.: Preliminary study of articulation training supporting system for hearing impaired using automated lip shape recognition. International Juornal of ARM 9(3), 70–78 (2008)
2. Park, H.M., Jung, J.W.: A study on lip-motion recognition algorithms. In: Proceedings of KIIS Spring Conference, vol. 18(1) (2008)
3. Yang, B.G.: A comparative study of American English and Korean vowels produced by male and female speakers. Journal of Phonetics 24, 245–261 (1996)
4. Yang, B.G.: A study on vowel formant variation by vocal tract modification. Speech Science 3, 83–92 (1998)
5. Yang, B.G.: 프라트(Praat)를 이용한 음성 분석의 이론과 설계 (2003)

Requirements for the Deployment of Sensor Based Recognition Systems for Ambient Assistive Living

Jit Biswas[1], Matthias Baumgarten[2], Andrei Tolstikov[1], Aung Aung Phyo Wai[1], Chris Nugent[2], Liming Chen[2], and Mark Donnelly[2]

[1] Institute for Infocomm Research, Networking Protocols Department, Singapore
{biswas,atolstikov,apwaung}@i2r.a-star.edu.sg
[2] Computer Science Research Institute and School of Computing and Mathematics, University of Ulster, Shore Road, Newtownabbey, BT37 0QB, UK
{m.baumgarten,cd.nugent,l.chen,mp.donnelly}@ulster.ac.uk

Abstract. The deployment, replication and adaptation of sensor environments at various scales and for various purposes is one of the challenges academia as well as industry are faced with today. Individual user requirements, the heterogeneity of devices, the often non-standardized communication protocols in addition to proprietary-related aspects are just some of the problems, which must be addressed in order to establish flexible, efficient and maybe most importantly, cost-effective smart environments that are capable to facilitate Ambient Assisted Living (AAL). This paper discusses some of the requirements for the design and deployment of activity recognition systems and also addresses some of the problems that arose during the replication and adaptation of such a system along with a reflection on the lessons learnt.

Keywords: Smart Environments, Ambient Assisted Living, System Deployment and Replication.

1 Introduction

The monitoring and recognition of behavior and activities is an important research topic in the domain of AAL and beyond. AAL is viewed by many as a potential cornerstone in enhancing daily life in addition to supporting communication activities between people and also between people and the environment they are in. This is of particular interest when considering the increasing use of technology that may be used to provide assistance, guidance as well as a general safety layer to the elderly or to the disabled who would otherwise not be able to live independently. Thus, within the context of this paper, the general aim of AAL can be summarized as to provide unobtrusive and user-centric support for all kinds of activities of daily living (ADL) through the provision of an intelligent environment that is capable of sensing "itself" as well as its current context of use; interpreting the sensed information and at least partially reason upon them to, ultimately, (re-)act to changes in order to enhance or assist the user's experience. This process is depicted in Fig. 1, which also highlights a

Y. Lee et al. (Eds.): ICOST 2010, LNCS 6159, pp. 218–221, 2010.

number of properties that can be monitored. Naturally, such properties are not limited to physical concepts such as light or temperature but also include social and device specific information. Similar, re-active measures can be provided in various ways such as through environmental adjustments, guidance, or automated alarms in case of emergencies. Naturally, both monitoring as well as re-action mechanisms need to be performed and delivered as inconspicuously as possible hiding both, the computational complexity as well as the hardware infrastructure, from the user.

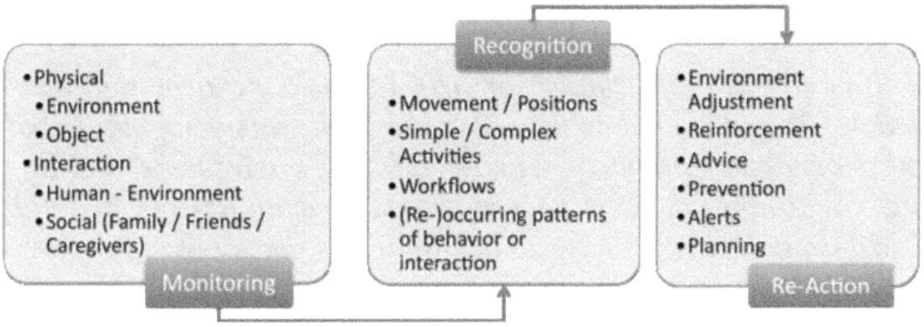

Fig. 1. Properties of Ambient Assisted Living

Recent advances in hardware technology have produced a large variety of sensors and actuators that can be deployed in various ways to perform specific monitoring as well as re-active tasks. Major approaches include attaching sensors to a person under observation or to objects that constitute the environment. Nevertheless, given the disparate and heterogeneous nature of such environments, sensor deployment as well as generic data processing algorithms that are capable of interpreting and reasoning upon such environments and also the deployment of such technologies and software components into different environments are very much an active research area. Efforts have recently been made to develop an integrated systematic framework to facilitate the sharing and reuse of data, processing capabilities and solutions. The OpenHome framework [1] has developed a common data model referred to as HomeML, a model of encoding processing rules HomeRuleML along with a suite of other tools for this purpose. The semantic smart home framework [2] proposed a semantically enabled solution for seamless integration and interoperability.

This paper discusses some of the requirements that need to be addressed for the design of generic activity recognition systems for AAL and the subsequent deployment thereof. In addition it discusses a number of the problems that occurred during the replication of such a system into a different environment and reflects on the lessons learnt.

2 Requirements for the Deployment of AAL Recognition Systems

This section discusses some of the specific requirements that have been found following working with a number of AAL based recognition systems that should be taken into account for the design and deployment of activity recognition systems. These requirements are mainly based on, but not limited to, the variations between installations and the inevitable need for the extensibility and flexibility of such systems to handle different technologies, for sensing different modalities, different use-cases, differences between end-users and the need for controlling performance parameters. In summary, the requirements can be presented as:

• *Spatial differences in the mutual positioning of functional areas: Although, different homes may have the same functional areas, their mutual positioning may differ. Regions of interest may appear in different rooms or even different floors altogether and sometimes they may be co-located. This dictates the choice of appropriate sensors for ADL detection and tracking. Moreover, this also affects the algorithms that work on prediction and other probabilistic phenomena that are based on the expected difference of event times between successive areas.*

• *The need for calibration: Distance or orientation dependent sensors such as PIR sensors need to be calibrated with a specific deployment in mind (both user and environment dependent). Similarly, video and image cameras need to be tuned to the e.g. lighting conditions, desired coverage and orientations of the subjects to be monitored; Microphone arrays have to be aligned to the source of origin and ambient noise needs to be identified. Calibration can be quite difficult but is essential for algorithms to accurately recognize the sensed concepts.*

• *Choice of sensor / platform / communication technology: Sensing technology is rapidly advancing and newer, more sensitive, more flexible and more robust devices are rapidly reaching the market. A good example for this constant technology improvement is object location with bar-code readers, RFID and UWB readers. Other examples are indoor RF based location tracking and outdoor GPS based location tracking. Similarly, various sensor platforms may be used (e.g. Sun Spots, Crossbow and others). It is unreasonable to expect another installation to change the underlying sensor platform technology in order to support a given algorithm. In fact, from our previous experience, it is more likely that software has to adapt to the underlying hardware architecture rather than vice versa.*

• *Differences in use cases: The need for personalization and the need for reproducibility at different locations are interrelated. These differences in ADL recognition strongly influence user modeling. It is easy to see that two end users in different locations may perform the same ADL in slightly different ways, or in a slightly different order to which algorithms need to adapt.*

• *Feature selection for micro-context: Algorithms that rely on personalized training for feature set recognition (such as the training of an accelerometer feature recognizer) must be retrained for new users. Furthermore, if the recognition algorithm makes use of additional accelerometer features, these must be exemplified (through training data generation) and the system must be re-trained or at least re-calibrated to produce the appropriate micro-context.*

• *Flexibility and adaptability of ADL algorithms: Ideally, an ADL recognition system should be made adaptive to multiple sensor platforms and sensor modalities and it should be able to distinguish between different feature sets and sensing modalities that may occur at different locations.*

• *Performance and resource related considerations: Algorithms that are meant to allow for resource conservation (through sensor selection, powering-down unused sensor assemblies, etc.) need to be highly flexible in order to encompass differences in system architectures and resource conservation strategies and need to feature autonomous reconfiguration to automatically adapt to new environments.*

3 Conclusions and Lessons Learnt

Proprietary related issues remain the biggest obstacle when deploying new hardware or software components or when replacing existing ones. Thus simple and, ideally, proprietary-free interfaces that connect the underlying sensor layer with various analytical components are highly desired. Similarly, platform and program independent communication mechanisms are desired to which components can publish or (un-)subscribe too in order to access individual services or to receive information or events they are interested in. Another aspect to be evaluated before system components are replaced is that of conformity of all relevant aspects of the target environment in dependence of the original environment. In most cases, it is not enough to simply provide a new sensor that is capable of sensing the same concept but more importantly, it is necessary to ensure that all characteristics of the sensor component(s) in addition to their communication functionality conform to that of the original system. This requires that sensors have the same e.g. sensitivity, responsiveness, range, physical dimensions, etc., which is of particular importance when downgrading from a more sophisticated research oriented hardware platform to a less powerful but more affordable commercially oriented hardware platform. Thus, before extending or replacing hardware components, a detailed mapping of the characteristics of the source and the target system needs to be performed, clearly identifying the differences between them and also outlining the requirements necessary to adapt to the new system. Other relevant lessons learnt largely correlate with standard system engineering principles and can be summarized as follows: it is paramount to have a clear and in depth understanding about the domain, the environment and the users a system is to be designed for; interfaces, workflows and test cases need to be as clearly defined as possible concentrating in particular on vendor specific hardware characteristics, which are often overlooked; simple, standardized and ideally proprietary-free communication interfaces should be used wherever possible; data security and privacy related problems should be addressed as early a possible as they largely impact the design of the overall framework.

Plans for future work will concentrate on the standardization and utilization of micro-contexts for AAL, which would allow for more flexible, independent and component based systems that would eventually be deployable and configurable in an plug and play fashion and the incorporation of various autonomic features that will improve the robustness of such systems and the dynamic configuration thereof.

References

1. Nugent, C.D., Finlay, D.D., Davies, R.J., Wang, H.Y., Zheng, H., Hallberg, J., Synnes, K., Mulvenna, M.D.: HomeML - An open standard for the exchange of data within smart environments. In: Okadome, T., Yamazaki, T., Makhtari, M. (eds.) ICOST. LNCS, vol. 4541, pp. 121–129. Springer, Heidelberg (2007)
2. Chen, L., Nugent, C.D., Mulvenna, M.D., Finlay, D.D., Hong, X.: Semantic Smart Homes: Towards Knowledge Rich Assisted Living Environment. In: McClean, S., Millard, P., El-Darzi, Nugent, C. (eds.) Intelligence on Intelligent Patient Management, pp. 279–296. Springer, Heidelberg (2009)

3D Matching applied ICP Algorithm for 3D Facial Avatar Modeling Using Stereo Camera

Hyo-seok Kang, Sung-hoon Yu, and Mignon Park*

ICS Laboratory(B723), The Department of Electrical and Electronic Engineering, Yonsei University, 134, Shinchon-Dong, Sudaemoon-Gu, Seoul, 120-749, Korean
khs3538@yonsei.ac.kr, mignpark@yonsei.ac.kr

Abstract. This paper is proposed by 3D facial avatar modeling using stereo camera. We use the adaboost algorithm for facial detection to get 3D facial data. We make the 3D facial modeling to match extractive 3D data with justified 3D facial avatar. We use ICP algorithm for matching 3D data and control the number of vertex and feature point for efficiency and accuracy. Feature point is selected within outline points using canny edge method. We propose to make personal 3D facial avatar for reducing expense and time.

Keywords: 3D facial avatar, Stereo camera, Vertex, Iterative Closest Point(ICP).

1 Introduction

Animation market has been getting bigger these days since the users want more reality in 3D animation. 3D avatar is used in the cyber space as a guidance for shopping and searching. The use of 3D avatar is increasing dramatically in a time of passing over from personal computer period to personal robot period because of developing humanoid robot. UI(User Interface) will be used to control robot easily and comfortably.

The growth of today's 3D avatar market shows that it's great potential. To create the Key Frame Animation discontinuously in 3D animation or 3D game, it requires much time and effort. Therefore, 3D modeling has been developed along with many other tools[1] [2]. It requires a long time to make the animation because current tools can only allow drawing motions one by one. This results the low rate of using avatar in the animation industry. Engineers need more capabilities in strong technology to improve the animation industry. This paper is shown 3D avatar modeling using stereo camera to create each Key Frame Animation. It creates intimacy and uses UI easily.

This work is organized as follows. In section 2, related works from the extraction of 3D data using stereo camera are discussed. Section 3 explains 3D Matching in justified model and extractive 3D data using ICP algorithm. Experimental results and discussions are presented in Section 4. Finally, conclusion is given in Section 5.

* Corresponding author.

Y. Lee et al. (Eds.): ICOST 2010, LNCS 6159, pp. 222–225, 2010.

2 3D Data Extraction Using Stereo Camera

Stereo camera can get 3D vertexes using disparity between two cameras. We obtain depth information to control disparity. It is available data in distance from 30cm and 3m for detecting a face[3]. In this paper, we need 3D facial vertex data. So we use to detect face using the Adaboost algorithm offered OpenCV. 3D data is provided (X,Y,Z) value of each pixel. we use Canny Edge extraction method for robustness in environment because extractive outline includes feature points. It is shown in Fig 1.

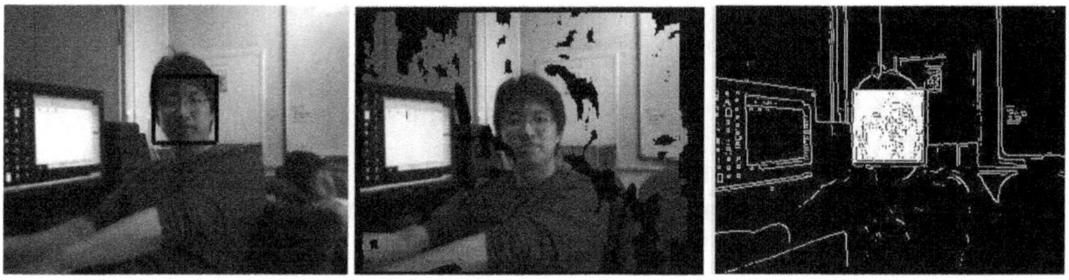

(*a*) (*b*) (*c*)

Fig. 1. Detection of face using Adaboost algorithm(*a*), 3D image in stereo camera(*b*), and feature vertexes using canny edge extractive method(*c*)

3 3D Matching Using ICP

We need 3D vertexes matching for merging extractive data with justified 3D facial data. In this paper, We use Iterative Closest Point(ICP) algorithm that is usually used to match 3D vertexes.

In summation, ICP Algorithm is as following:

1. Get the closest vertex set corresponded to each data Point in model.
2. Calculate the Registration between obtained vertex sets.
3. Apply a conversion for matching vertex sets from process 2.
4. Repeat from process 1 if Registration Error overflows an acceptable error range.

In process 1, we use an Euclidean distance when we calculate a distance.

$$d(P,M) = \|P - M\| = \sqrt{(x_p - x_m)^2 + (y_{p,} - y_m)^2 + (z_p - z_m)^2}, \tag{1}$$

where $P = (x_p, y_{p,}, z_p)$, $M = (x_m, y_{m,}, z_m)$.

We obtain the closest vertex set of model corresponded to each data point that is calculated for a distance from an image. In process 2, we get rotation matrix and translation matrix based on process 1. First of all, we define the number of data point(P) as N_p and model point(M) as N_m. The purpose of process 2 is to get minimization of q_R, q_T in equation 2.

$$f(q) = \frac{1}{N_p}\sum_{i=1}^{N_p} \|m_i - R(q_R)p_i - q_T\|^2 \tag{2}$$

The center of mess of data points and model points is represented by equation 3.

$$\mu_p = \frac{1}{N_p}\sum_{i=1}^{N_p} p_i,\ \mu_m = \frac{1}{N_m}\sum_{i=1}^{N_m} m_i \tag{3}$$

The cross-covariance matrix $\sum pm$ of data points and model points is equation 4.

$$\sum pm = \frac{1}{N_p}\sum_{i=1}^{N_p}[(p_i - \mu_p)(m_i - \mu_m)^t] = \frac{1}{N_p}\sum_{i=1}^{N_p}[p_i m_i{}^t] - \mu_p \mu_m{}^t \tag{4}$$

We define $A_{ij} = (\sum pm - \sum pm^t)_{ij}$ and $\Delta = [A_{23}\ A_{31}\ A_{12}]^T$ to determine equation (5).

$$\left(\sum pm\right) = \begin{bmatrix} tr\left(\sum pm\right) & \Delta^T \\ \Delta & \sum pm - \sum pm^t - tr\left(\sum pm\right) I_3 \end{bmatrix}, \tag{5}$$

where I_3 is 3×3 Identity matrix.

From equation (5), we can get q_R that is corresponding unit eigentvetor to the largest eigenvalue of matrix $Q(\sum pm)$.

$$q_R = [q_0\ q_1\ q_2\ q_3] \tag{6}$$

And then, q_T is defined in equation (7).

$$q_T = \mu_m - R(q_R)\mu_p, \tag{7}$$

where

$$R(q_R) = \begin{bmatrix} q_0{}^2 + q_1{}^2 - q_2{}^2 - q_3{}^2 & 2(q_1q_2 - q_0q_3) & 2(q_1q_3 - q_0q_2) \\ 2(q_1q_2 + q_0q_3) & q_0{}^2 + q_2{}^2 - q_1{}^2 - q_3{}^2 & 2(q_2q_3 - q_0q_1) \\ 2(q_1q_3 - q_0q_2) & 2(q_1q_2 - q_0q_3) & q_0{}^2 + q_3{}^2 - q_{21}{}^2 - q_2{}^2 \end{bmatrix}$$

In process 3, we convert data using q_T and q_R in process 2. In other words,

$$P_{k+1} = q_k(P_0) \tag{8}$$

We define threshold τ in process 4. And then we repeat from process 1 to 3 until satisfying $d_k - d_{k-1} < \tau$. We can know how many rotation and translation in these processes. Rotation matrix(R) and translation matrix(T) are defined as equation 9.

$$T = q_T = \begin{bmatrix} t_1 \\ t_2 \\ t_3 \end{bmatrix}, \quad R = R(q_R) = \begin{bmatrix} r_{11} & r_{12} & r_{13} \\ r_{21} & r_{22} & r_{23} \\ r_{31} & r_{23} & r_{33} \end{bmatrix} \tag{9}$$

4 Experimental Result and Consideration

In this paper, we extracted facial 3D point using stereo camera. Our purpose is that we make personal 3D facial avatar to match extractive data with some justified models. Detecting user's face using stereo camera and extracting 3D data are represented in Fig 4.

For matching extractive data from stereo camera with justified model, we used ICP algorithm in this experiment. We studied the number of vertex for applying ICP algorithm in real-time. Fig 2. is a result for error rate and computing time.

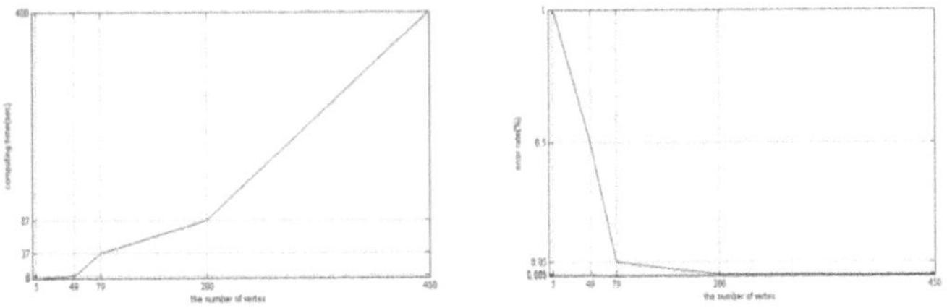

(*a*) (*b*)

Fig. 2. Computing time(*a*) and accuracy(*b*) for the number of vertex

We determined 200 feature vertexes and matched 3D facial data with justified model in Fig 3.

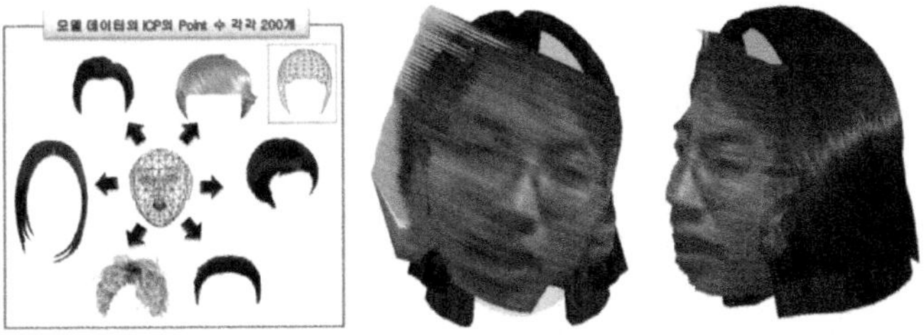

(*a*) (*b*) (*c*)

Fig. 3. Justified models(*a*) and matching 3D facial avatar in front of face(*b*)and side(*c*)

5 Conclusion

The object of this paper implements personal 3D face avatar. The modeling method using the stereo camera makes that the cost can be reduced and 3D avatar can be rapidly produced. However, implementation of the whole face is impossible. So we suggested the method to make completed 3D facial avatar, which was matched extractive data using stereo camera with modeled avatar. The number of a vertex and the abstraction of characteristic points are important for the matching about computing time and accuracy. The feature point and the number of a vertex were found with trial and error. The 200 vertexes have the best result at an accuracy and speed. The performing speed is about 87 seconds, and an error came out less than 0.01% without falling into Local minimum.

References

1. Noh, J.: A survey of Facial modeling and Animation Techniques, USC Technical Report, pp. 99-105 (1998)
2. Wen, Z., Huang, T.S.: 3D Face Processing: Modeling, Analysis and Synthesis Series. The International Series in Video Computing 8, 10–160 (2004)
3. Pollard, S., Mayhew, J., Frisby, J.: PMF: A stereo correspondence algorithm using a disparity gradient limit. Perception 14, 449–470 (1985)

System for Tracking Human Position by Multiple Laser Range Finders Deployed in Existing Home Environment

Hiroshi Noguchi, Ryo Urushibata, Takahiro Sato, Taketoshi Mori, and Tomomasa Sato

The University of Tokyo,
7-3-1 Hongo, Bunkyo-ku, Tokyo, Japan
{noguchi,urushib,takahiro,tmori,tomo}@ics.t.u-tokyo.ac.jp

Abstract. This paper describes construction of a system for measurement of human position from laser range finders (LRFs) deployed in real home environment. The system gathers and stores scan data from LRF modules equipped with room corners at different hip heights by network. We also develop a tracking method based on a particle filter framework. In the filter, after scan data is subtracted with background data and noise data is eliminated with grid map that represents room layout, the position is estimated based on detected scan points with the filtering framework. This method realizes robust tracking of the occupant in real cluttered environment. We demonstrated the system can measure human position accurately in real home environment.

1 Introduction

People tracking and measurement of people's trajectory in real home environments are important topics for location-aware system, intelligent support system, monitoring human activity of elderly people and automation system of home appliances. Currently, we have been developing the system for monitoring elderly people who live alone at remote area by using pyroelectric sensors[1]. The measurement of people position and analysis of trajectory are useful for optimization of the numbers and the locations of pyroelectric sensors.

Currently, some researchers utilizes laser range finder (LRF) for human tracking in indoor environments. Since the LRFs capture accurate distances on two-dimensional plane, it is suitable to measure accurate position of people and objects. Zhao[2] developed the method to measure people's positions in station with multiple LRFs at ankle heights by Kalman filter. Glas[3] realized tracking of people's positions and directions in hall with multiple LRFs at hip heights by particle filter. The targets of these researches are tracking people in crowded space. They assume the almost all outer shapes are captured with LRFs at the same heights in the space where no objects except people exists. However, in home environment, there are many occlusive objects such as walls and tables. Only fragments of outer shape are captured with LRFs. In real home environment, since deployment of fixed base is difficult, the heights of LRFs are various and integration of outer shape fragments is difficult. Thus, it is impossible to apply their approaches to real home environment directly.

Y. Lee et al. (Eds.): ICOST 2010, LNCS 6159, pp. 226–229, 2010.

We develop system for tracking person in real home environment with multiple LRFs. The system consists of the devices that are easily introduced into real environment and the software including the method to track the person in real home environment with multiple LRFs. In home environment, scan data at ankle height is very cluttered and occlusive with table legs and objects on the floor in real home environment. We assume the devices are deployed at hip heights and single person lives in home environment. Our tracking method measures person's position robustly in real home environment with grid map approach and design of tracking filter for fragmented contour data in real home environment where many occlusion objects exist.

2 Measurement System by Using Multiple LRFs

We develop the LRF module for easy introduction of LRFs into real home environment. The module is shown in the left upper part of Fig. 2. The module consists of the LRF and the microprocessor board. Specifications of the LRF are maximum range distance 5.6[m], range area 240[degree], angle resolution approx. 0.36[degree] and 10Hz sampling rate. The module's size is a cube whose edge length is about 15[cm]. The height is variable with spacers and horizontal angle of LRF is also variable in 45 degree unit.

The LRF scan data in each module is gathered by wired LAN for reliability of measurement. Electric power of the module is supplied with Power over Ethernet (PoE). This mechanism reduces wiring tasks and cost of deployment in real home environment. We also developed the management software for modules. The software automatically detects modules in network, gathers scan data and accumulates the data into the database system.

3 Person Tracking by Particle Filter

We utilized a particle filter similar to the Glas's approach [3]. In the particle filter framework, the filter is easy to design filtering model and the filter tracks targets robustly. We consider 2D position $x_t = (x, y)$ as a state in the filter. As transition model, we assume the occupants move in uniform speed. As for evaluation model, Since the heights of deployed LRFs are not equivalent, fitting of fixed shape to scan data is difficult. Thus, we have the simple approach that the particles are evaluated with distance between state (x, y) of particle and projected positions of scan data below the equation.

$$p(\boldsymbol{y}_t|\boldsymbol{x}_t) = \prod_{i=0}^{m} exp(\frac{-(d_i - R)^2}{\sigma^2})$$

Where m is number of foreground points. σ is distributed variance, defined empirically. R is distance from center of body to outer shape. We define $R = 15$[cm] in our method.

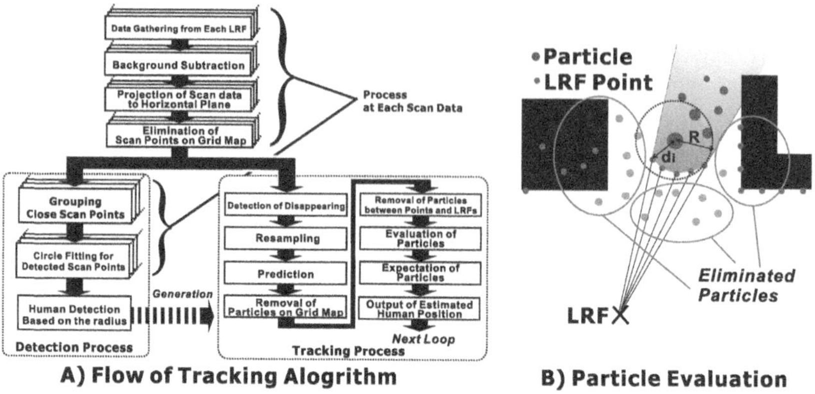

Fig. 1. Flow of Tracking Algorithm and Particle Evaluation

The flow chart of our method is shown in Fig. 1. At scan data of each LRF, background subtraction of distance and 2D projection of scan data to horizontal plane are calculated. The background distance is captured when the occupant is absent. The projected points that are not associated to body contour still remain by only background subtraction because the outer shape of objects on tables and door contour are frequently changes as human activity. For elimination of these scan data points, we utilize grid map of room layout. In mobile robot, grid map represents for room layout and obstacles. In our method, we prepare simple grid map. The occupied grid, which represents walls and fixed furniture and objects, is black and empty area is white. Scan point on the occupied grid is eliminated.

For detection of appearance, the filter detects clusters of projected scan points, fits the circle to detected points with least squares method and detects position of the habitant if the radius of fitting circle is within the range. As for detection of disappearance, when the filter misses the tracking in the several frames, the filter decides that the person has disappeared. In tracking, the particle on the occupied grid of the map are eliminated, which means the particles' weight become zero. The particle whose position is between foreground of scan points and LRF is also eliminated. This elimination improves tracking stability. Particle evaluation and removal is shown in the right of Fig. 1.

4 Experiment about Person Tracking

We introduce our system into the real environment (the left part of Fig. 2). The modules are deployed on the existing objects. The subject is 20's male. The scan data are stored during about 1 year without stopping the modules.

We evaluated tracking performance with typical trajectory data stored in the home environment. Since introduction of other position sensor into the home is difficult, we generated reference position manually by watching raw scan data of LRFs. The positions and directions of LRFs ware calibrated by hand. Grid map, which is shown in background of the experiment result, was written by hand with layout data of home environment. The number of total frames in the experiment was 709. The number of

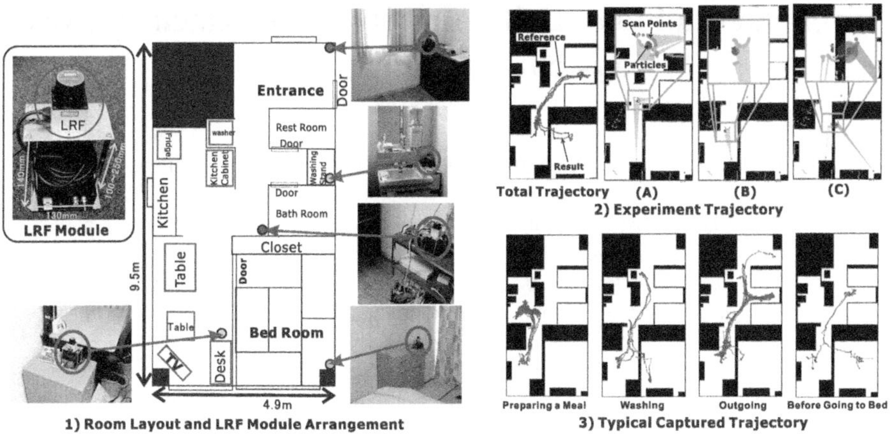

Fig. 2. Layout of Experimental House, Experiment Trajectory and Typical Trajecto- ries: 2-A) Positions is estimated accurately even if the outer shape at the different heights are different. 2-B) Contours of both body and arm are captured. The particles shift to arm positions. 2-C) the particles are separated because the particles exist over door position.

particles is 1000. In the experiment, the filter missed the occupant in no frame. The average of position error was 18 [cm]. Since this value is within radius of human body at hip height, the accuracy of tracked position is sufficient. The calculation time in one frame is within 50[ms], which is sufficient to track the person online. Tracking scene and captured trajectory is shown in the right part of Fig. 2.

5 Conclusion

We construct the system for measurement of human position with multiple LRFs. The system consists of measurement modules that are easily introduced into real home environment and the software that estimates human position with the filter. The filter based on particle filter framework estimates the human position robustly in cluttered real home environment. Grid map and design of evaluation model improve the tracking performance in scan data fusion from hip-height LRF scan data. We demonstrated that the system can measure human position accurately in real home environment.

References

1. Mori, T., Urushibata, et al.: Anomaly detection algorithm based on life pattern extraction from accumulated pyroelectric sensor data. In: IROS, pp. 2545–2552 (2008)
2. Zhao, H., Shibasaki, R.: A novel system for tracking pedestrians using multiple single-row laser-range scanners. IEEE Transacations on Systems, Man and Cybernetics Part A: Systems and Humans 35(2), 283–291 (2005)
3. Glas, D.F., Miyashita, et al.: Laser-based tracking of human position and orientation using parametric shape modeling. Advanced Robotics 23(4), 405–428 (2009)

Implementation of Daily Activity Management Service System with Smart Grid

Hyun Sang Cho[1], Tatsuya Yamazaki[2], Sung Eun Kim[3], and Minsoo Hahn[1]

[1] Digital Media Laboratory, IT Convergence Campus, KAIST,
517-10 Dogok-dong, Gangnam-gu, Seoul 135-854, S. Korea
haemosu@kaist.ac.kr, mshahn@ee.kaist.ac.kr
[2] National Institute of Information and Communications Technology (NICT),
4-2-1, Nukui-Kitamachi, Kogan, Tokyo, 184-8795, Japan
yamazaki@nict.go.jp
[3] Graduate School of Public Health, the Catholic University of Korea (CUK),
505 Banpo-dong, Seocho-gu, Seoul 137-040, S. Korea
sungeun.kim@samyang.com

Abstract. Health management is fundamental to enabling elderly people to 'age in place' in their homes, and health care services can help elderly people to manage their health. The number of elderly people who require such care services is increasing rapidly, causing a parallel rise in the need for expert care providers. One of the solutions to this demand for expert care is an automatic health care system that may be integrated into a residence, but installing and operating such systems can be prohibitively expensive. To solve this issue, a cost-effective activity monitoring based health care system is proposed in this study. The system uses the infrastructure of a smart grid and a home network system in order to reduce the costs of installation and operation.

Keywords: Activity Monitoring, Health Care, Smart Grid.

1 Introduction

In most modern countries the population is aging, and the pace of this aging trend has been increasingly accelerating [4]. In spite of their age, many senior citizens continue to work into their later years and to lend the benefit of their experience to society. For many seniors, however, aging leads to troubles such as cognitive decline, which may affect aspects of memory, reasoning faculties and the ability to focus, and to troubles such as increased vulnerability to disease and injury, declines in physical strength, and other age-related maladies. In addition, aging can cause economic problems for seniors and can pose communication challenges for seniors attempting to reach out to other generations [4][6].

Studies have found that the cognitive decline due to aging is not global, and that such decline affects some mental functions more than others. Certain types of memory (including short term memory, which may be affected by damage to the hippocampus or frontal lobe), the ability to build conceptual models of new mechanisms, and the ability to retrace one's steps and to navigate were found to be most affected

Y. Lee et al. (Eds.): ICOST 2010, LNCS 6159, pp. 230–233, 2010.

by the aging process [7]. In contrast to short term memory, long term memory is less affected by aging. Thus, appliances with advanced technology that are intended to be used by an aging population should maintain concept models like those of more conventional appliances. The best way of maintaining a concept model is by using conventional appliances in a familiar place, or at least maintaining the metaphor of such conventional appliances.

In this paper, we describe a service system that is integrated with a home network and smart grid in order to monitor and guide the daily activities of an aging resident. The service system is designed to share the existing infrastructure of the smart grid and the home area network (HAN) service system, which will already have access to information about the electric appliances in a home. Thus, the installation and maintenance costs of the proposed care system can be minimized. The system provides for a universal connection to the overall smart grid and HAN service system through a remote control device as well as automatic health management services that include activity monitoring.

2 Aging in Place

A home is a familiar place of psychological comfort that meets social and physiological needs, including privacy [5]. The GVU center at Georgia Tech in USA addressed three key problem areas of aging in place: recognizing crisis, supporting everyday cognition and providing awareness of daily life and long-term trends [6]. New types of multimodal user interfaces are being invented to enhance and assist declining physiological and psychological abilities. Awareness system are also being invented to connect individuals or groups to help people maintain a peripheral awareness of one another's activities and situations in order to balance the comforts of home with the need for intimate social relationships [2][6].

To live an independent life, an individual must be able to perform basic activities of daily living (ADLs) such as eating, bathing, using the toilet, and moving around, as well as instrumental activities of daily living (IADLs) such as preparing meals, using the telephone, and maintaining the household [6]. Thus, the ability of an individual to conduct such activities is a barometer of that individual's health condition. In modern life, most of these activities involve the use of electric appliances and therefore result in electric power consumption. This means that the monitoring of power consumption can be a general means of monitoring ordinary activities.

3 Smart Grid and Smart Meters

A smart grid is the combination of existing power generation and distribution systems with information and communications technology (ICT) in order to achieve the reliable and intelligent management of a complex power supply grid that includes distributed power generators and consumers. A home energy management system (HEMS) is a system that serves to optimize power consumption through using distributed renewable power generators & storages [3]. A smart meter is a component allowing the interaction of a HEMS and a smart grid. The smart multi-power tap

(SMPT) is the most advanced power strip type smart meter, and it can detect functional location information as well as temporal power consumption data and the identity of appliances [1].

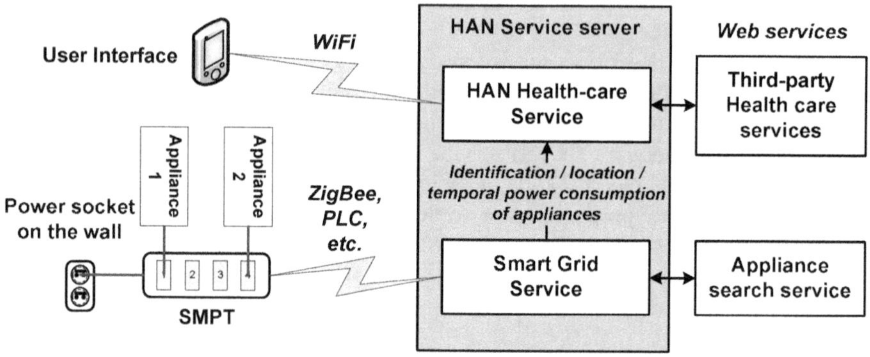

Fig. 1. System schematic with HAN service system and Smart grid

An in-home display (IHD) shows feedback on power consumption such as accumulating costs, real time prices and analysis of user power consumption in order to encourage users toward power-saving behavior. The common IHD format is a wall-pad display, but various species of displays such as handheld devices (PDA or smart phone), image projection onto a wall, sound and voice, and robots have been developed for convenient feedback and user interface. The proposed service system uses the infrastructure of the smart grid, including the electric power management features of the smart grid system.

4 Service System and Usage Scenario

In this paper, a new activity management system to allow the elderly to age in place is proposed. The system is to be implemented through an augmented convergence of the smart grid and the HAN service system. The smart grid is an emerging market that has being driven by global cooperation among many governments, and the infrastructure of the smart grid will be installed for most homes in the near future (many nations target the year 2030). Since the smart grid reduces power consumption in order to lessen the cost of power in a home, the infrastructure of the smart grid is an ideal means of addressing the economic problem of enabling retired elderly people to age in place.

One of the most difficult problems of the health care system is the legality of the diagnosis provided to a patient and actions taken on behalf of the patient. Most diagnoses and actions require certified experts, doctors, and the healthcare system itself cannot solve the lack of experts. The proposed system is focused on the prevention of crises by keeping long term records of activities in order to maintain the general health and quality of life (QoL) of the monitored patient, and thereby reduce the pressure for expert manpower. Figure 1 shows a schematic of the proposed system that includes the HAN service system, the smart grid, and third-party web services.

All activities including the operation of lamps, electric ovens, TVs and computers are monitored by the system. One of the basic services of the system is crisis detection. The system detects abnormal states of activity such as no activity for a certain time, and too many or too few activities of a certain category of ADLs. The system provides long term trends of the ADLs if the user permits the monitoring of their activities. Since the information is stored into databases, doctors or experts can analyze the activities if diagnosis of the activities becomes necessary. In addition, the system provides for the universal connection of appliances and third-party service providers.

5 Conclusion

In this paper, a new activity management system is proposed that would allow elderly people to more comfortably 'age in place.' The system is intended to be implemented through the existing infrastructure of a smart grid and the HAN service system. The system can help to prevent a user's health condition from reaching crisis by keeping long term records of user activities through monitoring the electric power consumption of appliances such as a treadmill, an auto drug dispenser, a TV, and the lamps in a home.

The system analyzes activity trends by means of a context-aware health management service in order to help maintain a user's general health and QoL. The system proposes a model combination of green technology and a health care system, and opens a low cost home health monitoring service market to third-party service providers that would not require those providers to buy new high cost facilities and instruments, enabling them to instead rely on the monitoring of existing appliances.

References

1. Cho, H.S., Kato, T., Yamazaki, T., Hahn, M.: Simple and Robust Method for Location Detection of Electric Appliances Using Markers and Programmable Logic Devices. In: ISCE 2009 (2009)
2. Cho, H.S., Lee, D., Lim, S., Hahn, M.: SoTong: An Aware System of Relation Oriented Communication for Enhancing Family Relationship. In: ISUVR 2008 (2008)
3. Kushiro, N., Suzuki, S., Nakata, M., Takahara, H., Inoue, M.: Integrated Home Gateway Controller for Home Energy Management System. In: ICCE 2003, pp. 386–387 (2003)
4. Lawler, K.: Aging in Place: Coordinating Housing and Health Care Provision for America's Growing Elderly Population. In: Harvard Joint Center for Housing Studies (2001)
5. Mitty, E., Flores, S.: There's No Place Like Home. In: Geriatric Nursing, vol. 30(2) (2009)
6. Mynatt, E.D., Essa, I., Roger, W.: Increasing the Opportunities for Aging in Place. In: CUU 2000 (2000)
7. Zajicek, M.: Interface Design for Older Adults. In: WUAUC 2001 (2001)

Gesture-Based Interface Using Baby Signs for the Elderly and People with Mobility Impairment in a Smart House Environment

Tae-Young Lee, Heon-Hui Kim, and Kwang-Hyun Park

Kwangwoon University, 447-1 Wolgye-dong, Nowon-Gu, Seoul, Korea
{taeng,heonhuikim,akaii@}kw.ac.kr

Abstract. We present a development of a gesture-based interface for the elderly and people with mobility impairment in a smart house environment. To reduce a burden of memorizing a variety of gesture commands, we introduce baby signs which are natural and easy-to-remember body signs without special education. The baby signs can be applied not only to communicate with others but also to interact with a computer for people with low level of proficiency in conventional peripherals. To achieve this purpose, we have attempted to create a real application working under illumination change and real-time requirement. The system observes the user's sign by a monitor-mounted camera and color gloves. Introducing a robust hand segmentation method against illumination change and adopting HMMs, our initial result shows 94.33% success rate for 6 sign words.

Keywords: Gesture-based interface, baby sign, hidden Markov model.

1 Introduction

Increasing population of senior citizens is considered as one of the serious social problems, and more helpful systems are required to improve their quality of life in daily activities. To support the elderly and people with disabilities to live independent life, a number of engineering approaches have been studied to develop assistive systems such as a bed-type robotic system [1], a welfare robot [2], and an Intelligent Smart Home system [3]. However, in many cases, their human-machine interfaces are very difficult to use specially for the elderly, since voice-based devices often fail to recognize voices of older people and gesture commands in vision-based interfaces are artificial and easily forgotten. In order to reduce a burden of memorizing a variety of gesture commands, we introduce baby signs which are natural and easy-to-remember body signs without special education. For example, a baby's intuitive gesture opening his/her arms corresponds to a sign word 'hug me'. This sign can be used and easily understood not only to babies but also to adults.

Baby signs have been studied since 1980s, and now become one of effective communication ways receiving wide attention from many parents [4]. In engineering point of views, the baby signs can be applied not only to communicate with others but also to interact with a computer for people with low level of proficiency in conventional peripherals. As a practical application, we developed a vision-based baby sign recognition system for a gesture-based interface in a smart house environment.

Y. Lee et al. (Eds.): ICOST 2010, LNCS 6159, pp. 234–237, 2010.

2 Baby Signs

In general, gesture commands are carefully defined considering how much simple, intuitive, and easy to understand for both users and machines [5]. This requirement restricts to define a proper gesture corresponding to a control command in task level (e.g. tasks for "going out", "delivering drink" in [6]), and results in implementing often these task-level commands by a voice-based interface in a practical application despite of its limitation.

As an alternative, baby signs (Fig. 1) are more intuitive to express the commands, and thus can reduce a burden of memorizing a variety of gesture commands. Among various baby signs [4], we selected 6 sign words for fundamental activities in daily life, so that the elderly and people with disabilities can easily control robotic systems in a smart house environment. Figure 1 shows the selected baby signs and their body motions, and corresponding control commands are described in Table 1.

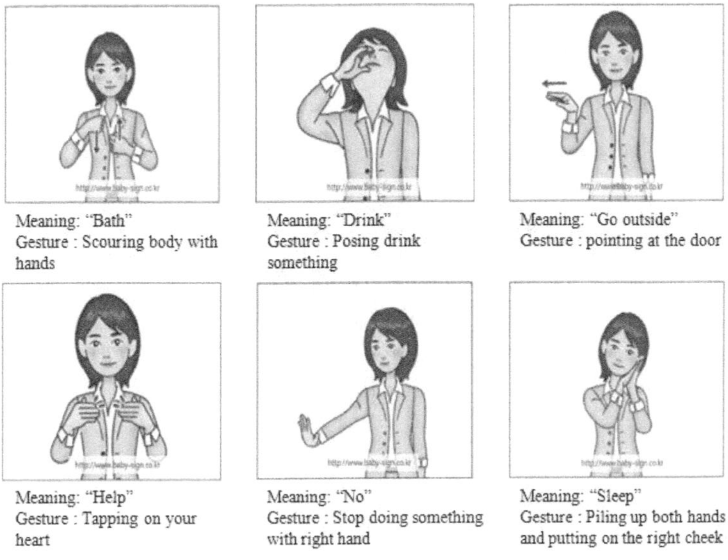

Fig. 1. Baby signs for daily activities

Table 1. Sign words and corresponding control commands for daily activities [6]

Sign Word	Situation/Need	Corresponding control commands
Bath	Dirty/Wash hands or a face	Preparing bath
Drink	Hungry/Meal or beverage	Delivering drink
Go outside	Go out	Going out
Help	Emergency	Calling someone
No	Reject or stop	Task Cancel
Sleep	Tire/Go to a bed	Preparing bed

3 Gesture Recognition System

Our system observes the user's sign by a monitor-mounted camera and color gloves. Even though this provides a bright color easily identified by a computer vision algorithm, a robust tracking of the hands is important due to the lighting effect of the room and the monitor. To segment hand region robustly even under illumination change, we adopt HSV histograms for color gloves and background [7]. These HSV histograms are used to produce a binary mask for hand region using a Bayes classifier, and small noises are removed by morphological filters including size filtering and hole filtering. We included a finding hand step in the loop of hand segmentation to enhance the discrimination of the color models of hand and background. This enables the hand color to be distinct from the similar color patterns in background. Considering the size of blobs and the distance between the center position of the candidate blobs and the hand positions in the previous image frame, we find hand regions and HSV histograms are updated based on the obtained mask.

The feature sets used for training and recognition consists of the following blob characteristics (Fig. 2): the change in x, y center positions between frames, mass, the length of the major and minor axes, eccentricity, orientation angle of the major axis, and x, y coordinates of the major axis.

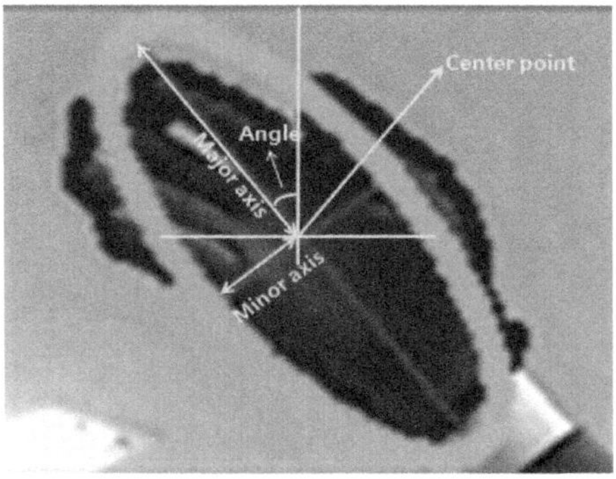

Fig. 2. Feature values for hand region

As a classifier we adopt left to right HMMs with 6state-2skip-12vec-2emmiting states implemented using HTK (Hidden Markov model Toolkit) [8].

4 Experimental Results

We experimented six sign words, "bath", "drink", "help", "go outside", "no", and "sleep" in a laboratory environment. For the test, all 150 gesture examples were randomly divided into a set of 80% examples and a set of 20% independent test examples. The test examples were not used for any portion of the training. We repeated this training and test cycle 20 times using HTK and calculated the average of the success rate. Table 2 reports the success rate of baby sign recognition, and our initial result shows 94.33% success rate for 6 sign words.

Table 2. Recognition result of baby signs

Word	Success Rate (%)
Bath	87.79%
Drink	91.25%
Help	97.50%
Go outside	93.44%
No	96.33%
Sleep	97.86%

5 Conclusion

This paper proposed a gesture-based interface using baby signs for the elderly and people with mobility impairment to enhance their quality of life. The developed system can be used as a human-friendly interface in a smart house environment. In spite of many advantages, we have further challenging works such as distinguishing each finger for more information of hand shapes to improve the performance. We also need to test our system with real end-users.

References

1. Seo, K.-H., Oh, C., Choi, T.-Y., Lee, J.-J.: Bed-type Robotic System for the Bedridden. IEEE, Los Alamitos
2. Lee, H.-E., Kim, Y., Park, K.-H.: Development of Steward Robot for Human-friendly Interaction. IEEE, Los Alamitos
3. Do, J.-H., Jang, H., Jung, S.H., Jung, J., Bien, Z.: Soft Remote Control System in the Intelligent Sweet Home
4. http://www.babysign.com/
5. Stern, H.I., Wachs, J.P., Edan, Y.: Optimal Consensus Intuitive Hand Gesture Vocabulary Design. IEEE, Los Alamitos (2008)
6. Kim, Y.-h., Lee, H.-E., Kim, H.-H., Park, K.-H., Bien, Z.Z.: A Task Planning System of Steward Robot for Human-friendly Human-Robot Interaction. In: Proceedings of the 5th International Conference on Smart Homes and Health Telematic (ICOST 2007), Nara, Japan, June 21-23, pp. 100–109 (2007)
7. Sigal, L., Sclaroff, S., Athitsos, V.: Skin color-based video segmentation under time-varying illumination. IEEE Transactions on Pattern Analysis and Machine Intelligence 26(7), 862–877 (2004)
8. http://htk.eng.cam.ac.uk

Quantitative Approach of Remote Accessibility Assessment System (RAAS) in Telerehabilitation

Shinyoung Lim[1], Jongbae Kim[2], Uzoh Ikpeama[1], Erik Porach[1], Robert Dale Lynch[3], and David M. Brienza[1]

[1] Department of Rehabilitation Science and Technology, Rehabilitation Engineering Research Center on Telerehabilitation, University of Pittsburgh, PA, 15260, U.S.A.
{sylim,uzoh,eap26,dbrienza}@pitt.edu

[2] National Rehabilitation Center - Research Institute, Seoul, Korea
jbkim@nrc.go.kr

[3] FAIA, Architectural Expert & Consultant, Haymarket, VA 20169, U.S.A.
bob@robertdalelynch.com

Abstract. Assessing the accessibility using 3D Virtual Reality and telecommunication technology has influenced home adaptation to improve accessibility in homes for individuals with disabilities, especially with Spinal Cord Injury. To provide clients with quantitative ideas on home adaptation with levels of accessibility, we propose a tentative method of measuring accessibility in home. There are a number of assessment protocols to assist rehabilitation professionals and architects in gaining wheelchair accessibility. In this paper, we briefly introduce quantitative assessment method of wheelchair accessibility in home. The feasibility of mathematical expressions of the quantitative accessibility was discussed.

Keywords: accessibility assessment; tele-rehabilitation; mobility issues.

1 Introduction

The motivation of quantitative approach in accessibility assessment is to provide rehabilitation professionals and architects with objective evidence for home adaptation or renovation to improve wheelchair accessibility in home while rehabilitation professional and architects are located remotely by using tele- rehabilitation technologies. Quantitative measurement methods of wheelchair accessibility in home provide rehabilitation professionals, architectures, and wheelchair users with an opportunity to verify space for renovation in their homes and eventually give a clear idea on investment and payment for enhancing accessibility for their Activities of Daily Living (ADL).

In this paper, we briefly introduce mathematical rationales that have been used to measure accessibility, proposed mathematical expressions, measuring accessibility based on a few activities of daily living (ADL) in home with small number of human subjects are also discussed.

Y. Lee et al. (Eds.): ICOST 2010, LNCS 6159, pp. 238–241, 2010.

2 Mathematical Rationale

Most of the evaluation items on the 'Evaluation Form for Accessibility Assessment' developed for conventional in-person assessment, require an answer of yes, no or not applicable. Architects and rehabilitation professionals depend on non-numerical expressions of accessibility assessment with a few activities of daily living (ADL). The motivation of quantitative approach stems from the needs of objective and reasonable facts of accessibility in home adaptation for individuals with mobility issues.

Assessing accessibility has been a long term issue in most accessibility protocols because each model is either too simple that leaves things out or too complex for most individuals to follow [1, 2]. After analyzing related numerical expressions of measuring accessibility, a relevant numerical expression for a quantitative approach of wheelchair accessibility is proposed as:

$$Accessibility = \sum_{I}^{J} \left(\frac{Distance * Time}{Routes}\right), \tag{1}$$

where I is the starting locations and J is the destination locations. Equation (1) measures distance in meters and time in seconds. Routes refer to the number of reasonably available paths to get from one location to another. With this simple equation, the measurement is an easier and more straightforward method when compared to the other methods. Distance and time are two vital components when determining accessibility, although the number of routes available to get from point A to point B should be considered critical as well. If there is more than one route from a starting location to a destination location, the distance and time values used need to be averages. The results of equation (1) are able to be applied to individuals in wheelchairs without further adjustments. A lower accessibility value means a greater accessibility gains. As equation (1) leaves a discrete number value, relative accessibility assists professionals to clearly understand its meaning of accessibility compared by regular division:

$$\text{Relative Accessibility (of A to B)} = (\text{Accessibility}_A \ / \ \text{Accessibility}_B) \tag{2}$$

3 Method

A photo and a floor plan, shown in figure 1, of the building were used to develop service scenarios in activities of daily living (ADL). The investigation was carried out at a smart house owned by Blueroof, an industry partner focusing on state-of-the- art living technology to provide a safer home environment as shown in figure 1. To collect data for assessing accessibility, a very small subject pool carried out the investigation. It consisted of two individuals with no mobility issues, one to navigate through the scenarios and one to measure the required data. Authors use a manual wheelchair to measure accessibility.

The route for the first scenario was marked on floor plan printouts in figure 2. This was transferred to the actual house using tape guidelines that indicated the desired path. After marking the house to comply with the marks on the floor plan, the total

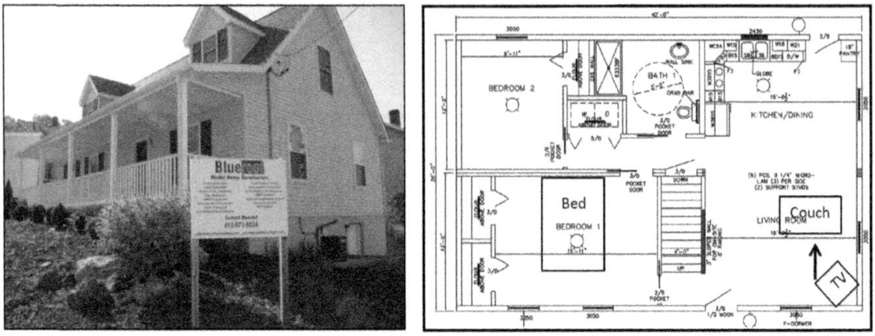

Fig. 1. Floor plan of Blueroof House located at suburban area of Pittsburgh, PA

distance of the route in the scenario was measured and recorded in meters. In this short paper, we introduce one scenario among six scenarios developed based on most frequent activities of daily living in home as described in table 1 and routings of the scenario is also shown in figure 2.

Table 1. A Scenario of Activities of Daily Living (ADL): Waking up, shower, and breakfast

Amy has just woken up to the aroma of blueberry pancakes floating through the house. Anticipating a delicious breakfast, she gets up and heads over to the bathroom to rinse her face and hands before ending up in the kitchen for breakfast.

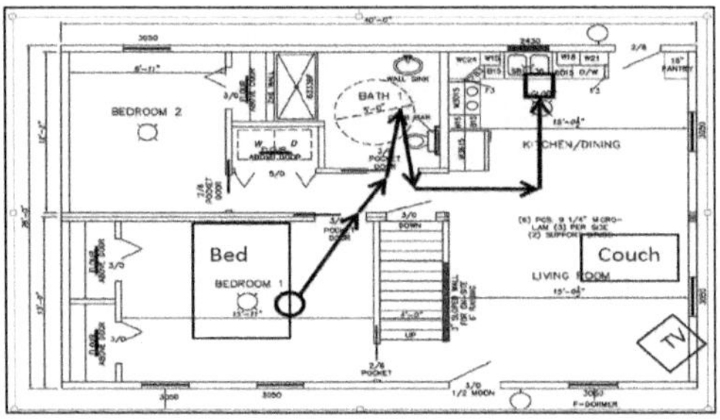

Fig. 2. Routing path with marked nodes

4 Results

Table 2 shows the results of measuring accessibility. The values were calculated using equations (1) and (2), with times and distances varying but the number of routes remaining constant at 1. On foot traveling was done with about the same ease throughout all areas of the house. However, differences were noticed during wheelchair travel. There was an issue that the maneuvering space available in the hallway, which didn't leave an adequate turning radius to get to the bedroom or bathroom in the wheelchair. The scenario had difficulty in making a "U" turn, and the carpet in the bedroom seem to create even more resistance than the one in the living room.

Table 2. Results of Accessibility Measurements

Wheelchair Accessibility (Subject A)	625.11
Wheelchair Accessibility (Subject B)	699.05
On Foot Accessibility (Subject A)	256.70
On Foot Accessibility (Subject B)	226.47
Relative Accessibility by Subject A (Wheelchair to On Foot)	2.44
Relative Accessibility by Subject B (Wheelchair to On Foot)	3.09
Routing Distance (m)	12.44
# of Routing Nodes	7

5 Conclusions

In this paper, we introduce a mathematical rationale for assessing quantitative accessibility and testing results using individuals in wheelchairs and individuals without disability in a home environment. A real world implication of this approach will be a cost effective method for measuring accessibility, as well as a way to determine to what extent modifications are needed in the home. The proposed expression will be assisting rehabilitation professionals and architects to assess accessibility using the telerehabilitation protocol. Further studies including a larger subject pool with actual users of wheelchairs in measuring accessibility as well as accessibility grades that will be acceptable and standardized to provide a threshold for home adaptation to improve wheelchair accessibility in homes.

References

1. Meyers, A.R., Anderson, J.J., Miller, D.R., Shipp, K., Hoenig, H.: Barriers, facilitators, and access for wheelchair users: substantive and methodologic lessons from a pilot study of environmental effects. Social Science & Medicine 55, 1435–1446 (2002)
2. Sakkas, N., Perez, J.: Elaborating metrics for the accessibility of buildings. Computers, Environment and Urban Systems 30, 661–685 (2006)

Indoor and Outdoor Localization Architecture for Pervasive Environment

Omar Chakroun[1], Bessam Abdulrazak[1], Mauricio Chiazzaro[1], and Mounir Frikha[2]

[1] Domus Laboratory, University of Sherbrooke, Sherbrooke QC, J1K 2R1 Canada
[2] Sup'Com, Ariana Tunisia
{omar.chakroun,bessam.abdulrazak,
mauricio.chiazzaro}@usherbrooke.ca
m.frikha@supcom.rnu.tn

Abstract. Location awareness is one of the key aspects for pervasive computing environments. It enables location data to be accessed and used anywhere by any application. Major challenges to design effective localization solutions are pervasive deployment and support for heterogeneous technologies. In our efforts to design an effective localization solution, we present a dynamic and efficient infrastructure independent layered architecture. The architecture is highly distributed, integrates inference engine to provide best location estimation for multiple technologies. Our architecture is efficient and comes across challenges in localization process such as computational power, reusability and components dependency.

Keywords: Hybrid Localization Architecture, Smart Spaces, Pervasive Computing.

1 Introduction

Today pervasive computing became an active research area. Researchers around the globe have presented several models and architectures to make Weiser vision practical [7]. Pervasive computing environments are context-dependent and sensitive to any change in context information. Since location information is considered as one of the important part of the context, therefore it has to be managed so that context integrity can be maintained for supporting location dependant applications. In our attempt to provide a global localization solution for pervasive environments, we present three layered dynamic and efficient Localization System (LocSys) architecture that is infrastructure independent and highly distributed to support multiple applications, frameworks and technologies. The remainder of this paper is organized as follows: in section 2, we summarize the existing localization researches on the domain. In section 3, we introduce our location solution architecture making the emphasis on each layer and component. And we conclude by focusing on advantages and features in our solution with opening to future works in section 4.

Y. Lee et al. (Eds.): ICOST 2010, LNCS 6159, pp. 242–245, 2010.

2 Related Work

The recent systems evolution and miniaturization led localization solutions migrate from telecommunication operators [3] to client side. These solutions present good positioning resolution and accuracy using their own beacons, receivers and specifying their own protocols and software [7, 1, 2] suitable in indoor environments. These solutions are one block designed and can't be upgraded or improved. They are sensitive to environment changes, costly, technology dependant and difficult to deploy. To overcome the above mentioned limitations, researchers provides solutions that take advantage of existing data and telecommunication infrastructure such as Wireless Local Area Networks (WLAN), Global System for Mobile communications (GSM). In such solutions, the position calculation is done in the client device [8, 7, 6, 5], not in dedicated servers. These solutions are Operating Systems (OS), wireless interfaces and/or internal components dependent, making them not suitable for heterogeneous components deployment. These solutions have computational power and memory limitations and were designed to perform maximum coverage without taking consideration neither on system complexity and dynamicity nor on internal components dependency.

3 LocSys Architecture

Our research objective is to provide a multi-technological localization solution that meets the requirements of end user applications in pervasive environments. Based on our observations, we took a hybrid approach and design a three layered architecture. This architecture supports already deployed infrastructure (infrared sensors and tactile carpets) in DOMUS laboratory and leverages wireless communication frameworks (Wi-Fi and Bluetooth). All LocSys components are implemented as OSGI services to support any environment change and facilitate their deployment and reusability. Fig. 1 shows Locsys architecture, which is composed of detection layer, decision and refinement layer, and presentation layer.

3.1 Detection Layer

The function of this layer is to collect, adapt and process information extracted from the environment. This layer is further divided in to three sub-layers.

Sensing: The sensing sub-layer contains functionalities to sense the real world and provides information of seen access points (APs) and their respective measured RSSI levels (Spotters). In this sub-layer, three types of technology can be distinguished; i) RF based technologies such as Wi-Fi and Bluetooth, ii) global technologies such as GPS, iii) close field technologies such as Infrared sensors, and tactile carpets that can provide relatively exact location information. Technologies management component is dynamic repository that provides functionalities such as installing, uninstalling, starting, stopping technologies and localization techniques.

Adaptation: The adaptation sub-layer transforms collected information to more useful data. This information is used to feed the trackers to provide location estimation. The adaptation sub-layer provides two major components; i) Distance

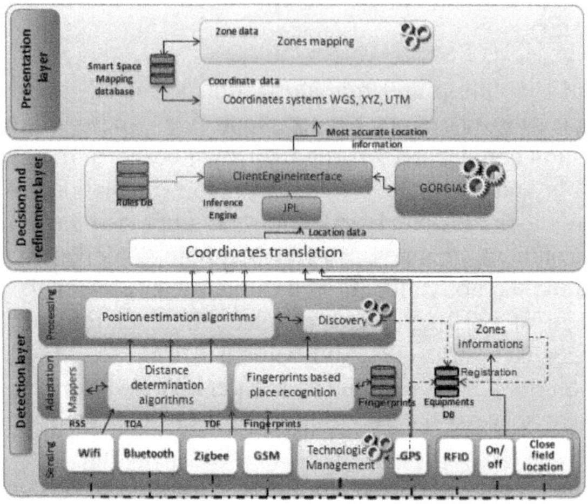

Fig. 1. LocSys architecture

determination algorithms; its function is to transform measurements (RSSI, Time of Arrival (TOA), and Time of Flight (TOF)) to ranging and distances estimation. ii) Fingerprints-based place recognition uses RSSI-based fingerprints to detect places by implementing data fusion and correlation to increase reusability and results pertinence.

Processing: The processing sub-layer contains components transforming adapted data to position estimations and discovery mechanisms providing functionalities to detect new reference points. i) Position estimation algorithms (Trackers), these algorithms are designed to be reusable and shared between different technologies. ii) Discovery module integrates mechanisms and techniques that collaborate with position estimation algorithms component to detect and store newly discovered reference points.

3.2 Decision and Refinement Layer

The main purpose of this layer is to put on equal footing all information recovered from the lower layer in coordinate systems point of view, and to extract the most accurate location information for each particular device; using predefined conditions based on researches on localization algorithms and technologies accuracies. This layer is divided into two major components;

Coordinate translation: Since we integrate different technologies suitable for various environments, we need to put all recovered location information on equal footing. This component prepares location estimation data so that the inference engine can perform the technology-technique combination choice, to support both indoor and outdoor environments and so that transfers between environments can be done in a smoother way.

Inference engine: Considering the system temporal constraint, the amount of data to process and dynamicity, an inference engine is integrated to extract the most accurate position estimation for each device. This task is done using prestored rules specifying algorithms and technologies combination accuracy. This component has an adaptative behavior; if some rules are added or modified, the engine operations will be modified to suit these changes.

3.3 Presentation Layer

For pervasive deployment and to meet application needs, LocSys provides location information with two different granularity levels; first, the coordinate data level provides components location information in different coordinates systems so that applications with interest to particular coordinates systems can be supported. Second, the zones data level provides more abstract location information using two methods; i) Using previously developed ontology [4] and by correlating coordinates-based location information and zones definitions, expressing referential and absolute localization. ii) Using geographic databases and correlating coordinates-based location information with areas geographic definition.

4 Conclusion and Future Work

In this paper, we proposed LocSys architecture for positioning systems to support location dependent applications in pervasive environments. In our design, the localization process is initiated in a collaborative mode between administrators and users to avoid privacy related issues. The distribution and dynamicity will lead to more efficient resources management and facilitate administration tasks. To support our architecture, a framework is under evaluation using real scenarios at Domus apartment. The results will be presented in future papers.

References

1. Ekahau, http://www.ekahau.com/products/positioningengine
2. Ubisense, http://www.ubisense.net/
3. Bellavista, P., Kuüpper, A., Helal, S.: Location-based services: Back to the future. IEEE Pervasive Computing 7(2), 85–89 (2008)
4. Chikhaoui, B., Benazzouz, Y., Abdulrazak, B.: Toward a universal onthology for smart environments. In: iiWAS (2009)
5. LaMarca, A., et al.: Place lab: Device positioning using radio beacons in the wild. In: Gellersen, H.-W., Want, R., Schmidt, A. (eds.) PERVASIVE 2005. LNCS, vol. 3468, pp. 116–133. Springer, Heidelberg (2005)
6. Sohn, T., et al.: Experiences with place lab: an open source toolkit for location- aware computing. In: ICSE, pp. 462–471 (2006)
7. Kolodziej, K., Johan, H.: Local Positioning Systems: LBS Applications and Services. Crc Press, Boca Raton (2006)
8. Reyero, L., Delisle, G.Y.: A pervasive indoor-outdoor positioning system. JNW 3(8), 70–83 (2008)

Undernutrition Prevention for Disabled and Elderly People in Smart Home with Bayesian Networks and RFID Sensors

Nathalie Cislo

PRISME Institute, University of Orleans,
63, avenue de Lattre de Tassigny, 18020 Bourges Cedex, France
Nathalie.Cislo@bourges.univ-orleans.fr

Abstract. Undernutrition prevention or detection for disabled or elderly people must be performed rapidly to avoid irremediable consequences. In this paper a classification of uncertainties centered on a meal notion is first proposed. Two of these uncertainties are developed in a smart home and homecare context. *Meal preparation* probability is evaluated by a simulation based on Naïve Bayesian Networks. To determine if a person is at risk of malnutrition or undernutrition, and to supervise prepared *meal quality and quantity* in terms of nutrients, the use of RFID tags is discussed, bringing many open issues for which additional sensors are proposed. This research work was initiated in a collaborative project called CaptHom.

Keywords: Smart Home, Undernutrition Prevention, Bayesian Networks, RFID Sensors, Gerontechnologies, Disabled People, Elderly People.

1 Introduction

If many works deal with smart home, especially for fragile people, few researches are focused on what happens particularly in the kitchen [1], [2], [3]. The nutrition issue for disabled or elderly people, from a physiological point of view, rather than from a cognitive point of view is still a research niche. However, malnutrition, an insufficient, excessive or imbalanced consumption of nutrients [4], is a major concern in geriatrics: many clinicians agree that 5 to 10% of elderly people at home, 50% in hospital and up to 70 to 80% in geriatric institution suffer from undernutrition [5].

The work on undernutrition presented in this paper was initiated in a collaborative project called CaptHom with an aspect dedicated to homecare for fragile people.

In the second section is presented a classification of uncertainties, centered on the notion of "meal", in order to avoid undernutrition. In section three undernutrition prevention is proposed with Bayesian Networks and results of a simulation to detect a meal preparation are presented. Then, the use of RFID sensors is discussed in the fourth section to identify what food was prepared and eaten, and which quantity and quality in terms of nutrients. Many open issues are listed, that introduce perspectives developed in section five after conclusion.

Y. Lee et al. (Eds.): ICOST 2010, LNCS 6159, pp. 246–249, 2010.

2 Undernutrition Prevention

Because undernutrition can be irremediate, the goal is undernutrition prevention or detection, as soon as possible. When elderly people or disabled people are at home, the issue is to deal with three uncertainties, centered on the meal notion (Fig. 1): (1) a meal was prepared, (2) the meal was really eaten, totally or partially, (3) the person does not suffer from undernutrition in spite of a sufficient quantity of food : meal quality is sufficient.

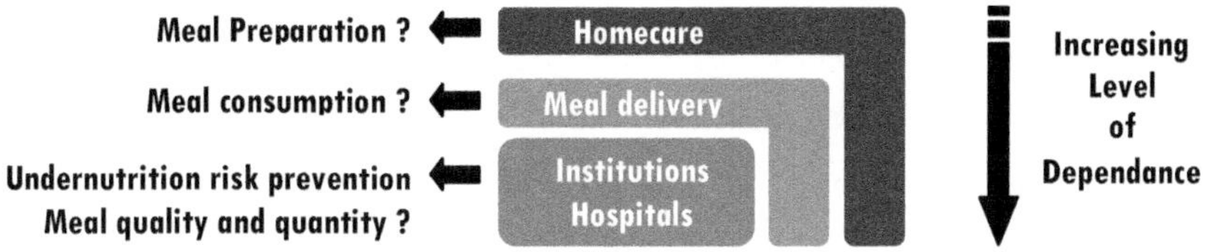

Fig. 1. Classification of uncertainties to verify in order to prevent undernutrition, corresponding to different levels of dependance

In institution or in hospital it is theoretically possible to prevent or to detect undernutrition. When meals are delivered at home, a human being can still verify if the patient eats. But when people are cooking, in a homecare context, control is difficult if a camera is out of question for ethics concern. Answers to issues occurring with less dependant people can be applied to more dependant patients (Fig. 1). For instance automatic weight control in homecare context can be exported to institutions or hospitals.

3 Bayesian Networks for Undernutrition Prevention

According to the State of the Art on existing IA or Control tools presented in [6], Bayesian Networks (BN) are a good solution to deal with uncertainty. DAGs (Directed Acyclic Graphs) have an additive advantage: they are *very easily understandable*, even by non-programmers, they can facilitate communication between researchers and clinicians.

An inconvenience, when a Bayesian Network is constructed, is that a *learning is needed, or an expert advice*.

We first focused on meal preparation, in order to know the probability that a person prepared a meal. The chosen Bayesian Networks are *naïve BN*, a very simple form of trees, where dependences between son nodes are neglected (which is not true in real life), avoiding then unnecessary computing, but giving good results.

To know if a meal is prepared a list of non exhaustive events are observed: presence in the kitchen, refrigerator opening, tap flowing, cupboard opening, garbage can opening, gas stove or electric cooker ON, time, duration…

To perform the *conditional probabilities learning*, for instance to know which is the probability to have a meal preparation according to the fact that the refrigerator is opened and closed, the person must be observed. The worst solution is to ask the person to write each action in the kitchen with date and time; the best one, but the most complex, is to automatically register this information with relevant sensors.

Key-actions (or key-events) have to be defined too, for instance, refrigerator opening. To have a significant information, a number of key-actions must be detected in a given time: if someone is present in the kitchen, opens the refrigerator, switches the cooker on, between 6 and 9 in the morning, in less than 60 minutes, one can conclude that the probability that someone has prepared a breakfast is very high.

A *simulation* of the situation described below was done with the Bayesian Network Toolbox (BNT) of Matlab. Table 1 gives a subset of conditional probabilities according to an evaluation of adults activities in a kitchen. The simulation result is a probability equal to 0.9 to have a meal preparation.

Table 1. A priori conditional probabilities for events in the kitchen

P(m=F)	P(m=T)
0,8	0,2

m: meal preparation, k: kitchen,
f: refrigerator, c: cooker, F: false, T: true

m	P(k=F)	P(k=T)
F	0,8	0,2
T	0,1	0,9

m	P(f=F)	P(f=T)
F	0,7	0,3
T	0,2	0,8

m	P(c=F)	P(c=T)
F	0,9	0,1
T	0,05	0,95

4 RFID Sensors for Undernutrition Prevention

In a Smart Home, to be sure that a fragile person really eats a prepared meal, and is not at risk of undernutrition, it is needed to know what food was prepared and eaten, which quantity and quality in terms of nutrients, and to keep weight records.

Control of events in smart kitchen is done with a high variety of sensors: opening and closing detectors (for refrigerator, cupboards, drawers…), presence sensors like the CaptHom device, flowmeters, accelerometers, supervisor, pressure sensors, thermometers, smoke sensors, light sensors, GPS devices, RFID sensors…

In order to keep track of different pieces of food in a kitchen, the proposal is to stick *RFID tags* [7] [8] on strategically chosen pieces of food, because these are either easy to tag or relevant (caloric food, with proteins, nutrients…).

RFID sensors in the kitchen bring many *open issues*:

1. A frequent inventory is needed and a human intervention is intrusive, high-cost.
2. The RFID system software must discriminate if articles out of a cupboard are needed in a recipe, or were momentarily out. The time record is not sufficient, because unneeded food can stay forgotten, and come back into place, many hours or days after. The software can be coupled with a cognitive deficiency assistance.
3. RFID loops location has to be optimised to detect food in motion.
4. In some pathologies, like diabetes, a complementary system must be able to evaluate exactly how much food was prepared and eaten.
5. Vegetables and fruit are large open issues. Ink RFID does exist [9], but for the moment it is used to tag cattle, not for eatable applications.

Beside these issues *weight control* is a relatively easy task, assuming that there are many pressure sensors existing, placed in sofa, chair, bed, to get automatic records.

5 Conclusion and Perspectives

To prevent or to rapidly detect undernutrition, a classification of uncertainties centered on a meal notion is first proposed. Two of these uncertainties are developed.

Meal preparation probability is evaluated by a simulation based on Naïve Bayesian Networks. But a learning, or an expert are needed, and events are detected by a series of sensors. Real time records have to be compared to a normal activity, in order to detect abnormal activities or a lack of activities, to raise the alarm.

To determine if a person is at risk of undernutrition, and to supervise prepared *meal quality and quantity* in terms of nutrients, the use of RFID tags is discussed, bringing many open issues for which additional sensors are proposed.

Encouraging results from simulation allow to begin a second phase, where conditional probabilities are learned from the records of disabled and elderly volunteers living in the 130m^2 fully equipped experimental apartment of GIS Madonah (Scientific Interest Group for Night and Day Homecare for Elderly or Disabled People), inside Bellevue Institution, in Bourges, France. Occupancy time of the kitchen is assumed to be different in adults group and in elders group, with individual variations: conditional probabilities personalization is then scheduled. The focus is made too on the comparison between recorded activity and normal activity.

Among issues presented in section 4, about RFID tags on food, on the one hand optimization for loops localization, and on the other hand smartness of the algorithm dedicated to follow up tags on food are the future goals, waiting for eatable RFID ink.

Aknowledgments. We especially thank all our partners involved in the CAPTHOM project of the S2E2 cluster (Sciences and Systems of Electrical Energy), and the French Industry Ministry and locale authorities for their financial help.

References

1. Groussard, P.Y., Pigot, H.: Cognitive modeling of a cooking activity: Integration of the Contention Scheduling Theory in the Cognitive Architecture ACT-R. In: NASTEC 2008, August 13-15, pp. 94–98 (2008)
2. Dion, A., Pigot, H.: Modeling cognitive errors in the realization of an activity of the everyday life. In: Cognitio 2007 (2007)
3. Vergnès, D., Giroux, S., Chamberland-Tremblay, D.: Interactive Assistant for Activities of Daily Living. In: ICOST 2005, Sherbrooke, Canada (2005)
4. Malnutrition, In: Dorland's Medical Dictionary
5. Martin, Y.: Malnutrition. In: IVème Journée Scientifique du Laboratoire Marcel-Mérieux, Lyon (2004)
6. Naïm, P., Wuillemin, P.-H., Leray, P., Pourret, O., Becker, A.: Réseaux bayésiens, 3rd edn., Eyrolles (2007)
7. Ho, L., Moh, M., Walker, Z., Hamada, T., Su, C.-F.: A Prototype on RFID and Sensor Networks for Elder Healthcare: Progress Report. In: SIGCOMM 2005 Workshops, Philadelphia, PA, USA, pp. 70–75. ACM, New York (2005)
8. Déploiement de solutions RFID: les bonnes pratiques pour mener à bien un projet. Rapport Ministériel, France, http://www.industrie.gouv.fr/pdf/deploiement_rfid_280206.pdf
9. RFID Ink, http://www.somarkinnovations.com

A Platform for a More Widespread Adoption of AAL

Diego López-de-Ipiña, Sergio Blanco, Ignacio Díaz-de-Sarralde, and Xabier Laiseca

Universidad de Deusto, DeustoTech – Tecnológico Fundación Deusto,
Avda. Universidades 24, 48007 Bilbao, Spain
{dipina,sergio.blanco,isarralde,xabier.laiseca}@deusto.es

Abstract. This paper describes an AAL-enabling platform which combines OSGi middleware, interactive TV, RFID and NFC in order to ease the day to day of not only dependant or semi-dependant elderly people (its main focus) but also their care takers and relatives. The end result is an affordable, unobtrusive, evolvable, usable and easily deployable ICT infrastructure which aims to approach the vision of "AAL for All".

Keywords: AAL, OSGi, interactive TV, RFID, NFC, Rule systems.

1 Introduction

Ambient Assisted Living [1] fosters the provision of equipment and services for the independent or more autonomous living of elderly people via the seamless integration of info-communication technologies (ICT) within homes and residences, thus increasing their quality of life and autonomy and reducing the need for being institutionalised or aiding it when it happens.

A common issue in AAL systems is that deployment is limited to premises where an important economic investment and cumbersome ICT deployment can be justified. The main aim of this work is to define an AAL-enabling platform, namely ElderCare, which addresses this limitation.

An important collective not usually targeted by AAL platforms is the people concerned with or interested in the elderly people, e.g. relatives or friends which are not directly involved in caretaking. Hence, this work proposes different access and notification mechanisms to keep them up-to-date.

Another hard issue to solve regarding AAL is adequate and timely care-related data management at residences and homes. In them, big amounts of data must be gathered and reported in real-time to be able to follow the progress and incidents regarding elderly people's daily routine. Thus, this work proposes to combine NFC mobiles and RFID tags to address this issue.

The structure of the paper is as follows. Section 2 gives an overview of related work. Section 3 presents the overall architecture of the ElderCare system. Section 4 offers more details on the three distributed component types conforming ElderCare's modular, extensible and intelligent architecture. Section 5 draws some conclusions and states some future work plans.

Y. Lee et al. (Eds.): ICOST 2010, LNCS 6159, pp. 250–253, 2010.

2 Related Work

In [2], Standford describes one of the first AAL solutions: an instrumented elderly home using pervasive computing to help the residence's staff to easily identify where they are needed and to give them support to increase their work efficiency. Information is acquired by the system via locator badges, weight sensors in beds and so on, enabling the staff to better study and react to the problems that arise. The main limitations of the system are the difficulty of integration of new hardware and the residence-centric design.

The GatorTech Smart Home [3] is a remarkable 5 year long project that led to the construction of a very advanced smart house. A modular OSGi-based service architecture is defined that allows easy service creation, context and knowledge intelligent management and the integration of some custom-built hardware. Unfortunately, this solution can only be deployed in residences willing to make a big investment and go through a heavy deployment process.

The combination of NFC technology and RFID tags has been used in several research projects related to medicine and caretaking [4][5][6]. However, none of them stores the most relevant caring information with the residents themselves.

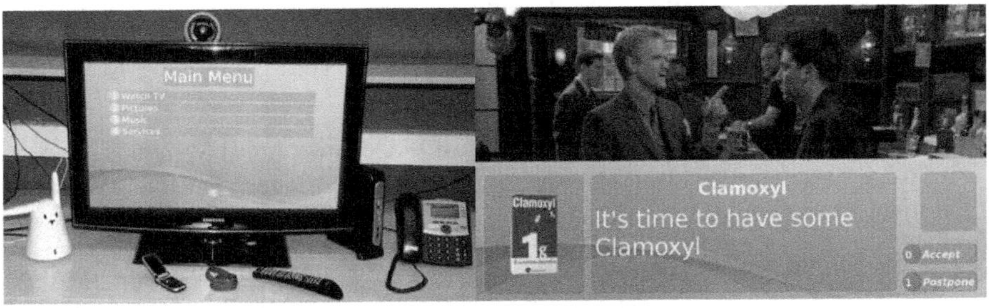

Fig. 1. AAL Kit (left hand side) and Interactive TV interface (right hand side)

3 The ElderCare Platform

This platform is devised to provide universal ICT support for friendly aging either at elderly people's own homes or in residences. In essence, The ElderCare platform aims to *provide a holistic ICT infrastructure for AAL that it is:*

- *Affordable* since it has to be offered at a low cost to ensure anybody can purchase it. In our prototype, the base system amounts to 265 €, a price that could be reduced significantly if such a product was to be produced massively.
- *Unobtrusive* so that it can be seamlessly integrated within a home or residence room, i.e. it should have the form of other common electronic devices.
- *Easily deployable* so that relatives or even elderly people can plug in the system and configure it.
- *Usable and accessible to any user collective.* The system must provide adequate user interfaces for Elderly people, care staff and family and friends.
- *Evolvable.* It should be easily integrated with any existing or emerging home automation devices, notification mechanisms and assistive services.

In summary, ElderCare addresses the aforementioned requirements proposing the following three distributed component type architecture:

1. *A bundle of essential hardware and software components known as* ***AAL Kit*** which can be deployed in any home or residence room to offer support for prolonging personal autonomy. A key part of this AAL Kit is a set-top-box enhanced DVB-T decoder. The set of default assistive services it provides are described in §4.
2. *A central remote management and service provisioning system*, namely ***ElderCare's Central Server***. It remotely manages and collects data from the Local Systems deployed in the rooms of a residence or in different homes, issuing notifications to staff and family alike when needed. It also offers an AAL service repository, something like an "AAL store", which can be accessed from a web browser to select, download and install new services.
3. *A mobile client to assist in care logging, namely* ***Mobile Care Logging System***. It is used by relatives and care staff to record, through NFC mobiles in elderly people's RFID wristbands, events and caring procedures performed over them.

4 ElderCare Internal Architecture

This section details the three distributed component types conforming ElderCare's system architecture.

1. **ElderCare's Local System:** Internally, an ElderCare's Local System is governed by an OSGi server (deployed on Equinox) which manages the following set of embedded default services:

   – *TV Tuning and Widget Manager*. It generates the interactive TV main interface offered by a Local System, using a in-house widget system that allows users to control the system using TV remotes and touch screens.
   – *Home Automation Manager*. This service allows communication with different widely available building automation standards such as X10, Zigbee or KNX.
   – *Alert Manager*. Alerts may be programmed locally or remotely. Generally, alerts will be rendered in the TV screen, although other alternative channels when the TV is off are possible such as TTS through TV's speakers.
   – *Elderly Vital Sign Monitor*. Vital sign data collection and analysis from a Zephyr HxM biometric wireless vest has also been integrated. Data is reported to the server, where health alerts are identified and forwarded to relevant people.
   – *Service Manager*. This core service provides the extensibility capability of a Local System. It allows to install/un-install services dynamically without system reboot.

2. **ElderCare's Central Server:** The Central Server offers a unique façade from which managers of Local Systems (relatives or staff in a residence) can control ElderCare deployments using an advanced web interface developed with GWT. Another interesting feature of the Central Server is its capability to react autonomously to unexpected or emergency aspects in Local Systems via a rule- based system that supports different rule engines.

3. **ElderCare's Mobile Client:** Recording caring logs *in situ* through an NFC mobile phone and an intuitive mobile logging application on HF RFID tags worn as wristbands or watches by residents is a very feasible approach for suitable care data logging. The most recent and relevant care information remains at all time in the resident's wristband, so that without a network link, any caretaker can quickly review a resident's care status, and all data is synchronised with the server by mobiles where all patient-related data is stored and published in the form of tweets or RSS feeds. A total of 34 and 164 messages could be stored in the 1K wristband and 4K watch RFID tags considered, after applying ElderCare's data encoding format.

5 Conclusions and Further Work

This work has shown a novel AAL infrastructure platform offering three main features: a) it is affordable and easily deployable at both elderly people's own homes or in their residences, b) it does not only primarily target elderly people's assistance but also helps caretakers in their work and properly keeps relatives and friends up-to- date and c) it alleviates data management in care taking by combining NFC mobiles and data storage on RFID tags. Future work will evaluate the ElderCare platform in a real deployment, a residence recently created which will be opened in May 2010.

References

1. Ambient Assisted Living Joint Programme (2009), `http://www.aal-europe.eu`
2. Stanford, V.: Using Pervasive Computing to Deliver Elder Care. IEEE Pervasive Computing 1(1), 10–13 (2002)
3. Helal, S., Mann, W., El-Zabadani, H., King, J., et al.: The Gator Tech Smart House: A programmable Pervasive Space. IEEE Computer 38(3), 50–60 (2005)
4. Bravo, J., López-de-Ipiña, D., Fuentes, C., Hervás, R., Peña, R., Vergara, M., Casero, G.: Enabling NFC Technology for Supporting Chronic Diseases: A Proposal for Alzheimer Care givers. In: Aarts, E., Crowley, J.L., de Ruyter, B., Gerhäuser, H., Pflaum, A., Schmidt, J., Wichert, R. (eds.) AmI 2008. LNCS, vol. 5355, pp. 109–125. Springer, Heidelberg (2008)
5. Mei, H., Widya, I., van Halteren, A., Erfianto, B.: A Flexible Vital Sign Representation Framework for Mobile Healthcare. In: Pervasive Health Conference (November 2006)
6. Tadj, C., Ngantchaha, G.: Context handling in a pervasive computing system framework. In: 3rd International Conference on Mobile Technology, Applications &Amp; Systems Mobility 2006, vol. 270. ACM, New York (2006)

A Guideline-Driven Platform for Healthcare Services in Smart Home Environments

Chun-Feng Liao[1], Shin-Chih Chang[1], Li-Chen Fu[1], and Ching-Yao Wang[2]

[1] Department of Computer Science and Information Engineering
National Taiwan University, Taipei, Taiwan
[2] Information and Communication Laboratory
Industrial Technology Research Institute, HsinChu, Taiwan
{d93922006,r97922122,lichen}@ntu.edu.tw, cyw@itri.org.tw

Abstract. This paper presents a guideline-driven healthcare service platform for smart homes. The clinical guidelines are usually established by medical experts according to the symptoms of diseases. Based on the biological and ambient information detected by sensors, the guideline-driven system makes the appropriate care decisions and then takes actions. In case of emergency, the platform uses the short message system to inform the relevant units immediately. The proposed service platform can therefore reduce the burdens of care and unexpected events in an effective way; therefore it enhances the quality of family care.

Keywords: Telecare, Guideline Interchange Format (GLIF), home healthcare.

1 Introduction

The population of elderly people is growing rapidly in recent years. Since aging in place and independent living at home are critical to improve the quality of elders' daily lives, the technologies of providing home healthcare services are getting considerable attentions. The increasing needs of home healthcare services usually add to the burden of medical experts. Many systems were proposed to automate the delivery of home healthcare services, but most of them are limited to data collection and uploading, which do not actually relief medical experts from heavy workloads.

Clinical Guidelines (CG) are the proven best practice documents of diagnosis and prescription, which are widely used in practice to improve the quality of care and to reduce the medical errors [5]. The GLIF (GuideLine Interchange Format) [3] is a CG encoding standard. GLIF consists of an extensible object model based on RDF (Resource Description Framework), by which guidelines become computer-interpretable and executable. One can perceive that the executable guidelines can facilitate the automatic delivery of home healthcare services. As a result, we propose a guideline-driven home healthcare services platform, namely, GHSP (Guideline-driven Home healthcare Service Platform). A typical use case of GHSP is that the medical experts encode their knowledge of care procedures or the advices to be delivered into GLIF documents, which are then deployed to an OSGi service gateway located at elders' homes. After that, a GLIF

Y. Lee et al. (Eds.): ICOST 2010, LNCS 6159, pp. 254–258, 2010.

execution engine, directed by the guideline, provides healthcare services automatically by coordinating sensor and actuator networks (see Fig.1). In this paper, we present the design rationale and implementation of GHSP, as well as some applications of guideline-driven healthcare applications based on GHSP.

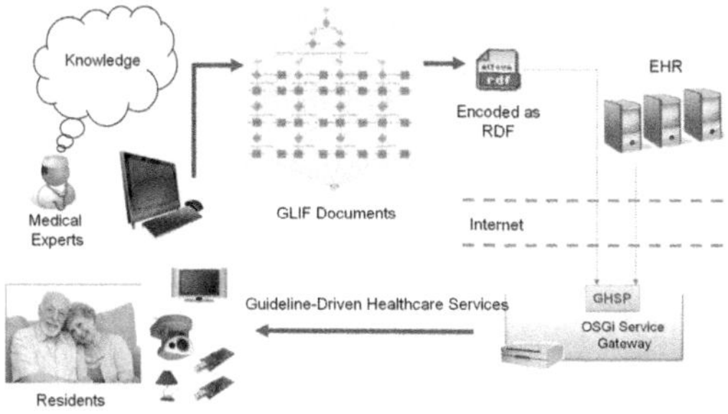

Fig. 1. Providing guideline-driven home healthcare services

2 Related Work

There are several existing healthcare systems that provide services based on CGs. GLEE (GLIF3 Execution Engine) [6] is based on an event-driven execution model, which is used to implement alerting services such as POES (Physician Order Entry System). EGADSS [2] is a clinical decision support system. The inference agent of EGADSS spontaneously pulls out the bio-information of user from electronic medical records and compares with guidelines in the database. After that, the system issues reminders. Most of current guideline-driven systems focus on providing services in hospitals or medical institutions. Furthermore, the end users of these services are mainly medical experts such as doctors or nurses. In this work, we concentrate on providing healthcare services to elders at home.

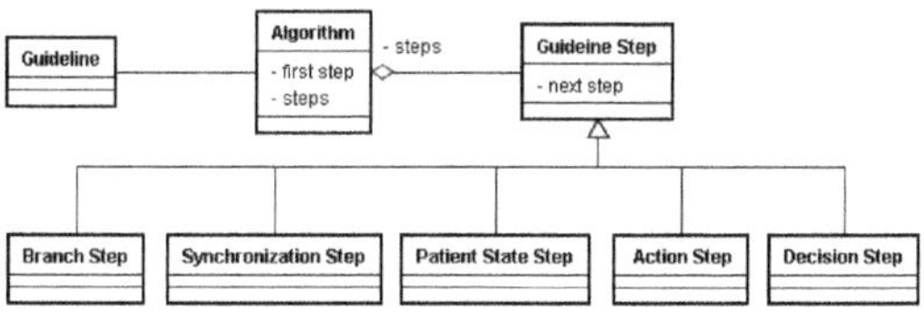

Fig. 2. GLIF object model

3 System Architecture

The guideline representation format used by GHSP is GLIF version 3 (GLIF3). It consists of three abstraction layers: Conceptual Level, Computable Level, and Implementable Level (see Fig.3). Conceptual Level defines conceptual mental model of clinical guidelines that are comprehensible to humans. GLIF 3 specification presents Conceptual Level in an object-oriented way. The most important ingredient of a Guideline is an Algorithm (see Fig.2). An Algorithm is very similar to a workflow, which composes of different types of guideline steps. From this point of view, we can observe that executing a guideline is analogous to executing a workflow in enterprise systems, except that information used for decision and the actions to be taken are different. In order to make guidelines interpretable by computers, the GLIF object models are explicitly defined by Core GLIF Ontology in Computable Level. By extending Core GLIF Ontology, guideline execution engine designers should define domain-specific ontology used by guideline developers. For instance, in GHSP, Home Context Ontology (HCO) and Home Appliance Ontology (HAO) specify common data models for home healthcare services (see Fig.3). Based on these data models, a medical expert specifies the decision criteria, which are indicated in the Decision Steps (Fig.2), by using expression languages. GLIF3 does not assume a specific expression language. In this work, we use Unified Expression Language (UEL) [1] to encode such criteria. For example, the expression ${user.name == 'Jason L.' and user.bdt >= 38} indicates the condition that Jason L. is having fever. If the contexts or situations of inhabitants match the criteria, the system issues commands to actuators in home network based on Ambient Control Directives (ACD, see Fig.3) specified in Actions Steps. For example, if Jason L. is having fever, an alert will be sent to his family as well as the healthcare service center.

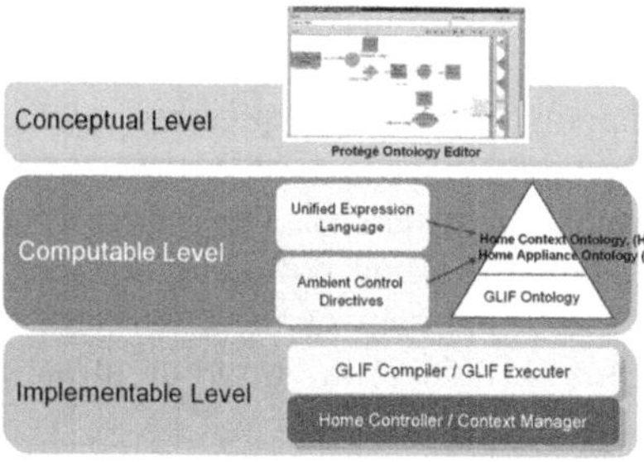

Fig. 3. Mapping GHSP core components to GLIF abstraction layers

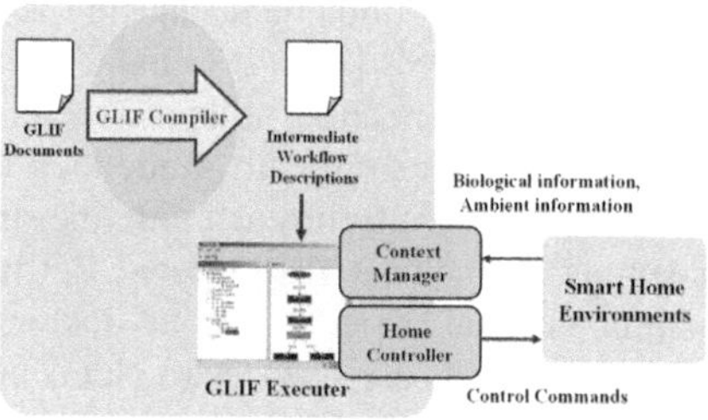

Fig. 4. System architecture of GHSP GLIF execution engine

The abstractions mentioned above are realized in Implementable Level. Fig.4 depicts the architecture of the GLIF execution engine of GHSP. In the first stage, the GLIF documents are transformed into internal workflow models, which is the input data model of GLIF Executer. The core procedures of the compiling process are shown in Fig.5. GLIF documents are first encoded into GLIF/RDF data models. After that, the ArqFacade component decomposes GLIF/RDF data modes into Step Descriptors. ArqFacade can extracts information from RDF data models efficiently by using SPARQL [4]. Finally, Step Generators generates workflow models according to the workflow graphs and directives indicated in Step Descriptors. In the second stage, generated workflow models are fed into the GLIF Executer. GLIF Executer is essentially a workflow engine that performs healthcare services by issuing commands to Home Controller (in HAO/ACD format) according to HCO-based sensor information gathered by Context Manager. Consequently, GHSP can provide

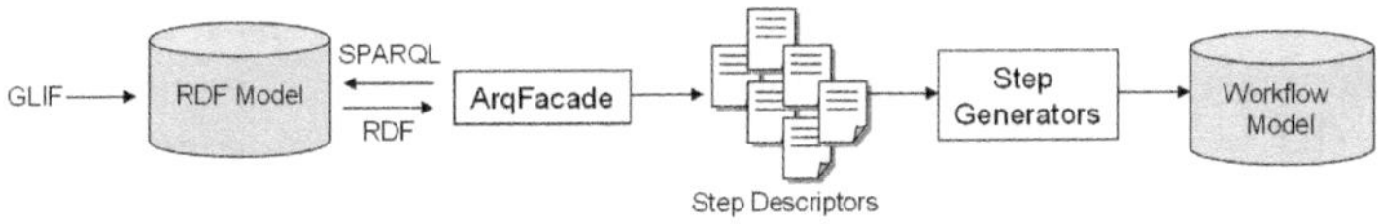

Fig. 5. GLIF Compiler

guideline-driven context-aware healthcare services, which adapts to ambient contexts as well as biological information.

4 Prototype Implementations and Application Scenarios

We investigate the feasibility of GHSP by implementing GLIF execution engine prototypes and two application scenarios. Components that comprise these prototypes and applications are implemented as OSGi bundles, which are deployed on a Knopflerfish 2.3.2 platform with JDK 1.6.0. The first scenario is a blood pressure monitoring service, which is triggered whenever users measure the blood pressure (via a FORA 3250 sphygmomanometer). If the results are not within an interval defined in the guideline (Fig.6), alerts will be issued by both sending SMS messages to the care center as well as text-to-speech voice prompts. The interval parameters and triggered actions can be adjusted on-line by revising and redeploying guidelines to the service gateway. For instance, an action that plays relaxing music to stabilize the user mood can be added. The second scenario is a diet suggestion service, which consists of an RFID reader attached on a smart refrigerator. The refrigerator is able to record consumed foods. The service summarizes and analyzes the nutrition of consumed food daily. According to the guideline, a daily report of diet suggestions is automatically generated and is displayed on the screen of refrigerator every morning.

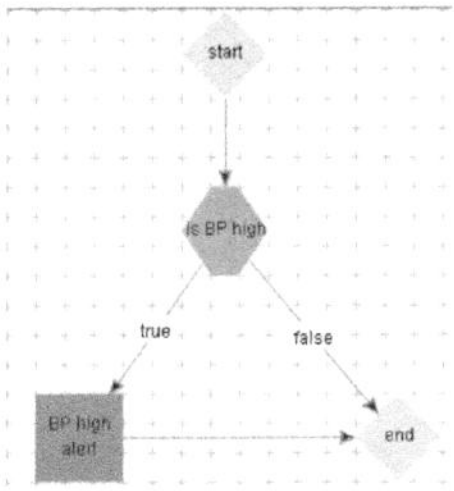

Fig. 6. Graphical view of the blood pressure monitoring service guideline

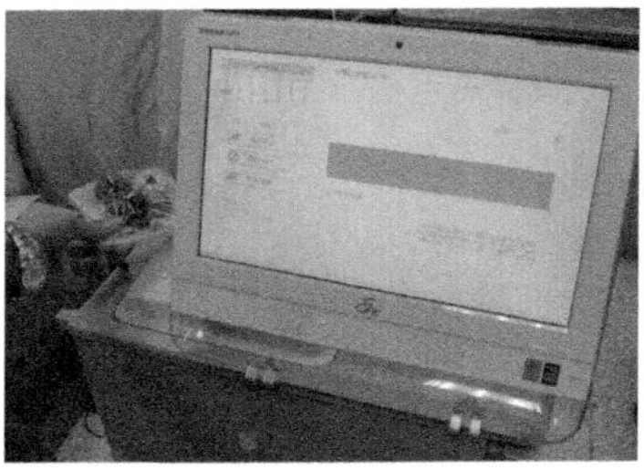

Fig. 7. Smart refrigerator attached with an RFID reader and a touch screen

5 Conclusion

In this paper, we propose to extend the uses of executable clinical guidelines from medical institutions to home environment since these guidelines preserve valuable domain knowledge of medical experts. Specifically, we have designed and implemented a guideline-driven home healthcare platform, namely, GHSP, which delivers context-aware care services to inhabitants at home. GHSP is able to interpret GLIF documents and to trigger appropriate care services according to ambient contexts and biological information of inhabitants. The components of GHSP are implemented as OSGi bundles and therefore they are modularized and reusable. When developing application scenarios, we notice that authoring GLIF documents is a great barrier even for medical experts. Hence, we will develop GUI for authoring GLIF documents in more intuitive way in the future.

Acknowledgement

This research is supported by the Industrial Technology Research Institute, under Grant NO.99- EC-17-A-05-01-0626, and by National Science Council, under Grant NSC 97-3114-E-002-002.

References

1. JSR 245 Part I - Expression Language (EL). Java Community Process (2009)
2. McCallum, G.: EGADSS: A Clinical Decision Support System for use in a Service-oriented Architecture. MSc. Thesis, Computer Science, University of Victoria (2006)
3. Peleg, M., Boxwala, A., Tu, S., Wang, D., Ogunyemi, O., Zeng, Q.: Guideline Interchange Format 3.5 Technical Specification (2003)
4. SPARQL Query Language for RDF, W3C Recommendation (2008)
5. Woolf, S.H., Grol, R., Hutchinson, A.: Potential benefits, limitations, and harms of clinical guidelines. Br. Med. J. 318(7182), 527–530 (1999)
6. Wang, D., Shortliffe, E.H.: GLEE: a model-driven execution system for computer-based implementation of clinical practice guidelines. In: Proc. AMIA Symp. (2002)

Virtual MIMO Based Wireless Communication for Remote Medical Condition Monitoring*

Joonhyung Kim, Donghyuk Han, and Jong-Moon Chung

Communications and Networking Laboratory
School of Electrical & Electronic Engineering, Yonsei University
262 Seongsanno, Seodaemun-gu, Seoul 120-749, Republic of Korea
{jh.kim,asrun,jmc}@yonsei.ac.kr

Abstract. Remote medical monitoring services for elderly people is necessary, especially for societies where the population of elderly people are rapidly increasing and healthcare costs are increasing due to lack of human resources. Wearable health-monitoring systems (WHMSs) can provide real-time medical condition monitoring using multiple biosensors attached to the human body. In this paper, virtual multiple input multiple output (MIMO) is proposed as a suitable technique for biosensor networks as it enables higher throughput capacity and less energy consumption than conventional schemes. The performance analysis of the proposed system shows that the lifetime of the virtual MIMO-based system outperforms existing systems.

1 Introduction

Wearable health-monitoring systems (WHMSs) [1] are representative technologies that offer real-time health condition monitoring and reporting to the user and the user's desired medical center. In WHMSs, multiple biosensors attached to the human body detect physiological signals such as heart rate, blood pressure, body temperature, and oxygen level. Detected signals are transmitted to a medical center through a central node (CN), so the user and the remote medical center can check the user's health condition.

Biosensors for WHMS are equipped with small batteries. For reliable and continuous support, energy-efficient transmission techniques are essential in extending the system's lifetime. Multiple input multiple output (MIMO) transmission ensures lower energy consumption compared to conventional transmission through long-haul wireless communication channels that experience fading conditions. However, MIMO transmission is not appropriate for small wireless sensor network (WSN) devices. In

* This research was supported by the National Research Foundation (2009-0088423) of the Ministry of Education, Science & Technology (MEST) and by the Ministry of Knowledge Economy (MKE) under the Information Technology Research Center (ITRC) support program supervised by the National IT Industry Promotion Agency (NIPA-2009-C1090-0902-0038) of Korea.

Y. Lee et al. (Eds.): ICOST 2010, LNCS 6159, pp. 259–262, 2010.

the paper, Virtual MIMO (V-MIMO) [2] is proposed to be used for WHMS applications. V-MIMO technology provides an enhanced performance by using the spatial diversity gain of the signals in a fading environment.

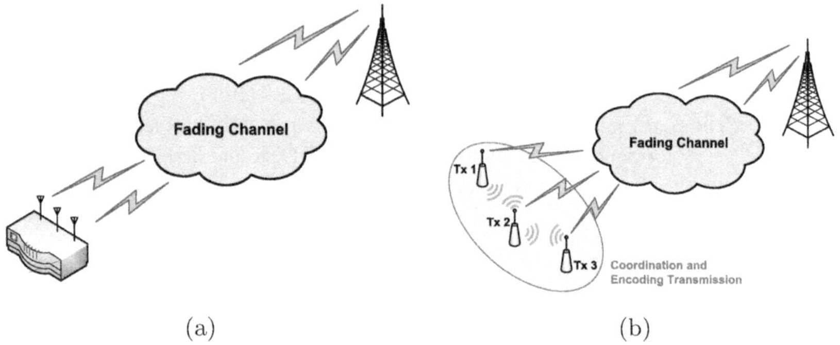

Fig. 1. Concept of MIMO and Virtual MIMO Transmission

This paper is organized as follows. In chapter 2, MIMO and virtual MIMO techniques are explained. In chapter 3, we propose a virtual MIMO-based wireless medical monitoring system and evaluate its performance. Chapter 4 concludes the paper.

2 MIMO and Virtual MIMO Techniques

Fig. 1 shows a general concept diagram of MIMO and Virtual MIMO transmission. MIMO is a transmission technique that uses antenna arrays to obtain diversity gain. Virtual MIMO technique is an alternative solution that realizes cooperative MIMO transmission on WSN devices which each consist of single antennas. As shown in fig. 1 (b), each sensor node acts as an antenna of an entire virtual antenna array. V-MIMO also obtains MIMO diversity gain, which results in minimizing transmission energy. However, compared to MIMO system, V-MIMO requires additional energy consumption due to local data exchange between the CN and sensor nodes.

3 Virtual MIMO-Based Wireless Communication for WHMS

Fig. 2 shows an example of the proposed V-MIMO based medical monitoring system. As shown in fig. 2, V-MIMO use various types of biosensors attached on the human body to monitor the user's health condition. For example, V-MIMO nodes can be a pacemaker, a glucose meter on user's wrist, and an in-shoe sensor such as Nike+ [3]. Health-monitoring data from each biosensor is sent to CN which conducts data collection and processing. After the CN finishes data processing, the processed data is transmitted to a medical center.

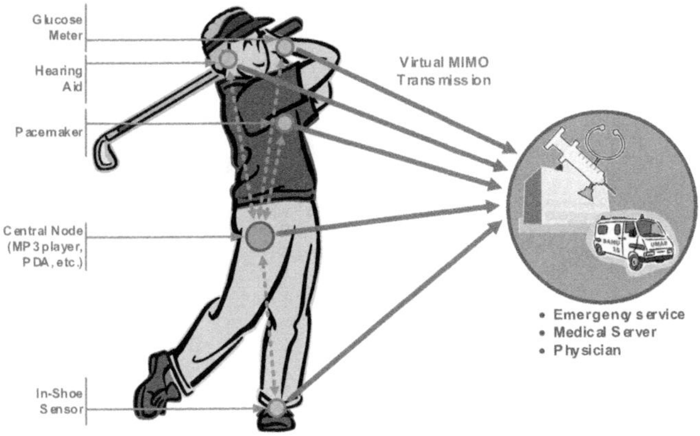

Fig. 2. Virtual MIMO-based wearable health-monitoring system

Biosensor data communication consists of two transmission phases: local transmission and long-haul transmission. First in local transmission, each biosensor sends perceived physiological data with a central node. Then, the CN processes the data and performs space-time block coding (STBC). Afterwards, the coded data is transmitted to the biosensors which take part in V-MIMO transmission. After finishing local transmission, the CN and the biosensor nodes can transmit the coded data simultaneously to a remote medical center, which is commonly a long-haul transmission. In long-haul transmission, not only the CN but also the other biosensors participate so that they form a virtual antenna array to accomplish MIMO diversity gain.

In general, WHMSs regularly report user condition to the medical center. According to user condition changes, however, the report interval can vary. For example, when biosensors detect significant changes in a person's body condition (such as irregular heart rate or blood glucose), the system should begin to send the monitored health data more frequently. In this case, frequent data monitoring and transmission will lead to a more significant energy consumption of each biosensor. To be able to estimate the lifetime of the health monitoring devices, the varying energy consumption rate caused by the transmission interval changes needs to be considered.

Performance analysis of the proposed V-MIMO transmission system is conducted as follows. There are two types of nodes, a central node and a biosensor, at each transmitter and receiver side, which consist of a 2×2 virtual antenna array. For simplicity, it is assumed that all nodes are the same. Each biosensor has single transmission antenna, and is equipped with a lithium coin battery ENERGIZER CR2032 [4] which has a capacity of 480 mWh.

Fig. 3 (a) illustrates the lifetime of WHMS system where 10,000 bits of body information is transmitted periodically. Fig. 3 (b) shows four representative simulation results from Fig. 3 (a). Despite of additional energy consumption for local data exchange, V-MIMO consumes less energy than conventional method for transmission distance longer than 33 m. The effect of energy efficiency improvement from using

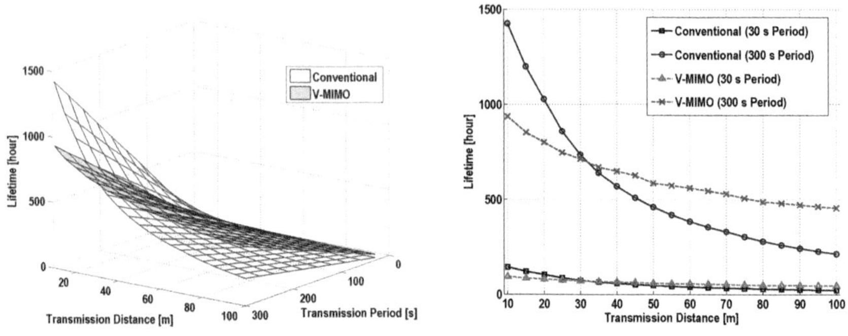

(a) Simulation Results (Transmission Periods 0 ∼ 300 s)

(b) Representative results (Transmission Periods 30 and 300 s)

Fig. 3. System Lifetime Comparison (Conventional vs. V-MIMO Transmission)

V-MIMO becomes apparent as the transmission period becomes longer. As a result, we can conclude that V-MIMO transmission is more energy-efficient transmission mechanism which shows significant gain in throughput and power consumption as the transmission distance becomes longer.

4 Conclusion

In this paper, a V-MIMO based wireless communication system for remote wireless medical monitoring is proposed. The results show that V-MIMO transmission can provide large advantages in transmission distance and energy consumption at the cost of additional control to coordinate the individual wireless health monitoring devices.

References

1. Pantelopoulos, A., Bourbakis, N.G.: A Survey on Wearable Sensor-Based Systems for Health Monitoring and Prognosis. IEEE Trans. Sys. Man and Cyber. 40(1), 1–12 (2010)
2. Cui, S., Goldsmith, A.J., Bahai, A.: Energy-Efficiency of MIMO and Cooperative MIMO Techniques in Sensor Networks. IEEE J. Sel. Areas Commun. 22(6), 1089–1098 (2004)
3. Nike+, `http://nikerunning.nike.com`
4. Energizer CR2032 Product Data Sheet, `http://data.energizer.com/PDFs/cr2032.pdf`

HealthQuest: Technology That Encourages Physical Activity in the Workplace

Hyungsin Kim[1,3], Matthew Swarts[2,3], Seunghyun "Tina" Lee[2,3], and Ellen Yi-Luen Do[1,2,3]

[1] School of Interactive Computing, [2] College of Architecture
[3] GVU Center, Georgia Institute of Technology
85 5th Street, Atlanta, GA 30332
hyungsin@gatech.edu, matthew.swarts@coa.gatech.edu, tinalee@gatech.edu, ellendo@gatech.edu

Abstract. To offset sedentary lifestyles, physical activity is widely promoted in the workplace. In this paper, we present HealthQuest, a mixed reality system to motivate employees' physical activity. HealthQuest leverages a company facility's existing physical infrastructure augmented with distributed kiosks. Users engage in wellness learning quests by walking from kiosk to kiosk in the environment. The system assists in achieving company health promotion goals.

Keywords: Health Promotion, Physical Activity, Smart Environment, Kiosk.

1 Introduction

The World Health Organization (WHO) emphasized that the workplace is a priority setting for health promotion [1]. The workplace directly influences the physical, mental, economic, and social wellbeing of workers. However, the sedentary nature of this work can contribute to employees' unhealthy habits [2]. Research shows that people who are physically active can reduce their risk of developing major chronic disease such as coronary heart disease, stroke, and type 2 diabetes by up to 50% and the risk of premature death by about 20~30% [3].

The goals of HealthQuest are to (1) encourage employees to increase everyday steps by walking around the existing physical environment, (2) educate employees on wellness awareness through kiosk-based quests, and (3) stimulate social interaction through team activity. We believe that technology can play a significant role in helping all employees to develop healthy behaviors, including older adults.

2 HealthQuest System

The HealthQuest System uses a combination of spatially distributed interactive kiosks and personal monitoring via the web through an easy to follow points system. By taking a few extra minutes on their usual walk to the coffee machine or trip to the restroom, employees are encouraged to take the recommended 30 minutes of physical activity per day. Quests lead users from kiosk to kiosk, learning about wellness.

Y. Lee et al. (Eds.): ICOST 2010, LNCS 6159, pp. 263–266, 2010.

During quests the system forms maps of employees' wellness knowledge and traces their physical activity. HealthQuest extends existing web-based personal health recording systems by integrating knowledge maps and physical activity. A point system allows individuals to compare their progress with their team member and all other employees at their company.

2.1 System Architecture

The HealthQuest System is composed of a set of kiosk terminals, which are wirelessly connected to databases and central server through a wireless infrastructure (Figure 1). It also coordinates a learning management system, a content delivery system, and a web server. The user interacts with the system on two ends. The primary interface is through the spatially distributed kiosks. Users track and set goals for their personal performance through the web. The touch screen kiosk consists of a touch screen monitor embedded or offset from a wall in a shared environment. A thin client processes information from the touch screen monitor and provides graphics back to the monitor. The thin client connects to an existing wireless network in the work environment. A barcode reader, magistripe reader, or RFID reader is attached next to the touch screen monitor and connected to the thin client to provide identification. The selection of reader depends on the existing identification system in place. Before a user can log into the system, they must first register their company identification number with the system by swiping or scanning their ID card at the kiosk. They choose a login and password for later access through the web for custom settings and performance tracking.

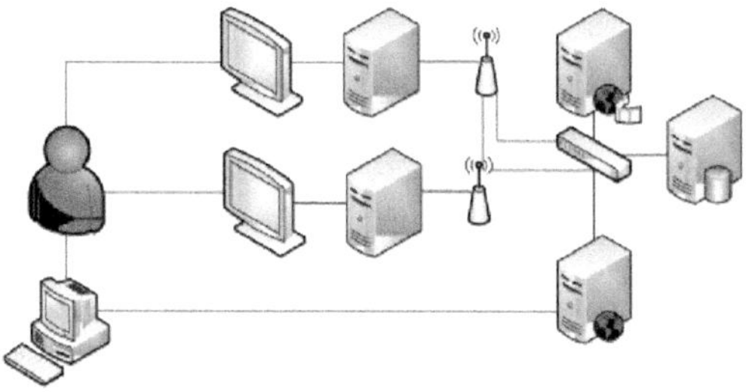

Fig. 1. System Architecture

A user begins a quest by swiping or scanning their ID card using the reader next to the touch screen. The system authenticates the user and loads the content for that user. Upon completion of an individual learning object the quest directs the user to their next target kiosk location. The system stores the network of kiosk nodes and links that represent trips between pairs of kiosks. A link table stores each link between a pair of nodes and the distribution of times taken for all users. The time distributions are used to automatically weight each node link.

2.2 Network Weights

The system stores the activity distribution between every two nodes. Bi-directional links (Link A to B and Link B to A) exist between each pair of nodes (Node A and

Node B). Suppose Node A is on the second floor and Node B is on the first floor with a stairwell in between. More effort, and therefore more time, is required to move up from Node B to Node A than down from Node A to Node B. Figure 2a (Group_AB) shows the distribution of times for all users of the 'downhill' Link AB. Now suppose that an individual is less able to apply effort. This individual's time distribution could be shown in Figure 2b (Individual_AB). Notice that the mean of the Individual_AB time distribution is higher than that of Group_AB. That is, the system knows that on average our user takes longer to go from Node A to Node B than other members of the group. However, we cannot immediately conclude that the individual is applying less effort than others.

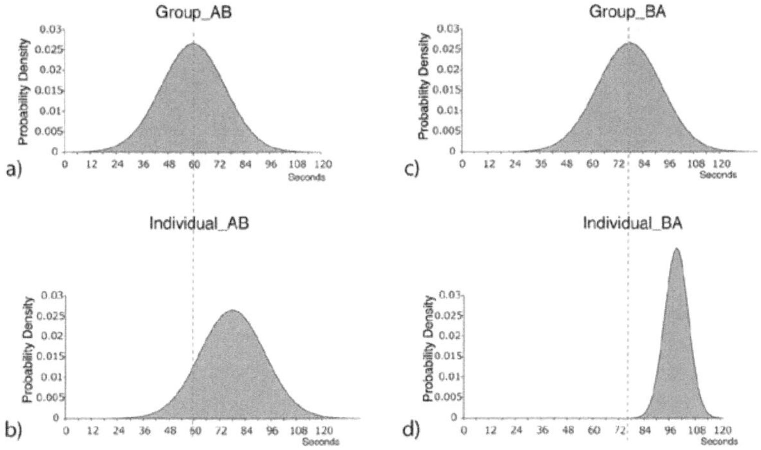

Fig. 2. Time Distribution

As users must go up stairs to travel from Node B to Node A, the time taken will likely be greater than from Node A to Node B. Therefore the hypothetical distribution of Group_BA (Figure 2c) shows a higher mean value than that of Group_AB. The time distribution from Node B to Node A for the user is shown in Figure 2d (Individual_BA). Comparing these linked time distribution we see that the user is generally slower than the group.

Users receive points for traveling from one node to another in a quest sequence. The points depend on both the group weighting as well as the individual user weighting of links. This method allows the system to award points based on individual effort, taking into account user impairment. Finally the system allows users to view their results on the web. In the web-based monitoring, users view their points, graphs of their individual and group effort, and their web of knowledge based on their responses to the quest knowledge questions. This passive method of data collection allows users to focus on their activities rather than the recording of their activities.

2.3 Accessibility Features

To increase the potential number of users in the workplace, HealthQuest is designed for the elderly and people with functional limitations such as visual impairment and poor mobility. For the elderly and visually impaired users, our visual icons are as large as possible and have high contrast between touch areas, text, and background color (shown in Figure 3). In particular, following accessibility guidelines [5], we provide larger type, a minimum of 18 point, which significantly improves legibility for most people. Our wall-mounted kiosk (shown in Figure 4) is placed in the workplace for both standing users and wheelchair users to access the screen.

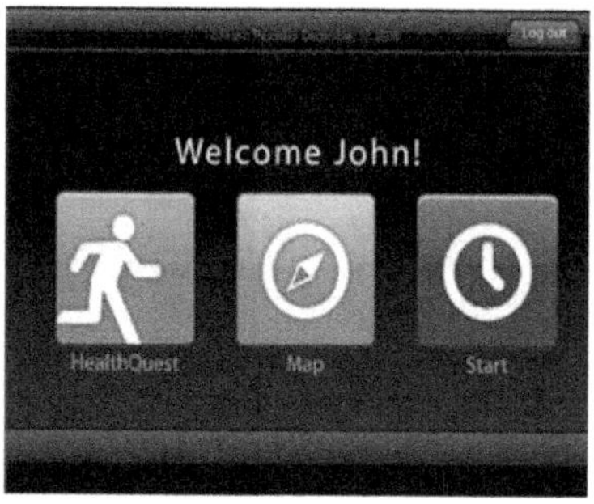

Fig. 3. A sample touch screen interface

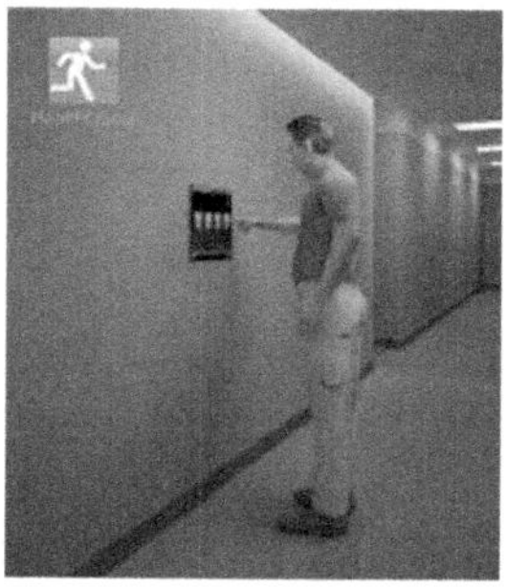

Fig. 4. Screenshot of the mockup system

4 Conclusion

In this paper we have presented the HealthQuest System for encouraging physical activity and wellbeing in the workplace. Our system adjusts the point weights for those with mobility issues including older adults. Future studies will explore other interaction techniques to maximize the simultaneous use of the system by multiple users. We also plan to address specific group interaction apart from general socialization through movement in the building environment.

References

1. Watson Wyatt Worldwide, Realizing the Potential of Onsite Health Centers (2008), http://officemdsf.com/files/2008-US-0025_Watson_Wyatt_report.pdf
2. Brunner, B.: Worksite Health Promotion - Online Research (2003), http://www.esdproj.org/site/DocServer/Worksite_Health_Promotion_2003.pdf
3. USA Department of Health and Human Services. Physical activity and health: a report of the Surgeon. Pittsburgh, PA (1996)
4. Gill, J.: Access Prohibited, Information for Designers of Public Access Terminals, Royal National Institute for the Blind, 224 Great Portland Street, London (1997)
5. Chisholm, W., Vanderheiden, G., Jacobs, I.: Web content accessibility guidelines 1.0. interactions 8(4), 35–54 (2001)

A Reliable Fall Detection System Based on Wearable Sensor and Signal Magnitude Area for Elderly Residents

Guan-Chun Chen, Chih-Ning Huang, Chih-Yen Chiang, Chia-Juei Hsieh, and Chia-Tai Chan

Institute Of BioMedicl Engineering, National Yang-Ming University,
155, Li-Nong St., Sec.2, Peitou, Taipei, Taiwan, R.O.C.
{g39704021,g39604001,g39504021,g39804012,ctchan}@ym.edu.tw

Abstract. Falls are the primary cause of accidents for elderly people and often result in serious injury and health threats. It is also the main obstacle to independent living for frail and elderly people. A reliable fall detector can reduce the fear of falling and provide the user with the reassurance to maintain an independent lifestyle since the reliable and effective fall detection mechanism will provide urgent medical support and dramatically reduce the cost of medical care. In this work, we propose a fall-detecting system based on a wearable sensor and a real-time fall detection algorithm. We use a waist- mounted tri-axial accelerometer to capture movement data of the human body, and propose a fall detection method that uses the area under a signal magnitude curve to distinguish between falls and daily activities. Experimental results demonstrate the effectiveness of proposed scheme with high reliability and sensitivity on fall detection. The system is not only cost effective but also portable that fulfills the requirements of fall detection.

Keywords: elderly people, fall detection, wearable sensor, accelerometer.

1 Introduction

Over the last 30 years, developed countries have experienced the problem of an aging society because the population of aged 65 and above has steadily increased [1]. The major causes of severe injury in the elderly residents (above 65 years old) are falls. Approximate 25~35% of elderly residents experienced fall-related injury more than one time per year [2]. Most notably, nearly 3% of the fallers lie without help more than 20 minutes [3]. Such situations may lead the fallers in danger no matter the falling is severe or not. The fall-related cost forecasting of medical care for elderly residents goes to $43.8 billion by 2020 [2]. Accordingly, a reliable fall detection system is essential for independent living elderly people with high risk of falls. The assessment of falls is difficult due to the subtle and complex body movement which requires precise and reliable measuring techniques. Several fall detecting approaches are exploited to distinguish human movements, such as camera, gyroscope, and accelerometer [4]. The accelerometer-based fall detecting sensors have many advantages like low cost and convenience in the independent living environment.

Y. Lee et al. (Eds.): ICOST 2010, LNCS 6159, pp. 267–270, 2010.

Additionally, the wear position of the fall detection sensor is critical since the same posture in the different wear position, such as hip, trunk, wrist or head, will result in different signal patterns. The measurements of falls incline to "whole-body" activity instead of the peripheral movements, such as arm movements. In order to monitor the whole body movements the device needed to be put around the pelvis which is close to the center of the mass [5]. In this paper, we use a waist-mounted tri-axial accelerometer to capture the movement data of human body that not only is easy and convenient to wear but also provide the reliable fall detection.

The waist-mounted fall detection sensor can provide urgent fall alarm to the medical personnel in time that reduce the fear of falling and provide the user with the reassurance to maintain an independent lifestyle. The rest of this article is organized as follows. Section 2 introduces the proposed methods. The experimental results are addressed in section 3. Section 4 concludes and discusses the work.

2 Materials and Method

This study focus on the falls caused by faint or weakness that make resident from the daily activities to falling on the ground unconsciously. We classifies falls into 8 major types, and the postures before falls are stand, sit to stand, stand to sit, walk, walk backward, stoop, jump, lie on the bed. On the other hand, we also select 7 types of daily movements to verify the system wouldn't detect the daily activities as falls. The 7 types of daily activities include standing, sitting down, lying down, walking, jumping, going up (down) stairs, and jogging.

A 6*G* tri-axial accelerometer is placed on waist to measure three axial accelerations with 200Hz sampling rate and transform the values into voltage, and then stored in the embedded flash memory. According to sensor's orientation, the x-axis is frontal direction, the y-axis is vertical side, and the z-axis equals to sagittal side. Three criteria of fall detection are proposed in this paper:

1) Sum vector magnitude of acceleration $SVM_a = \sqrt{a_x^2 + a_y^2 + a_z^2}$, where *ax*, *ay*, and *az* are the acceleration of x-axis, y-axis, and z-axis respectively. It is used to describe the spatial variation of acceleration during the falling interval. The first threshold, *SVMa*, is set to 6*G* because the *SVMa* of the daily activities is smaller than 6 times of gravity (G) [6].

2) Acceleration on horizontal plane $S_h = \sqrt{{a_x}^2 + {a_z}^2}$. It means the body tilts forward or backward acutely. During the fall, S_h will larger than *2G*. In order to distinguish ordinary daily activities, like standing, sitting down, lying down, and walking, the second threshold, S_h, is set to $2G$.

3) Reference velocity $V_{ref} = \int_{T_{rs}}^{T_{ti}} |SVM_a(t) - 1| dt$, where T_{ti} is the time when the body tilts, and T_{rs} is the initial time that body is at rest [7]. As soon as S_h is bigger than $2G$, we set this point as T_{ti}, on the other hand, we use the continuous 60 data of stable SVM_a to estimate the faller is at rest or not, and set the time of first continuous data as T_{rs}. Before the integration, it needs subtract one time of acceleration of gravity from SVM_a. Certain daily activities may be misdetected as falls since the sudden motion

makes S_h exceed $2G$, such as the act of jump, go up (down) stairs, and jog. However, the V_{ref} of those daily activities are smaller than $1.7\ m/s$ that is experimental evidence. Daily activities can be successfully discriminated from falls through the V_{ref}.

As soon as SVM_a is lager than $6G$, the alarm will be sent out directly. While SVM_a is less than $6G$, S_h will be immediately checked to ascertain that the body tilts forward or backward acutely. Then we use the continuous 60 data of stable SVM_a to estimate the faller is at rest or not after S_h is lager than $2G$. If the faller is at rest and V_{ref} is over $1.7\ m/s$, fall alarm will be sent out that can distinguish between normal activities and falls.

3 Results

There are three 24-year-old males participate in the fall detection experiment. They fall on a 30 centimeter height soft bed with no impact from other forces. Figure 1 is the box plot of SVM_a, S_h and V_{ref} of falls and daily activities. Most of falls can be detected by the first case that SVM_a satisfies $6G$. However, some SVM_a of fall movements don't reach $6G$ that are judged by that S_h is larger than $2G$ and V_{ref} is over $1.7\ m/s$.

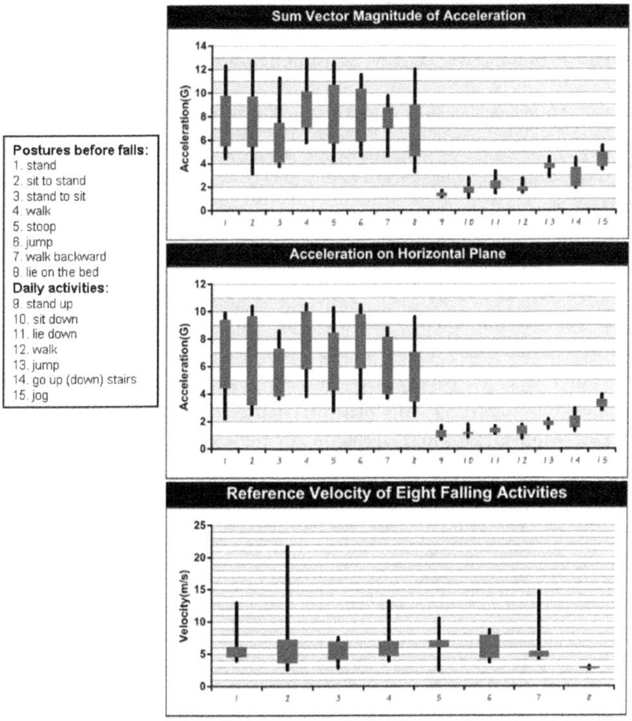

Fig. 1. Sum vector magnitude of acceleration (SVM_a), acceleration on horizontal plane (S_h) and reference velocity (V_{ref}) of eight falling activities

As shown in Figure 1, the SVM_a of daily activities are all smaller than $6G$. Then the fall detection algorithm used threshold S_h and V_{ref} to determine the movement is fall or not. Some specific movements, such as jump, go up (down) stairs, and jog, can easily be categorized to fall, and Figure 1 represents S_h of those severe daily activities is over $2G$. But these activities are not at rest, so they would not be detected as falls. As mentioned above, fall detection algorithm could detect falls precisely.

4 Conclusions

Precise distinguishing the eight types of fall and seven daily activities through the proposed algorithm had been accomplished. In the future work, the fall detection algorithm will perform in the micro-controller on circuit board and transmitted through the ZigBee module to the remote server to notify the related medical staffs. With the wireless sensor networks, the location-aware application is accomplished based on ZigBee. The advanced results will be demonstrated soon in the future discussion.

References

1. Zweifel, P., Felder, S., Meiers, M.: Ageing of Population and Health care Expenditure: a Red Herring? Health Economics 8, 485–496 (1999)
2. Brewer, K., Ciolek, C., Delaune, M.F.: Falls in Community Dwelling Older Adults: Introduction to The Problem. In: APTA Continuing Education Series, July 2007, pp. 38–46 (2007)
3. Lindemann, U., Hock, A., Stuber, M.: Evaluation of a Fall Detector Based on accelerometers: a pilot study. Medical & Biological Engineering & Computing 43, 1146–1154 (2005)
4. Alwan, M., Felder, R.A.: Eldercare Technology for Clinical Practitioners. Humana Press, Totowa (2007)
5. Mathie, M.J.: Monitoring and Interpreting Human Movement Patterns Using a Tri-axial Accelerometer. Ph.D. Thesis, New South Wales, Sydney, Australia (2003)
6. Bouten, C.V.C., Koekkoek, K.T.M., Verduin, M., Kodde, R., Janssen, J.D.: A Triaxial Accelerometer and Portable Data Processing Unit for the Assessment of Daily Physical Activity. IEEE Transactions on Biomedical Engineering 44(3), 136–147 (1997)
7. Wang, C.C., Chiang, C.Y., Huang, C.N., Chan, C.T., et al.: Development of a Fall Detecting System for the Elderly Residents. In: IEEE Proceeding, The Second International Conference of Bioinformatics and Biomedical Engineering, pp. 1359–1362 (2008)

Author Index

GPSR Compliance

The European Union's (EU) General Product Safety Regulation (GPSR) is a set of rules that requires consumer products to be safe and our obligations to ensure this.

If you have any concerns about our products, you can contact us on ProductSafety@springernature.com

In case Publisher is established outside the EU, the EU authorized representative is:

Springer Nature Customer Service Center GmbH
Europaplatz 3
69115 Heidelberg, Germany

Batch number: 10844619

Printed by Printforce, the Netherlands